EMPIRICAL STUDIES IN HEALTH ECONOMICS

HERBERT E. KLARMAN, Editor
with the assistance of
HELEN H. JASZI

EMPIRICAL STUDIES IN HEALTH ECONOMICS

Proceedings of the Second Conference on the Economics of Health

The Johns Hopkins University Press
Baltimore and London

The Johns Hopkins University Press, Baltimore, Maryland 21218
The Johns Hopkins University Press Ltd., London

Library of Congress Catalog Card Number 74-101646
ISBN 0-8018-1134-1

Originally published, 1970
Second printing, 1974

CONTENTS

*Not presented at the Conference.

ACKNOWLEDGMENTS

The Second Conference on the Economics of Health was held December 5-7, 1968, in the new Ernest L. Stebbins Building of the School of Hygiene and Public Health, The Johns Hopkins University, in Baltimore, Maryland. A grant from The Ford Foundation helped pay for the planning of the conference, the attendance of one hundred participants, and reproduction and editing of the papers, and provided a publication subsidy to reduce the price of the present volume. The Johns Hopkins University sponsored the conference and participated actively through its President, Lincoln Gordon, the Dean of the School of Hygiene, John C. Hume, and the Department of Political Economy. To all these sources of support the Planning Committee for the conference expresses its gratitude.

Planning Committee
Herbert E. Klarman, *Chairman*
Rashi Fein
Victor R. Fuchs
Selma J. Mushkin
Helen H. Jaszi, *Executive Secretary*

PART I

INTRODUCTION

Herbert E. Klarman
The Johns Hopkins University

TRENDS AND TENDENCIES IN HEALTH ECONOMICS

Research in the field of health is comparatively new as a specialized area of activity for economists. The Conference on the Economics of Health Services in 1962 at Ann Arbor, Michigan, brought workers in this field together for the first time. The papers in the proceedings volume of that conference are representative of the work completed in 1961-62.[1] At the end of 1968, the Second Conference on the Economics of Health in Baltimore once again brought together a similarly constituted group for intensive discussion of research completed in 1967-68.

DIFFERENCES BETWEEN THE TWO CONFERENCES

Several major differences between the two conferences are discernible. No longer is it necessary to discuss the distinctive economic characteristics of the health services industry and the unique opportunities it affords to the economic analyst. His potential contribution is now accepted, sometimes beyond his ability to deliver. The number of economists working in the field has become large enough to allow the planning committee for the second conference to select from among more than fifty potential contributors. Also noteworthy is the sizable number of new investigators. The list of contributors to this volume does not contain even one name listed in the proceedings of the Ann Arbor conference. Another difference in the papers reflects the accumulation in the 1960s of a substantial body of completed research and empirical findings on which to build. By 1968 it had become possible for one author to take as a matter of course the probable optimum size of hospital (Carr). An even more striking feature, which I shall discuss later in more detail, is the widespread reliance upon econometrics in the papers in this volume.

3

In inviting contributions the Planning Committee was heavily influenced by the probability that a particular paper would be completed prior to the target date, December 1968. Consequently, research for most of the papers was already under way in the spring of 1967, and only a few studies were, in effect, newly commissioned for the conference. Of the eighteen papers invited, fifteen were completed and fourteen are published here;* problems with data prevented completion of the other three in time for the conference. However, three other papers are included that were not prepared for delivery at the conference; they are based on work for recently completed doctoral dissertations.

The decision to build the second conference around ongoing work is the major reason for the large diversity of subject matter displayed in this volume, ranging from an analysis of the replacement demand for children following an epidemic in eighteenth-century New England to the very timely problem of the nature of the production function in the group practice of medicine. Another reason for this diversity, however, was the judgment of the Planning Committee that the time was not yet ripe to select a single problem for intensive exploration.

EMPIRICAL ORIENTATION

As Fein observes, the Baltimore conference may represent a watershed in health economics. The papers are, by design, empirically oriented. The contributors aim to answer certain questions, not merely to ask them. They try to make quantitative estimates of the importance of the independent variables, not merely to identify the direction of the change that the latter induce in the dependent variable. This common characteristic of the papers should not occasion astonishment, since it derives directly from an early decision of the Planning Committee to invite only reports of quantitative investigations. Speculative papers, "think pieces," were deliberately excluded. In the opinion of some observers this decision may have been unduly restrictive and therefore unwise.

The result is that a rather high proportion of these papers contain mathematical symbols, equations, and numbers, at the expense of text. While some papers combine economic theory and data analysis, many present models and concentrate on estimating parameter values through econometric techniques. The papers offer examples of principal components analysis, stepwise regression analysis, two-stage instrumental variable analysis, and single- and multiple-equation models of first and higher orders to which multiple regression analysis is applied. Included is a general market model for medical care

*Martin S. Feldstein's paper, "Health Sector Planning in Developing Countries," will appear in *Economica* in the spring of 1970.

services consisting of forty-seven equations with forty-seven endogenous variables and thirty-three exogenous variables (Feldstein-Kelman).

Several discussants are critical of this phenomenon: the decisionmaker does not know how to apply the findings yielded by these complex techniques unless they are translated for him (Fein); the approach adopted is too broad, too general, to be fruitful (de Janosi); the variables studied are ill chosen and not relevant to the solution of public policy issues (Ginzberg). There are clear instances where technique and substance are not well synthesized. In part, this defect stems from the fact that some of the authors are economists without prior experience in, or even exposure to, the health services field. In a few instances the papers represent first exercises, which tend to contain a heavier dose of technique than would a second or third study in this field by the same author.

Related perhaps, but not anticipated by the Planning Committee, is the adoption of econometric tools by some contributors whose previous work relied on other analytical approaches. It is possible that authors with prior experience in health economics may have traded away some of the advantages of a concrete knowledge of problems and institutional arrangements for the sake of acquiring and applying sophisticated statistical techniques. It remains to be seen whether this change will enhance their power to explain and predict events.

It is noteworthy that along with models and mathematical symbols has appeared the careful description of data and data sources. Perhaps this task warrants a more complete and more systematic exposition than it can receive in the papers in this volume, owing to limitations of space. Interested readers are referred by some contributors to longer versions of their work (Feldstein-Kelman, Yett) or to detailed descriptions of the total data on which the paper draws (Rosenthal).

DIVERSE FINDINGS

A small sampling of the more suggestive and interesting findings and hypotheses is presented here.

1. Changes in the death rate did lead at one time to adjustments in the birth rate. Children who died during the New England diphtheria epidemic of 1734–40, which was not anticipated and therefore could not be discounted in advance, were in part replaced (Stettler).

2. The hypothesis is advanced that age and poverty interact in such a way in this society that, among the poor, health may start to worsen at a younger age than among the more prosperous, that is to say, the poor tend to age at a faster rate. At relatively young ages (seventeen to forty-four) the health status of poor persons appears to be not very different from that of well-to-do persons (Newhouse).

3. Without standardization for age, families with a lower permanent income have more illness than families with a higher permanent income. Those with a lower income spend less per unit of illness (Andersen-Benham).

4. When physicians combine in larger units (and are paid fee for service), they produce more ancillary services per physician but not more physician visits (Bailey). Constant productivity in physician visits may thus coexist with increasing returns to scale for all services of the medical firm. The possibility that in the early years of practice physicians organized as a group may have a fuller utilization of capacity than solo physicians was not raised.

5. Economies of scale obtain in small hospitals but not in larger ones (Francisco).

6. Not only are the markets for physician services and for hospital care interdependent, but an understanding of the former may possibly afford a full explanation of the latter via the system of hospital staff appointments for attending physicians (Stevens).

7. Income is to be viewed not as a single economic variable, as is customary, but as perhaps four separate variables. First, income measures ability to pay for health care, except when superseded by health insurance status (Andersen-Benham). Second, income is an index of the style of life associated with the production and consumption of that income, and hence of health status. Infant mortality is inversely related to income; adult mortality may be directly related to income at certain ages.[2] Permanent rather than observed income is the valid measure for this purpose. Third (and somewhat related to the second point), income is an index of socioeconomic and cultural status and of attitudes toward health and medical care. For this purpose educational level may be a more valid single measure. Fourth, income, or rather earned income, is an indicator of the value of time. In producing health for himself a person with a higher earnings rate may be encouraged to substitute more and better health services for his own recovery time (Silver).

PERVASIVE AND RECURRING THEMES

Certain themes recur throughout the papers and the discussants' remarks. Indeed, they pervaded the floor discussion at the conference. Several of the leading themes follow.

1. The importance of the value of time has already been alluded to in one context, that of an individual's production function for health. Another application of time is in planning health facilities, when the travel cost of consumers and providers is allowed for (Carr).

2. Coming into focus is the distinction between medical care and health. When health status is neglected, the income elasticity of the demand for medical care is underestimated where gains in income are associated with health improvements, and conversely (Leveson). A valid measure of health is

by no means obvious; for example, work-loss days are a poor measure (Silver).

3. Although the quality of care is a complex matter and is generally intractable to measurement, it was discussed repeatedly in response to authors' acts of commission or omission. When a paper explicitly developed measures of hospital quality, the discussant asked whether the extra cost really pertained to quality care or to affiliation with a medical school (Feldstein). In the discussion of group practice the failure to measure quality of care was seen as a possibly serious oversight, since the group form of organization facilitates patient referral (Reder).

4. As expected, economists are preoccupied with the nature of markets — their structure, function, and performance. Markets are for goods and services or for factors of production. In the health services industry the significance for performance of the non-profit ownership of the short-term hospital is frequently discussed. Determining whether hospitals act as monopsonists or oligopsonists in the local area is vital for evaluating the acceptability of some of the explanations offered for the behavior of the market for the services of registered nurses and of the educational network that trains them (Altman, Yett). The discussants were not convinced that non-profit hospitals behave as monopsonists, both because motivation is lacking and because alternative explanations are available (Hansen, Rosen). That physicians behave as profit maximizers concentrating on marginal revenue is offered as a plausible explanation of differences in hospital and surgical use rates between subscribers to prepaid group practice plans and subscribers to other forms of health insurance (Monsma).

It was not practicable to pursue these questions of market structure and performance to the point of resolution at the conference, and to attempt to do so now may seem unfair. Yet it is important to make at least a few observations. Even non-profit hospitals *may* behave as monopsonists or oligopsonists in order to keep down expenditures, and evidence that hospitals engage in collusion on salaries is ample, both in terms of Yett's voluminous examples and my own experience. As for the effect of prepaid group practice on the use of services, it appears that more is often claimed on its behalf than may be warranted by available data.[3]

5. Empirical workers are concerned with the existence of data, access to them, and the availability of descriptive materials to define terms and help explain discrepancies in findings. For international comparisons, data are not plentiful and vary in quality (Malenbaum). Frequently they must be developed by the investigator himself, particularly for historical studies and for local areas. Sometimes the investigator draws on data that he initially helped develop, which he now offers to the public domain (Rosenthal). Unpublished data from household surveys, both occasional and repeated ones

such as the National Health Survey, are coming into increasing use. While certain data sources are expanding, others, such as the United Hospital Fund of New York, are contracting and will not be available for future years.

6. Several papers referred to the issue of the relationship, if any, between the supply of hospital beds and demand. The question that interests economists is this: when hospital bed capacity is increased under conditions of prepayment, is there a tendency to clear the market at a lower price or is the demand curve shifted upward? The controversy stems from Roemer and Rosenthal;[4] subsequent major participants in the discussion are Reder and Martin Feldstein;[5] other contributions and policy implications are analyzed by Klarman.[6]

Carr refers to this issue in his paper and adopts Rosenthal's position that supply responds to the same forces as demand, so that a change in supply does not lead to a shift in demand. Stevens examines the problem at greater length because he rates it highly important. His discussant points out that if supply exerts an influence on demand, then one cannot infer from the full utilization of existing facilities the need to expand them (Mills).

It seems to me, upon further review of the papers, that what Stevens views as a change in price, namely, the change in physician behavior subsequent to an expansion in bed supply, can also be viewed as a change in taste, an adjustment in the criteria for bed use. While a lower price follows a given demand curve, a change in taste would be manifested on a different curve. Elsewhere it recently has been suggested that possibly the demand curve changes it shape, becoming more elastic, when bed supply increases.[7]

RESEARCH AND POLICY

The theme that recurred with the greatest frequency was that research should be useful in making policy decisions. Every speaker who touched on the matter favored this position, none opposed it, and several papers explicitly state it. Such a consensus in favor of useful research will astonish those who believe that most economists working in the health field are not concerned with contributing to the solution of real problems but prefer to pursue the abstruse implications of abstract models. I have heard this view expressed on numerous occasions, and I seldom am successful in refuting it. Allowing for individual differences among economists, based on temperament or experience, I should still conclude from personal observation that this complaint of indifference to real problems is not well founded.

Most economists in the health field know that expenditures for health services approximate $60 billion annually, amounting to 6.5 per cent or more of the gross national product. It is also well known that the industry has been growing rapidly in terms of dollars and more slowly in relative size. Problems in the health services – including discussions of prices, incomes of providers, adequacy of manpower and of facilities, forms of organization for services and training, regulation, etc. – are lively public policy issues.

On the average, economists who work on health services problems display a high level of interest in public policy, often a far higher level than prevails in other applied areas of economics. Indeed, in my judgment, the economist is sometimes far too eager to propose solutions after a hasty or sketchy examination of a problem as presented to him by concerned health professionals. His desire that there be adequate provision of appropriate health services may be so intense, because it is so personal, that he may neglect to subject the problems of the health services and the proposed solutions to the critical scrutiny that he would ordinarily bring to bear on a public policy problem.

The important question, in my opinion, is not whether economists are interested in real problems of the health services but whether a given set of findings is ready for application. The answer to the first question is simply "Yes" for economists as a group. The content and flow of the discussion at the conference on such matters as the production function for group medical practice or the effects on demand of an increase in hospital bed supply, though couched in the formal language of economic theory, are impressive evidence that an active interest exists.

To the second question the answer is more problematic and must depend on specific circumstances. Sometimes it may be wise for the economist to advise the decisionmaker that the requisite evidence is lacking or that the import of the available evidence is unclear or that conflicting findings exist. As he often has in the past, the decisionmaker will use judgment, his own or an expert's, to reach the best decision possible. On the evidence in this volume it is possible to list some reasons why it may be premature to adopt some of the findings presented here in formulating policy decisions and why caution is always indicated in applying research findings to policy formulation.

Usually the findings are based on a complex process of statistical calculation and analysis beset by technical difficulties. In econometrics there is the basic problem of identification – does an equation deal with demand or supply? Problems of multicollinearity appear in most multiple regression analyses. Frequently the coefficient of determination is small and the residue of unexplained variation is large. Questions can be raised about possible biases in the computed estimates (Fuchs, Grossman, Leveson). Problems exist also in defining variables and in measuring them accurately (Goode, Grossman).

Even when the quantitative findings of two studies are identical, the investigators may differ in interpreting their meaning. A good example is Francisco's work, whose findings closely follow those of Ralph Berry.[8] While Berry emphasizes the large number of identical signs of coefficients, Francisco stresses the lack of statistical significance for the calculated values.

Choosing between the two interpretations calls for the exercise of experienced judgment.

A given locale is studied and yields different results because one investigator has analyzed a cross-section of the data while another looked at observations over time. Pauly-Drake find that the reimbursement mechanism does not influence hospital cost, while Klarman presents some evidence that it does. It is important that in this case the discussant attempted to explain why the authors' approach was likely to lead to negative findings.

Sometimes the basic model employed or developed by the author is criticized as inappropriate. One example of complete rejection of a model is Rosen's challenge of Yett's basic assumption that, in the market for nurses, hospitals behave as oligopsonists. Many of us know what the discussant could not know, namely, that what is asserted in Yett's paper represents a great deal of hard data, marshalled in his forthcoming monograph. Nor has the discussant yet offered an elaboration of his proposed alternative model in empirical terms. Nevertheless, it is not clear how firm a base Yett's findings afford for policy formulation at this time.

Occasionally the discussant approves of a paper but successfully casts doubt on the applicability of its findings. An example is Rothenberg's critique of Carr's paper: he finds the approach original and the execution excellent but questions the conclusion that there is little, if any, difference in outcome between central planning and market mechanisms. Rothenberg's reservations are that certain basic problems, such as a small number of hospitals in the local area and externalities, are assumed away and that asymptotic behavior is not relevant when the adjustment process is very long. Nor is it reasonable to assume, says Rothenberg, that central planners will not learn by doing.

Sometimes the estimates of parameters for a given variable differ widely between papers for reasons that are not apparent. For example, Silver calculates much higher values for the income elasticity of demand for physicians' services than do Andersen-Benham, whose findings fall within the range reported by previous investigators. Only a small part of the difference is accounted for by recognizing that elasticity is higher when calculated as the response of a percentage change in expenditures to a percentage change in income than if calculated as the response of a percentage change in the quantity of services taken to such a change in income. The differential narrows appreciably when Silver takes account of consumers' earnings. At present it must be concluded that this set of discrepant findings cannot yet be reconciled.

As Newhouse observes, when only some of the effects of health services are measured and others, like the intangible aspects of health, are not, the measured numbers alone do not necessarily lead to optimum policy recommendations. Items that escape measurement must not be treated as if their value were zero. Important institutions and arrangements may have been overlooked, and they do make a difference in determining sound policy. This point deserves to be qualified, however. The usefulness of a model lies in its predictive power, not in the realism of its assumptions; the ability to predict can be tested only in the course of time.

For all these reasons I believe that not all research findings should be applied promptly. They cannot be said to be wasted, since reversals in findings are known to take place. Indeed, the above comments and criticisms are consistent with a view that research is a cumulative process in which some questions are answered while new ones are being raised. It seems to me that some of the differences and discrepancies in findings described above were bound to occur. As more research is performed on a problem, the range of empirical findings tends to widen. One is less sure of the answer after the new research is completed than before. It is hoped that this phase will be followed by one of comprehensive review and by efforts to compare and reconcile the existing diversity of findings, and that in such a review the influence of the special assumptions associated with a technique and the peculiar characteristics of the data will be separated from real structural and behavioral differences.

Accordingly, I am not perturbed that we do not yet know what is the true income elasticity of demand for health services. Policymakers have made decisions in the past without this precise knowledge and will continue to do so in the future. It would be unfortunate, however, if a wide range of findings were accepted as fact without any attempt at reconciling them with each other and, more important, arriving at a new synthesis. It is important, therefore, that additional research be undertaken.

RESEARCH AGENDA FOR THE FUTURE

The research priorities of investigators often differ from those of policymakers. The principal reason is not, however, that the former are uninterested in policy. There may be legitimate differences of opinion concerning what public policy issue is important at a given time or is likely soon to become so. Sometimes investigators fail to work on a problem because data are lacking or their tools are inadequate. Often they wish to clarify problems that arose in the course of previous research. In the final analysis, they must feel free to pursue their own inquiries, while decisionmakers must be in a position to initiate research or to extend invitations to investigators to work on specified problems that they deem to have priority.

A partial research agenda in health economics can be drawn from the problems, qualifications, and uncertainties discussed in the preceding sections. Elements of such an agenda were also suggested by the papers that were invited for this conference but could not be completed in time, by papers that were not invited because it was not practicable to bring together topic and author, and by the existence of several problem areas that clearly enjoy a high priority today but have been neglected by academic economists.

Papers Not Completed

The Planning Committee invited papers on physicians' earnings, hospital productivity, and the changes in the use of services attributable to the introduction of deductible and coinsurance provisions in a health insurance plan. The invitations were accepted. In each instance the data did not materialize in time to permit the completion of a paper for this conference.

Excluded Topics

The Planning Committee recognized that it would be worthwhile to investigate certain other topics. It was not known, however, who would be able and available to undertake such work. Papers on drugs, supplies and equipment, paramedical health personnel, nursing homes, mental health services, and the economic effects of pollution in the environment would have been of definite interest. Approaches to measuring the value of intangible health benefits would have been welcome.

Neglected Topics

Most striking perhaps is the absence of papers on the recent increase in health services costs and expenditures (except tangentially) and on the sources and mechanisms of financing health services. For papers on the trend in cost, technical difficulties loom large. Over a period of time it simply is not possible to describe cost trends accurately without a stable measure of output. As a result, the tendency is not to deal with the problem of rising cost in the absence of urgency. When the papers for this conference were commissioned, the marked and prolonged acceleration in hospital cost and physician fees characteristic of recent years had not yet become manifest.

The cost problem has assumed increasing prominence, and the technical difficulties remain. However, the need to cope with the problem has become inescapable. The technical difficulties can be either overcome or sidestepped. The latter alternative is a realistic possibility, owing to the drastic discontinuity in cost trends introduced by the events centering around July 1, 1966, when Medicare went into effect and Medicaid became operative in several states. In effect, when all other things, including the composition and quality of output, were held more or less constant, a natural experiment took place.

It has not been within the tradition of economics to take advantage of natural experiments, let alone to design experiments deliberately. However, as economists are exposed to the other disciplines working in the health field, they abandon exclusive reliance on statistical devices for holding factors constant and resort to other sources of data, including both natural and artificial experiments. The increased availability of funds for health services research will make it possible to adopt these tools in the future.

The reasons for the absence of papers on financing are somewhat different. A paper on health insurance was commissioned but could not be completed in time, while a paper on the price elasticity of length of hospital stay is included. The basic reason, however, is the belief among many economists that for a long time medical economics overemphasized the problem of finances and the distribution of the financial burden of medical care expenditures at the expense of the more central problem of the allocation of scarce resources among competing wants.

Whatever may have held true in the past, there is no such emphasis today. There is reason to believe that as the issue of universal health insurance moves to the fore economists will perform some of the analyses that sound formulation of public policy requires. When they do, they are likely to review the various effects of service benefits, which health professionals are less inclined to question. They may be expected to inquire into the effects of insurance, sources of funding, and reimbursement mechanisms on the level of use of services, as well as on the distribution of use. They may distinguish between minimum or basic plans and additional, optional programs designed to cater more closely to consumers' desires. Plainly, the treatment of health insurance by economists in the emerging scene may depart from what is traditional not only in terms of the technique applied but also in terms of the questions asked, the assumptions made explicit and reviewed, and the data examined.

For the not distant future, it may be desirable to consider the advisability of conducting a conference that would concentrate on a single problem or policy issue. To be specific, a health economics conference could deal with costs or with demand for several types of service; with the supply and demand factors operating for a single product, such as hospital care; with a single factor of production; or with the structure and performance of specific sub-markets. How soon such a conference can be held will depend in part upon the vigor with which graduate departments of economics cultivate this field among students and faculty and in part on the development of devices and arrangements for financing focused research. It is likely that the latter would provide for something intermediate between the investigator's full freedom, under the existing grants mechanism, to choose both subject matter and approach and the government's total initiative and control, which prevails under the contract mechanism.

NOTES

1. S. J. Axelrod, ed., *The Economics of Health and Medical Care* (Ann Arbor: The University of Michigan, 1964).

2. Victor R. Fuchs, *Some Economic Aspects of Mortality in the United States* (New York: National Bureau of Economic Research, 1965); Herbert E. Klarman, "The Contribution of Health Services to Economic Growth and Well-Being," in U.S., Congress, Joint Economic Committee, *Federal Programs for the Development of Human Resources, A Compendium of Papers*, vol. 2 (Washington, D.C.: Government Printing Office, 1968), pp. 451-68.

3. Herbert E. Klarman, "Effect of Prepaid Group Practice on Hospital Use," *Public Health Reports* 78, no. 11 (November 1963):955-65; and "Approaches to Moderating the Increases in Medical Care Costs," *Medical Care* 7, no. 3 (May–June 1969):175-90.

4. Milton I. Roemer, "Bed Supply and Hospital Utilization: A Natural Experiment," *Hospitals* 35, no. 21 (November 1, 1961):36-42; Max Shain and Milton I. Roemer, "Hospital Costs Relate to the Supply of Beds," *Modern Hospital* 92, no. 4 (April 1959):71-73, 168; Gerald D. Rosenthal, *Hospital Utilization in the United States* (Chicago: American Hospital Association, 1964).

5. Martin S. Feldstein, *Economic Analysis for Health Service Efficiency* (Amsterdam: North-Holland Publishing Co., 1967); Melvin W. Reder, "Some Problems in the Economics of Hospitals," *American Economic Review, Papers and Proceedings* 55, no. 2 (May 1965):472-80.

6. Klarman, "Moderating the Increases in Medical Care Costs."

7. Louise B. Russell, *Regression Analysis of Medicare Admissions: Preliminary Report* (Washington, D.C.: Social Security Administration, 1969).

8. Ralph E. Berry, Jr., "Competition and Efficiency in the Market for Hospital Services: The Structure of the American Hospital Industry" (Ph.D. diss., Harvard University, 1965).

PART II

POPULATION, HEALTH, AND PROGRAM PLANNING

H. Louis Stettler III
The Johns Hopkins University

THE NEW ENGLAND THROAT DISTEMPER AND FAMILY SIZE

Standard evaluations of health measures by economists tend to emphasize the number of deaths that were averted as a result of these activities.[1] Such a simple calculation may easily overstate the effect of such programs on population size. This overstatement may be particularly serious in attempts to evaluate the impact of sanitary and medical activities in pre-modern or underdeveloped economies.

Consider as an illustration a variation on the Malthusian example: a closed economy with a fixed food production potential and smallpox. Assume further that the birth rate and death rate (from causes other than hunger) are given. If the birth rate exceeds the death rate, then the population will expand until all food is currently consumed. After such a position is attained, the death rate will adjust to equal the birth rate as surplus births cause an equal number of starvations. If at this time a smallpox inoculation program is instituted, smallpox deaths will diminish; however, the death rate from starvation will increase in direct proportion to the decline in the smallpox death rate. In fact, in such an economy, no program designed to reduce deaths by eliminating the medical causes of death will yield net increases in population. Only programs that lower the birth rate or alleviate the food constraint will bring about changes in population size.

Demographers and historians have often speculated that changes in the death rate stimulate adjustments in the birth rate. In particular, it has been

The research work underlying this paper was sponsored by Public Health Service Grant H.30.6092. The research effort was aided by the thoughtful comments and help of Margaret Bright and Herbert Klarman of The Johns Hopkins University and Robert Higgs of the University of Washington.

17

conjectured that the secular decline in the death rate over the past one hundred and fifty years has been, in part, responsible for the secular fall in the fertility rate. Specifically, it has been argued that the decline in the child mortality rate or the increase in the child survival rate decreases the number of births per family required to achieve some optimal or contemplated family size.[2]

If families actively seek to attain a given size, increases in child mortality, on the other hand, ought to lead to replacement of children or increased births per family.* The evidence to support such a conjecture is sparse and unconvincing. Basically, there are two bits of relevant data. First, studies have demonstrated that as family size increases, the incidence of child mortality increases more than proportionally.[3] The direction of causality is not clear in this case. In the generally unhealthy conditions of the past century, members of larger families were more exposed to the carriers of disease. Second, parish registers and family lists yield many instances in which children were given the name of deceased siblings. It would seem extremely hazardous, however, to suggest that only those children named for a departed brother or sister were replacements.† Perhaps the important question is not whether a few families replace deceased children, but rather whether families increase births in anticipation of a higher death incidence.

The validity of the concept of a "replacement demand" for children or a target family size depends entirely upon evidence that family births increase in response to increases in child mortality, actual or anticipated. Without such evidence it would be difficult to accept the proposition that the decline in the fertility rate is associated with a decline in the number of births required to attain a given family size. It is particularly difficult to accept such a proposition in view of the appealing alternative that the changing socioeconomic environment (rising incomes, urbanization, and industrialization) was conducive to lower fertility, and perhaps to a smaller optimal family size.

I

The experience of New England families during and after the severe outbreak of "throat distemper" during the years 1734–40 provides an unusually fine opportunity to test the hypothesis that changes in child mortality bring about adjustments in births. The period 1720-60 is quite suitable for such a test since the social, political, and economic environment was relatively

---

*This specifically assumes that the demand for children is perfectly inelastic or that changes in mortality, which are changes in the cost of obtaining a target size, do not change the target. It is clear that in certain cases an increase in the death rate reduces the number of births.

†Of the recorded births used in this study about 2 per cent were registered under the name of a deceased sibling.

stable. Certainly there were unsettling influences — the Great Awakening and the episodic contests with the French and their Indian allies.* The epidemic itself is also quite suitable.[4] Throat distemper, or diphtheria, as it has been identified, was a lethal affliction. Hence, its presence in a community can be easily and precisely identified from the death lists. In Kingston, New Hampshire, the site of the initial outbreak, 102 deaths were recorded in 1734; prior to that date, in no year had deaths exceeded 25, and they averaged less than 10 per annum. In the villages selected as a sample for this study, in the epidemic year, with one exception, deaths numbered at least twice those in prior years. The disease fell heavily upon the young. In New Hampshire 82 per cent of the victims were under ten years of age and another 14 per cent were under twenty. In the sample communities 85 per cent of the deaths occurring in the epidemic years were children. Another epidemiological characteristic of the throat distemper was the multiple-death family; 40 per cent of the families which lost one child lost more than one. On the other hand, of those families which did not lose a child during the epidemic, less than 5 per cent ever experienced a year in which more than a single child died. Perhaps the most important aspect of the epidemic is that before 1734 diphtheria, at least in its most virulent form, was almost unknown.[5] Consequently, it is unlikely that the disease's impact on child survival rates was adequately discounted by families prior to the epidemic, and it is unlikely that its impact could be ignored by families after the epidemic.

If families can and do adjust their births to yield an expected number of mature children, it would be expected that (1) families losing a child to the distemper ought to have more births than other families, and (2) the number of births per family ought to be greater for families formed after the epidemic than for families formed before the epidemic which did not lose a child to the distemper. To test these propositions, it is necessary to have information on deaths and births by family for a sample of New England communities.

II

Birth, death, and marriage registration was required by statute in most New England areas.[6] Baptismal records were also maintained in these semi-theocratic villages as a necessary administrative detail. During the late nineteenth century many of these registers were compiled and published for genealogical purposes. In some instances, the published compilations included additional material drawn from diaries, family bibles, and tombstones. In

*It may not be coincidence that the Great Awakening began in New England at the time of the epidemic. The French wars did not put severe demands on the colonials outside the border regions. New Englanders, however, were the main participants in Pepperill's Louisburg campaign of 1745, and a number of the sample families lost a father at Lake George during the final war.

some cases the published version was little more than a transcription of the original registers; in other cases the birth, death, and marriage data have been grouped by family name. The birth entry typically includes the names of the parents; the death entry, in the case of a child, usually includes the names of the parents and occasionally the child's age at death. The marriage lists include all marriages performed in the community and an occasional notation that an individual was married elsewhere. The baptismal registers include the names of the newborn, older children, and adults admitted to the faith in the community church.

The completeness and accuracy of the various registers can only be inferred from their contents and the legal nature of their mandate, since there are no prior evaluative studies of the American vital registers.[7] There are, of course, a number of inaccuracies, many of a clerical nature. The lists for Lexington, Massachusetts, fail to specify the exact year of death for those dying during the period 1753–55. There are a small number of birth entries for siblings supposedly born within six months of each other. There are also a few notes by the compilers that the handwriting in the original lists was illegible or that no date was affixed to an entry. The notations concerning cause of death are in many cases ludicrous.* It was assumed, nevertheless, that the dates and names listed in the registers were accurate and that the event registered did occur.

There are three pieces of internal evidence which suggest that the birth registers are relatively complete.† First, births whose registration might be considered a formality are often listed: there are numerous entries for stillborns and live births, named and unnamed, who died within a month of birth.[8] Second, births carrying with them a moral stigma also appear on the lists: there are many entries for children who were either illegitimate or were born less than six months after the parents' marriage.[9] Third, birth entries are lacking for only 12 per cent of the children who died during the epidemic. Many of these children may have been born elsewhere before their parents moved into the village; in fact, 80 per cent of these unregistered children are of parents who were not married in the village.

The death registers are less reliable. The main evidence of under-reporting is an unusually high vital index (births divided by deaths). For the sample communities, the index typically exceeds 4.[10] For the United States in 1800 a birth rate of 53 per thousand is a common estimate. If the death rate were underestimated at 18.6 per thousand (the 1860 value for Massachusetts), the

---

*For example: "Congestion of the Brain" (Marlborough); "Their lamps went out for want of oil" (Shrewsbury); "Pulmonary consumption caused by blowing a bugle" (Southborough).

†Completeness means here only reporting by families that reported marriages or deaths. There may well have been families who reported nothing.

vital index would stand at 3. In the late nineteenth century the index for northern European nations rarely exceeded 2.[11] Although, in general, there was under-reporting, it is conjectured that reporting was complete during the epidemic.

III

The thirteen towns for which data were collected are listed in Table 1. These towns were selected because they were known epidemic towns, their published registers were available at the Peabody Institute and Maryland Historical Society libraries in Baltimore, and their registers had been compiled by family. The last stipulation was made in order to minimize the probability of committing a clerical error in recording and assigning births to families.

From the registers two classes of statistics were collected, annual deaths by town and family births. Annual deaths were used only to identify the epidemic years. Family births were collected only for those families thought to be permanent residents of the community. Evidence of permanence included a registered marriage, a series of births, a registered death of a parent, or a registered death or marriage of a minor child. Family births include all children born to a father and his legal wives. Births out of wedlock are specifically excluded; they are, however, of only minor importance since only one father in the sample is known to have had an illegitimate son. Also excluded are the wife's children (if any) from a previous marriage; in fact, families containing a widow known to have children by a previous marriage are not considered. It should be noted that remarriage was an important aspect of life in colonial New England. In some communities fully an eighth of the sample families included a second wife and a few included a third.

Table 1: The Sample

Town	State	Epidemic	Families
Brookfield	Mass.	1738	33
Coventry	Conn.	1739–40	70
Gloucester	Mass.	1738	47
Haverhill	Mass.	1736–37	119
Lexington	Mass.	1740	19
Mansfield	Conn.	1739–40	29
Marlborough	Mass.	1740	34
Middletown	Mass.	1739–40	24
Oxford	Mass.	1740–41	46
Salisbury	Mass.	1736–37	69
Shrewsbury	Mass.	1740	29
Southborough	Mass.	1740	26
Wenham	Mass.	1736–38	44

Two basic samples of families were selected, epidemic and non-epidemic families. The sample of epidemic families is composed of all acceptable family units which experienced a death of a child under twenty during the epidemic year(s). Needless to say, not all such deaths are attributable to the distemper; in fact, in some communities 15 per cent of the families lost an infant less than six months old – an unlikely age to die of diphtheria. On the other hand, 40 per cent of these families lost more than one child – a distinctive feature of diphtheria.

The sample of non-epidemic families was selected from all other families meeting the marriage and residence requirements. There are two groups of non-epidemic families, (1) contemporary families, those whose first marriage date preceded the epidemic year, and (2) post-epidemic families, those whose first marriage date followed the epidemic year. An attempt was made to stratify the contemporary families so that the distribution of their marriage dates was approximately the same as that of the epidemic families; however, this was not always possible. The sample of post-epidemic families was stratified so that (1) for each community, the number of families selected equaled the number of contemporary families, and (2) the distribution of marriage dates by five-year periods was approximately uniform. Again, this was not always possible.

The sampling procedure and assumptions obviously introduce elements of bias. First, it was assumed that all deaths inflicted by the throat distemper were reported. If some were unreported, it is possible that a contemporary family might have experienced a diphtheria death. If this were the case, then the measured difference between family size of the epidemic and non-epidemic groups would be smaller than the true difference. Second, it was assumed that all deaths occurring in the epidemic years were attributable to distemper. Again, the bias is toward a measured difference smaller than the true difference, since families losing children to known and expected perils would be less apt to adjust their birth patterns. Third, the residence requirement tended to reduce the probability that small families would be included in the non-epidemic samples. Hence, the bias is again toward observing larger family size in the control sample.

IV

Table 2 presents the distribution of family births for each of the three samples. A cursory glance will suggest that the epidemic families in fact did tend to have more births per family than the non-epidemic families. Further, there appears to be no similar difference between the two non-epidemic samples. Standard statistical tests corroborate this impression. Considering only the epidemic and contemporary families, the difference in the means (1.10) is in excess of three times the computed standard deviation of the

Table 2: Family Births

Births per Family	Number of Families		
	Epidemic	Contemporary	Post-Epidemic
0	0	0	0
1	2	3	1
2	10	7	8
3	14	13	17
4	17	21	17
5	19	20	23
6	42	17	20
7	34	16	19
8	29	22	15
9	38	12	12
10	26	7	8
11	19	8	9
12	12	7	3
13	4	2	2
14	6	0	0
15	3	1	2
16	2	0	0
Total	277	156	156
Mean	7.64	6.54	6.43
Sample variance	9.07	8.44	8.18

difference distribution (.294). Hence the first hypothesis — that families losing a child to distemper have more births — would be accepted in a standard T test at the 99 per cent level. On the other hand, for the contemporary and post-epidemic families, the difference (-.11) is not only in the "wrong" direction but is also less than a third of the standard deviation (.326). Hence, under a standard T test, the second hypothesis — that post-epidemic families increase the number of births — would be rejected. Similar results are obtained from non-parametric goodness of fit tests, which are, perhaps, more appropriate. The Kolomogorov-Smirnov statistic is significant at the 99 per cent level for the first hypothesis but is *not* significant at the 40 per cent level for the second hypothesis.[12]

The results of the comparison of epidemic and contemporary families are not altogether unexpected. If the throat distemper tended to afflict the larger families, then the observed difference in family births might reflect differences existing prior to the epidemic. To test this hypothesis, seventy-one pairs of families were chosen. Each pair consisted of an epidemic and a contemporary family from the same village. The marriage dates of both families were either in the same calendar year or the marriage date of the epidemic family was earlier by no more than three years. Two types of tests were performed. First, the average number of births per family prior to the epidemic was computed for both groups of families, and a standard T test was performed. For the epidemic families the mean was 4.38 and the sample variance was 8.89; for the contemporary families the mean was 4.24 and the sample variance was 5.88. The difference of the means (.14) was less than a third as great as the combined standard deviation (.456), and the hypothesis that the means are equal would not be rejected. Second, to test whether families of one sample were typically larger than their paired counterparts, the Wilcoxon sign-rank test was used.[13] For samples with more than twenty-five pairs, this test statistic is approximately standard normal. The computed value of the statistic is .72; consequently, the hypothesis that the families were of the same size would not normally be rejected.

The results of the comparison of contemporary and post-epidemic families are also not unexpected. The bias induced by the sample and test design is apparently in the direction of the conclusion obtained.* Also, the implementation of a program of family planning based on changing child survival expectations may be a larger assumption than one can make about the colonial parent. The replacement of a child already dead is one matter; the replacement of a child not yet dead is another. There is, nevertheless, one piece of information that does conform to the initial hypothesis. Post-epidemic families had a larger average number of births in the first five and first ten years of marriage (Table 3). Although these differences are not statistically significant, they are of the expected sign. The post-epidemic families may have attempted to increase the number of births in the early years of marriage but,

Table 3: Births in Early Years of Marriage

	Contemporary Families	Post-Epidemic Families
Number of families	136	141
Mean number of births in first five years	2.35	2.48
Sample variance	.35	.66
Mean number of births in first ten years	3.94	4.16
Sample variance	3.07	2.41

*As contemporary families may have increased their births in anticipation of future deaths, it is even less likely that significant differences would be found.

finding that the distemper did not reappear, may have limited their births in later years.[14]

V

If families tended to replace dead children, as it appears that they did, then Chadwick, Shattuck, and other leaders in the nineteenth-century sanitary movement may have overestimated the benefits to be gained, in terms of mature workers, from widespread public health activity.[15] There are, however, some further questions concerning the applicability of the experience of the throat distemper of 1734-40.

First, how complete was replacement? If economic historians are to estimate net benefits, the extent of replacement must be known. In the sample communities, 493 children died during the epidemic. Of these, 443 belonged to sample families. It would seem, therefore, that about 68 per cent of the victims were replaced. Subjectively, this is a high replacement rate. The rates at which populations replace is likely to vary significantly. The relatively young age at marriage, the heavy incidence of the epidemic among children under ten, the presence of economic opportunity, and the general good health of the population suggest that New Englanders might have been better able and more willing to replace than other groups.

Second, were there differences between rural and urban families in replacement activity? Between New England and European families? To these questions there are no answers. The throat distemper in Boston, the only urban community in New England, took the milder form of scarlet fever. As for international differences, most recent work has indicated substantial similarities in family structure and demographic experience in New England, Normandy, and England.[16] Hence it may not be unreasonable to expect that replacement was as much a demographic feature of the English village of Clayworth and the Norman village of Crulai as it was of the New England community of Wenham.

Third, do families react differently to epidemic disease than they do to endemic disease, to new killers and to expected killers? It could be argued that a death attributable to an epidemic, especially a new epidemic, immediately changes the probability that a family will attain a given size with a set number of births. The family may then decide to replace. If the epidemic were prevented, the deaths would not occur and the replacements would not be born. On the other hand, it could be argued that a death attributable to an endemic situation is expected; hence its occurrence does not change the family's subjective probability that a given size will be achieved with a given number of births. If the endemic situation were ameliorated, the death would not occur; yet the replacement might still be born if the family did not recognize that a change in the probability of a survival had occurred. The recognition lag, of course, could persist for a generation or two.*

VI

The demographic experience of New England families during the diphtheria epidemic of 1734–40 supports the speculation that changes in the death rate stimulate adjustments in the birth rate – that children who died during the epidemic were, in part, replaced. The evidence, however, is not strong enough to support the hypothesis that families adjusted their births in anticipation of higher mortality rates.

NOTES

1. Selma J. Mushkin, "Health as an Investment," *Journal of Political Economy* 70, no. 5 (October 1962), pt. 2, pp. 143–45; Herbert E. Klarman, "Syphilis Control Programs," in Robert Dorfman, ed., *Measuring Benefits of Government Investments* (Washington, D.C.: Brookings Institution, 1965), p. 402; and Dorothy P. Rice, *Estimating the Cost of Illness* (Washington, D.C.: U.S. Department of Health, Education, and Welfare, Public Health Service, 1966), pp. 16–19.

2. United Nations, *The Determinants and Consequences of Population Trends*, Document No. St/SOA/Series A, Population Studies no. 17 (1947), p. 81; E. F. Penrose, *Population Theories and Their Applications* (Stanford, Calif.: Food Research Institute, 1934), pp. 115–20.

3. R. von Ungern-Sternberg, *The Causes of the Decline in Birth Rate within the European Sphere of Civilization* (Cold Spring Harbor, N.Y.: Eugenics Research Association, 1931), p. 40.

4. For a comprehensive medical and historical description of the epidemic, see E. Caulfield, *A True History of the Terrible Epidemic Vulgarly Called the Throat Distemper, Which Occurred in His Majesty's New England Colonies Between the Years 1735 and 1740* (New Haven, Conn.: Yale University Press, 1939).

5. John Duffy, *Epidemics in Colonial America* (Baton Rouge: Louisiana State University Press, 1953), pp. 113–16.

6. Nathaniel B. Schurtleff, ed., *Records of the Governor and Company of the Massachusetts Bay in New England (1626-86)*, 5 vols. (Boston: William White, 1853–54), 1:172, 276; 2:15; 3:426–27; *The Public Records of the Colony of Connecticut* (Hartford: Brown and Parsons, 1850), 1:47–8, 105–6, 551–52.

7. The registers and their limitations are more fully discussed in a paper currently being prepared with Robert Higgs. The legal background may be found in Robert Gutman, "Birth and Death Registration in Massachusetts," *Milbank Memorial Fund Quarterly* 36 (1958):59–74. A more general study of the uses of the registers can be found in Robert Greven, "Historical Demography and Colonial America," *William and Mary Quarterly* 24, no. 3 (July 1967):438–54.

8. See, as an example, S. W. Dimock, *Births, Baptisms, Marriages, and Deaths in Mansfield* (New York: Baker and Taylor, 1898), under family names Balch, Barrows, and Basset.

9. *Ibid.*, under family names Arnold, Morey, and Royce. Demos finds that almost half of the firstborn babies in Bristol after 1740 were born less than eight months after marriage (John Demos, "Families in Colonial Bristol, Rhode Island: An Exercise in

---

*In a modern developing country, where medical technology may be more advanced than other technologies, "replacement" may continue not as a result of a recognition lag but rather as a result of skepticism that the change in the death rate is permanent.

Historical Demography," *William and Mary Quarterly,* 3d ser., 25, no. 1 [January 1968]:56).

10. It is recognized that the vital index is not an ideal measure. It has been suggested that a high vital index might be found in various communities if their age and sex structure were significantly different from that of the rest of the population. Little is known about the age and sex structure of colonial society; however, what little evidence exists suggests that the sample communities were probably representative. According to the Massachusetts census of 1765, 47.7 per cent of the white population were under sixteen years; in the eleven sample Massachusetts towns, 47.5 per cent of the population were under sixteen. According to the same census, 52.5 per cent of the adult white population and 49.2 per cent of the total white population were female; in the sample towns, 52.1 per cent of the adult white population and 50.2 per cent of the total population were female. Twenty-five years later, according to the first federal census, 49 per cent of all whites were under sixteen, while 45.5 per cent of Massachusetts whites were under sixteen. In the same year, 49 per cent of all whites were female, while 51 per cent of Massachusetts whites were female (U.S. Bureau of the Census, *A Century of Population Growth* [Washington, D.C.: Government Printing Office, 1909], pp. 93–95, 158–61, 208).

11. Jacob Sander, *Comparative Birth-Rate Movements among European Nations* (Cold Spring Harbor, N.Y.: Eugenics Research Association, 1929), pp. 32–49.

12. A description of the test can be found in Sidney Siegel, *Non-Parametric Statistics* (New York: McGraw-Hill Book Co., 1956), pp. 127–36. Essentially, this test focuses on the maximum difference between two cumulative distribution functions. In the first case, the maximum difference occurs at family size five. For the contemporary sample, 41 per cent of the families have five or fewer children, while only 22 per cent of the epidemic families have five or fewer children. If the underlying distributions of family births were the same for both samples, then the probability that the cumulative distribution function would differ by as much as 19 per cent is less than .001.

13. This test was suggested by Joseph Gastwirth of The Johns Hopkins University. A description may be found in *ibid.*, pp. 75–83.

14. Family limitation cannot be ruled out. There is questionable evidence of family limitation in rural England at this time, and there is good evidence of deliberate family limitation in rural France during the early nineteenth century (see E. A. Wrigley, "Family Limitation in Pre-Industrial England," *Economic History Review* 19, no. 1 [April 1966]:82–109).

15. H. Chadwick, "The Opening Address of the President of Section F of the British Association for the Advancement of Science," *Journal of the Statistical Society* 25 (1862):505–7.

16. K. A. Lockridge, "The Population of Dedham, Massachusetts, 1636–1736," *Economic History Review* 19, no. 2 (August 1966):343. It should be noted that there were significant differences among these countries in ages at marriage.

Mark Perlman
University of Pittsburgh

COMMENT

This paper, which partakes of a current trend, attempts to answer questions about the stability over time of demographic behavior, using old demographic data. More specifically, it attempts to answer the question whether in the eighteenth century families had target sizes and whether, faced by new kinds of mortal epidemics, they adjusted their targets accordingly.

Dr. Stettler's method is to compare epidemic-hit families with contemporary non-epidemic-hit families during and subsequent to the epidemic, and non-epidemic-hit families who lived through the epidemic with familes formed after the epidemic was over.

Dr. Stettler in his description of epidemic families does not indicate whether maternal mortality occurred due to the epidemic. If it did, he apparently assumes that the father was the guardian of the target and that his subsequent wives were allowed only to fulfill the husband's original plan. Dr. Stettler further assumes that all mothers retained fertility potential, although no data are given to substantiate this assumption. Dr. Stettler has no information regarding child spacing (and presumably can get none), which is probably the one answer which could most easily confirm or reject his point.

His conclusions are: (1) that epidemic families had more children than did the luckier (non-epidemic) families; (2) that the post-epidemic behavior re-

	Epidemic	Contemporary
Mean births (total)	7.64	6.54
Pre-epidemic births	4.38	4.24
Epidemic and post-epidemic births	3.26	2.30

28

vealed a significant difference between afflicted (epidemic) and non-afflicted (contemporary) families and no significant differences between the non-afflicted contemporary families and the post-epidemic (non-afflicted) families.

My major question concerning Dr. Stettler's paper was that he seemed to use "target" and "replacement" concepts interchangeably in his discussion, even though at times he notes the distinction, as on page 25. His evidence does show the existence of a replacement concept. However, it gives no insight one way or the other regarding the existence of targets. Thus, he can conclude only that the epidemics led to replacements for children lost, and that there was no evidence regarding people making plans (*ex ante*) for the probable loss of children in future diphtheria epidemics. With reference to replacement, Dr. Stettler, unlike Lösch,[1] Habbakuk,[2] and most demographers, uses the father rather than the mother as the unit. Was this due to the form in which the data were available, or does he think it is a preferable measure?

As for the target concept, Dr. Stettler's data may not be suited to demonstrate much about it. His concept of target is too gross and does not reflect what it should include – (1) sex distribution, (2) number of children per subsequent wife, and (3) spacing and wife's fertility. The target concept, insofar as any such thing can exist (and he certainly suggests that it may not exist), may not be affected by any unplannable risk ("unplannable" in the sense that Frank Knight[3] and G. L. S. Shackle[4] discuss uncertainty). It may be that, from the standpoint of planning, epidemics are too uncertain to be assigned any appropriate probability risk.

In sum, the paragraph on page 18 beginning "The validity of the concept" contains the ambiguity which, in my opinion, should be removed from the paper. Dr. Stettler has shown that there was a replacement for children lost in the epidemic. He has not shown that this replacement was related to an *ex ante* plan ("target") which any family had. Instead, the replacement was an *ex post* remedy for an unpredictable risk. Dr. Stettler's findings suggest that the validity of the "target" concept is yet to be determined. Some may argue that the study of other periods may resolve his as yet unresolved question. However, I am not ready to agree that the concept of target can be tested by his method because Dr. Stettler's perception of target was, I suspect, too crude. In any event, it is not a situation consisting of only two alternatives, an inflexible target opposed to what Dr. Stettler calls "the appealing alternative that the changing socioeconomic environment (rising incomes, urbanization, and industrialization) was conducive to lower fertility, and perhaps to a smaller optimal family size." Whether the targets exist or not, they are subject to change, and the direction of the change caused by rising income, etc., is not clear cut, as has been indicated by postwar studies of American women.

NOTES

1. August Lösch, "Population Cycles as a Cause of Business Cycles," reprinted in *Population and Policy: Selected Readings*, J. J. Spengler and O. D. Duncan, eds. (Glencoe, Ill.: Free Press, 1956).

2. John Habbakuk, "English Population in the XVIII Century," *Economic History* 6 (1953):117–33.

3. Frank H. Knight, *Risk, Uncertainty, and Profit* (New York: Houghton Mifflin Co., 1921).

4. G. L. S. Shackle, *Decision, Order, and Time in Human Affairs* (Cambridge: Cambridge University Press, 1961).

REJOINDER

In the light of the major thrust of Dr. Perlman's comment, it seems best to let the original paper stand intact. In response to his criticism, I should now be inclined to emphasize the matter of the "replacement demand for children," de-emphasizing or perhaps even deleting the notion of "target family size." The immutability of a target size has been seriously challenged; the finding of a positive replacement demand remains unscathed.

H. L. S.

Wilfred Malenbaum
University of Pennsylvania

HEALTH AND PRODUCTIVITY IN POOR AREAS

This paper explores aspects of the relationship between health and production in less developed areas. It seeks support for the hypothesis that programs for health improvement are important components of a program for the expansion of output per man in poor lands. Inasmuch as resource limitations generally restrict the scope of a nation's development effort, choices must be made among alternative methods of promoting economic growth. In seeking the combination of inputs that lead to optimum development, how should a nation assess the gains from additional inputs in the health area as compared with additions to other economic inputs, including alternative investment, quantity of labor, education, or improved skills?

Some answers emerge from our exploration, but they are more suggestive than definitive. It is clear that there is both scope and need for further study of the economic consequences of efforts to improve health in low-income societies. The first section discusses the type of model through which the effects of greater health inputs on economic productivity can be traced. Empirical evidence on the relationship is presented in the second section. Finally, in III, the way in which a health-productivity relationship might fit into the economist's production functions for output and growth in poor lands is discussed.

Research for this paper has been financed in part by Grant CH 00294-01(2), Health Services and Mental Health Administration, U.S. Department of Health, Education, and Welfare. I am happy to acknowledge the assistance of Laura Rubin and German Otalora, graduate students at the University of Pennsylvania.

31

I

Improved health may be considered a *result* of improved productivity, a part of the product of growth rather than one of its causes. Only a rich nation can afford programs to assure its population's health. In the same vein, a poor nation cannot afford improved health. Lower death rates and the higher birth rates which tend to accompany them, at least initially, spur the rate of population growth. The result is more people to feed, more children to educate, less income per person, and a lower ratio of savings to total income. Reduced infant mortality is an important component of any reduction in the death rate. Hence the additional mouths to feed are those of children which, initially, are not accompanied by additional hands for work. It is not that "hands for work" are in short supply; poor countries maintain that capital shortages render the current labor supply relatively excessive. Unemployment and especially underemployment are too high. However much the supply of labor may gain in numbers or in quality from improved health and reduced death rates, there may be no corresponding gain in output. Thus, improved health in poor societies can lead to larger population, greater poverty, and eventually to deterioration in health.

All this is familiar and conventional lore on health-output relationships, and it does not augur well for our hypothesis. Also familiar is a health–development tautology. Obviously, a healthy worker is a more productive worker; at least he is absent from his job less often. Equally obvious is the proposition that any measure of development achievement in a nation must reflect the state of personal health in the nation. Further, an expansion in agriculture that provides more food per person for self-suppliers is considered, appropriately, a health measure. In addition, perhaps development activities such as improvement in quality of worker housing, in skill training to ease effective farm-factory transition, and, indeed, any movement of per capita income above subsistence level can also be termed health activities.

The numerous and diverse possibilities for the health-productivity relationship call for care in any statistical interpretation. Wealth and health are fairly closely related,[1] and there is some evidence that the relationship changes at a per capita income threshold of $400 to $500.[2] As the present work is limited to poor areas of the world, some of the uncertainties may be reduced. Also, the concept of a "health input" may create problems of statistical interpretation. We are interested in measures of health as independent variables that influence some such concept as output per man, the dependent variable. Health measures might be programs that lead to an improved state of health such as malaria eradication, protected wells, and medical facilities; they might be indications of the actual state of health, such as infant mortality, malarial incidence, and morbidity rates.

One difference between the two categories could be in their effect on the timing of the output. But the difference can be much more than that attributed to time lag, for some health programs do not have predictable health consequences. A government program for new latrine pits in villages may not alter personal habits. There is also evidence that major health programs in poor lands do not always pay off in indexes of improved health, even over a period of years. Thus a recent and extensive study casts doubt upon the ability of United States-sponsored health programs to achieve significant health gains in Ethiopian villages, as compared with control villages without the special health programs.[3] It is true that in Ethiopian society magic and traditional healing have long provided solutions for problems of the body and mind, but this situation is not unusual in the complex social and institutional structures of many other poor nations. Time lags can be long indeed; it may be necessary to continue programs for years before effects on health can be detected.

Yet there is the possibility that a health measure can produce economic gains without or before improving health. Increased agricultural productivity could come simply from the establishment of a nursing center in a village from which men go to the fields to work for the day. Even though the nurse may not be called upon by his family, the worker knows that they will receive medical aid if needed. The health-productivity link here is attitudinal. What, then, are the possible types of input-output sequences (models) that relate health and productivity? Three come readily to mind: first, the worker's increased energy potential, as a consequence of greater vigor and fewer sick days lost from work; second, the increased availability of other factors of production, such as access to agricultural land, forests, and resort areas, previously unusable because of insects, pollution, and other health menaces; and finally – already mentioned and perhaps least easily defined – gains through an enhanced response by labor to opportunities for expanding its contribution to production. This last sequence probably encompasses a range: at one extreme, enlarged health activities might serve directly to create higher motivation toward self-fulfillment and achievement; at the other, more mundane, extreme the health program might serve as a prerequisite to effective use of existing or newly available economic facilities.

These causal sequences can tell only a partial story in a real economy. From a technological point of view, improvement in a worker's health will increase his work potential. Whether the total output, or even the product per day or week of the healthier worker himself, will increase depends upon the labor supply in the region or industry. In many poor countries labor is already underemployed, at least for some part of the year. If the value of labor's marginal product is zero or below the average (institutional) wage, greater worker energy may simply be offset by greater underemployment ratios. In a Mexican village, workers in household pottery production suffered lead intoxication through absorbing oxide used for glazing. When treatment was provided, improvement in health did not expand output because the market was already too limited even for the product of debilitated workers. If in poor lands improvements in health do not expand output because of underutilization of labor, the potential relationship between health and output is difficult to discover.

With respect to the causal flow through the accessibility of new resources, the effect of better health conditions on land (capital) is properly analyzed as one of several possible technological advances affecting non-human factor supply. Production becomes possible on new lands if new methods of transport or new, faster-maturing seed varieties become available or if new health measures permit man to work the land. Whether such extensive possibilities are exploited depends on the demand for the product and on the alternative ways in which the demand can be met. For example, intensification of the productive process in areas now cultivated may be more efficient than putting more land under cultivation. The output gain through this particular sequence may be of importance in the real world, but it is not the kind of response with which we are concerned here. Resource expansion may also be accompanied by increased energy of workers whose health has been improved along with the land – for instance, through malaria eradication. Perhaps a separate study of the effects of human improvement and of land improvement is needed, with the former primarily relevant here.

Difficult to trace, but perhaps most important in real life in poor countries, is the causal sequence which stems from changes in worker attitudes. Here there may be a reversal of technological and economic considerations. Not many economists today question the key importance to economic growth of worker attitude in poor countries, where most workers are self-employed. If the worker is highly motivated, opportunities are created not only for greater physical output but also for expanded economic output. (Such a motivated worker in our Mexican village would find new markets, would adapt his product to capture more of existing markets, or would shift to a new enterprise.) More difficult is the "technological" basis of the transfer from events associated with health measures to a new approach to work and to greater productivity. The logic seems clear,* but the evidence from anthropological and other intensive studies is mixed at best. In some economically backward areas modern health measures are unwanted. But there also are societies where medical treatment extended by technical workers seems to be

_____

*As in the case of the nursing program in villages mentioned above. More fundamental, perhaps, health improvement through some specific health program attests to the power of man in contrast to the power of the mystical and the supernatural.

a prerequisite for the effectiveness of technical assistance programs. There are other reports, however, of persistent opposition to such ministrations outside the mystical and traditional witchcraft patterns.[4] Yet, as in the Indian examples cited, persistence succeeded in making health services an effective tool for action programs directed toward economic betterment. Current experience in the Tufts-Delta Health Center in Mount Bayou, Bolivar County, Mississippi,[5] provides evidence of the potential gains from health programs as a first and priority input on the road to economic progress.

The logic of this demonstration effect of health inputs and the reality of the links between health programs and other programs, combined with the fact of labor underutilization in poor countries, suggest that the statistical relationships discovered between health inputs and product outputs in such countries may be attributable in large part to the third causal sequence. It is with this expectation that efforts were made to identify statistical relationships in the present study.

II

Relevant statistical material is scarce. Emphasis was to be put on productive processes in which labor is the primary input factor. Although this is true in a general way for the world's less developed lands, averages even in these nations are composites of relatively small but relatively rich modern centers and relatively large but relatively poor traditional rural areas. Under such circumstances, national differences in output per man are influenced by the relative importance of modern capital-intensive production. Therefore, it seemed preferable to focus investigation, insofar as possible, on reasonably small and homogeneous rural groups at the village level. Reliance was to be placed upon existing research materials and operating programs. However, extensive examination of the pertinent professional journals and similar publications, as well as considerable correspondence, made it clear that studies made on a village or local basis do not provide significant information on health, and very little on economic product. This statement is true even for studies such as the evaluation of India's community development operations and for the vast number of village studies in Latin American countries, including Mexico. If a study contained reasonably relevant material, it covered only a single period and did not record a pattern of change. This broad generalization on the unavailability of materials stands even though the search for additional research findings continues, largely in Latin America (especially in Brazil and Colombia) and in the Near East (especially Syria and Egypt).

Accordingly, reliance had to be placed much more on macroeconomic material than was originally anticipated. Information was sought on a regional basis. Interregional comparisons replaced intertemporal comparisons. In India, for example, recent information on outputs, inputs, health, education, and the like was found in the field records of another study,* which provided comparable data for 1960 for twenty *taluka* in two states of India, ten in Maharashtra and ten in Uttar Pradesh. A second collection was composed of data relating to fifty provinces (*changwads*) in Thailand, all essentially rural and agricultural, which had already been subjected to intensive analysis for other purposes.[6] These convenient data could be broadened by adding some information on health and education. It was also possible to use data for the states of Mexico. Although some useful information could be obtained from publications for 1940, comprehensive data have recently become available in an agricultural census volume for 1960.[7] From data assembled through the United Nations and its specialized agencies about the statistical relationships between health and agricultural production for a number of poor countries, relevant measures for thirty-five nations could be analyzed. This writer's expectations were not high; it was contemplated from the start that certain nations would be eliminated in the course of the analysis precisely because the complex and heterogeneous information available about them could not be adequately summarized by the average statistics to which we were limited.

The following pages present brief summary accounts of the statistical analysis and results for these four regional groups — India, Thailand, Mexico, and the thirty-five developing nations. The pertinent statistics are presented in the tables. In all cases output in agriculture was employed as the dependent variable, with various economic and other measures serving as independent variables. The specific variables used for the different cases depend upon data availability. Among the agricultural-economic independent variables are labor, fertilizer, irrigation, new plows, and the like. For measures of health or health services there are such variables as infant mortality, incidence of malaria or other diseases, population per physician, new drinking wells, new latrines, vaccinations, and others. Finally, there are variables of labor quality, such as schooling and literacy. The variables were usually entered as an index, rate of use, or percentage, as appropriate and available. Needless to say, many of the measures used pose conceptual as well as enumerative problems. It is difficult to compare labor in agriculture in one country with another — even to compare regions in the same country. So much depends upon what labor participation is locally "customary" on the part of women and children. Infant mortality and morbidity data are often questionable, particularly when only the figures for a single year are used. There are similar problems with other statistics. Nonetheless, all have been used here with the hope that at a later date more selective statistics and improved procedures can be developed.

*International Studies of Values in Politics, a research program focused on political aspects of modernization, especially in developing nations. The study was conducted by scholars from research institutions in several countries — India, Poland, Yugoslavia, and the United States — in a general framework formulated by a central group at the University of Pennsylvania.

In each case the data were processed through a system of stepwise regressions which determined, independent variable by independent variable, those factors which contributed most to the explanation of the variation in the dependent (output or productivity) variable.* In this program,[8] the independent variables enter the analysis in the order of their correlation with the dependent variable.† The program provides a constant re-examination of the interplay of the independent variables and terminates when all statistically valid relationships with the dependent variable have been exhausted. In the present study, t values were also computed for the final coefficients; these are shown on the regression equations.

To illustrate the method, in the case of the thirty-five poor countries in Africa, Asia, and Latin America for which UN data were assembled, a preliminary trial was made with the following variables:

a, output: value of agricultural output in a recent period as a ratio (real change) of a postwar base
b, input, labor: percentage of labor force in agriculture
c, input, fertilizer: pounds of commercial fertilizer per acre
d, input, health: infant mortality rate
e, input, health: population per physician
f, input, health: dysentery, cases per 100,000
g, input, health: malaria, cases per 100,000
h, input, education: literacy rate

The hypothesis was that we would find negative (net) relationships between each of the variables d–h and the dependent variable a. Most of the variation in the latter was expected to be associated with the economic variables, labor and fertilizer, b and c, with positive regressions anticipated for both. Although the reasons for this assumption are obvious with respect to fertilizer inputs, they may not be so clear regarding the percentage of labor in agriculture. However, it will be recalled that the comparisons are among nations or regions and not over time. In comparing poor areas, is the size of increase in agricultural output in recent years likely to be greater in regions where a relatively large percentage of the labor force is agricultural than in regions where that percentage is small? The answer is not unequivocal. Structural shifts out of agriculture pose great difficulties in a poor, predominantly agricultural nation; they proceed at a slow pace even under very favorable circumstances. These considerations suggest that the regression coefficient is

*The program is the BMD02R-Stepwise Regression, developed in the Health Sciences Computing Center of the University of California at Los Angeles (version of May 2, 1966).
†Actually, partial F values provide both the order of entrance of the independent variables and the criteria for retention of a variable ($F \geqslant 0.01$) and for its subsequent exclusion ($F \leqslant 0.005$).

probably a positive one. An agricultural labor force that is large in relation to the total labor force means greater scope for intensification of output – the route for agricultural expansion which has been pursued in poor countries in recent years. However, the arguments are not definitive, nor is the evidence, as some of the work below indicates.

These expectations concerning the regressions were in fact supported by the statistical analysis of the UN data. Of the total variation in agricultural change accounted for by these independent factors, labor and fertilizer levels accounted for less than half (43 per cent), health variables for more than half (54 per cent), and literacy for the remaining 3 per cent. However, the standard errors of the regression coefficients of individual variables indicated doubtful statistical significance. Moreover, the coefficient of multiple determination, R^2 (the extent to which variations in the dependent variable are associated with variations in the independent variables), is very small (17 per cent). This certainly raises the major question of whether the group is sufficiently homogeneous to serve the purposes of this analysis. In subsequent work Argentina, Cuba, Israel, and Japan were eliminated as not being comparable to the other developing nations. For Ethiopia and Libya certain figures, especially for health measures, were far out of line with what is generally considered to be the situation.* In still another group, notably Iran and Iraq, there seemed to be internal inconsistencies in the available materials. Eventually, analyses were made for twenty-seven countries and then for twenty-two countries. Here results are presented for twenty-two countries, still selected from those in Africa, Asia, and Latin America. Use was made of all the above variables except f and g; for many countries these measures of dysentery and malaria were not reliable enough for use.

The regression analysis gives the following relationship:

$$X_1 = 133 + 0.344X_2 + 0.038X_3 - 0.13X_4 - 0.00095X_5 - 0.024X_6$$
$$[2.2] \quad [0.73] \quad [2.7] \quad [3.8] \quad [0.25]$$

X_1 refers to our measure of output; X_2, agricultural labor; X_3, commercial fertilizer; X_4, infant mortality; X_5, the population-physician ratio, and X_6, illiteracy. The net relationships between the agricultural inputs and the output are positive: greater illiteracy, higher infant mortality, and higher population per physician ratios show in each case a negative net relationship with output. The five independent variables, with twenty-two cases, account for over 62 per cent of all the variation in output among the countries, in contrast to the 17 per cent for seven variables and thirty-five countries. Of the total variation explained, about one-fifth comes from the agricultural inputs proper and almost four-fifths from the health variables; less than 2 per cent

*See, for example, the limited data published for them by the World Health Organization.

Table 1: Data for Selected Developing Nations

Country	X_1	X_2	X_3	X_4	X_5	X_6	X_7	X_8
1. Brazil	139.0	48.2	2.1	112.0	3,620	1.2	131.9	38.5
2. Chile	124.5	28.0	7.6	99.8	1,810	3.6	–	16.4
3. Colombia	129.0	41.8	7.2	82.4	2,270	475.4	89.0	37.7
4. Honduras	136.5	61.5	8.5	45.1	8,870	891.8	309.8	55.4
5. Panama	137.5	43.3	–	44.7	2,260	106.1	194.7	19.7
6. Peru	127.5	49.6	–	88.5	2,230	209.6	14.8	39.8
7. Burma	128.0	62.0	–	109.3	9,360	–	–	42.3
8. Ceylon	134.0	55.4	19.2	52.8	4,640	215.7	0.9	32.3
9. China (Taiwan)	146.5	46.9	135.8	22.2	2,420	0.6	0.3	46.1
10. India	128.0	70.0	2.6	72.8	5,780	–	–	72.2
11. Indonesia	107.5	66.9	5.4	74.7	40,740	0.3	–	57.1
12. Korea, Republic of	135.5	54.9	88.3	115.6	2,850	2.9	5.0	29.4
13. Pakistan	129.5	74.0	2.9	130.4	6,430	–	–	81.2
14. Philippines	133.5	57.9	6.3	72.9	1,390	49.6	103.6	28.1
15. Thailand	159.0	78.1	1.1	37.8	7,560	87.4	78.6	32.3
16. Cyprus	149.5	38.7	24.8	28.2	1,380	5.2	–	24.1
17. Morocco	119.5	54.6	1.9	149.0	9,930	617.1	149.3	86.2
18. South Africa	129.5	29.1	–	128.9	1,900	–	1.1	68.5
19. Syria	156.5	55.0	1.3	28.1	5,110	2.6	13.0	64.6
20. Tunisia	125.5	59.7	1.3	74.3	10,010	–	6.1	86.6
21. Turkey	142.5	72.9	1.5	165.0	3,220	0.7	13.6	61.9
22. U.A.R.	140.0	55.2	85.0	118.6	2,380	1.0	92.2	73.7

Source: see text

X_1, output: value of agricultural output in a recent period as a ratio (real change) of a postwar base
X_2, input, labor: per cent of labor force in agriculture
X_3, input, fertilizer: pounds of commercial fertilizer per acre
X_4, input, health: infant deaths per 1,000 live births
X_5, input, health: population per physician
X_6, input, health: dysentery, cases per 100,000
X_7, input, health: malaria, cases per 100,000
X_8, input, education: percentage literate among heads of agricultural households

comes from the degree of literacy. Moreover, as the absolute *t* values (brack-
eted) indicate, the coefficients for labor use, infant mortality and population
per doctor differ significantly from zero, at least at the .02 probability
level.*

The data for the developing areas as national units do seem to provide
evidence of statistically significant relationships between production and
health; moreover, the influence of health factors on output appears to be
quantitatively large relative to the influence of other factors, including the
familiar agricultural inputs. The degree of intercorrelation among the independent variables is small. There is no basis – in the time sequence of the
data or in the literature available on the individual countries, for example –
for attributing the level of infant mortality or of population per physician to
the degree of change in agricultural output over these years. Specific programs for improved health were not adopted in any pattern related to the
degree of change in output actually achieved over this period. In any event,
no such sequence is discernible. One is tempted to say: expand public health
activities (the infant-mortality rate was used as a ready, albeit crude, index of
over-all health status), expand the relative number of medical practitioners,
and there will be positive effects on output. True, there will also be reductions in death rates and perhaps even some expansion in birth rates over a
period. These variables were not introduced into the present analysis.† It is
clear, however, that, if the drive to greater output is attitude-based as well as
resource-based, the growth of population will not automatically offset the
expansion of output. Indeed, attitudes favoring individual progress should
gradually serve to slow down the rate of population growth.

With so much variation in agricultural output (38 per cent) not associated
with any of the independent variables, much stress cannot be placed upon the
specific quantitative form of the health input-agricultural output relationship.
For our purposes it is sufficient that it is present – that it reveals an output
gain along with an improvement in the health position. Additional tests were
made with the same UN materials, using somewhat different measures of
output, different numbers of independent variables, and, as indicated above, a
total of twenty-seven as well as twenty-two and thirty-five countries. These
consistently supported the relevance of health factors in accounting for variations in economic output.

The data for Mexico were obtained primarily from census materials. The
dependent variable had to be constructed from individual crop production

*For data, see Table 1.
†For the twenty-two countries, indeed for thirty-two for which reasonably adequate
data were available, the dependent variable was not correlated with the rate of population growth.

Table 2: Data for Mexico, 1940

State	X_1	X_2	X_4	X_5	X_6
1. Aguascalientes	163	50.8	151	3,609	44.6
2. Campeche	359	62.4	77	3,097	50.0
3. Coahuila	592	54.8	122	2,845	38.0
4. Colima	200	60.6	140	3,632	41.9
5. Chiapas	135	85.8	94	6,237	78.8
6. Chihuahua	242	63.0	114	3,389	38.9
7. Durango	202	76.8	96	5,739	50.1
8. Guanajuato	169	71.4	146	4,371	71.2
9. Guerrero	84	87.4	75	6,603	80.8
10. Hidalgo	105	76.4	118	6,280	72.4
11. Jalisco	132	64.4	143	2,347	52.5
12. Mexico	103	78.6	146	6,252	69.1
13. Michoacan	133	75.8	109	4,657	70.1
14. Morelos	181	77.3	107	1,554	55.9
15. Nayarit	198	73.4	112	7,767	51.0
16. Nuevo Leon	144	54.8	107	1,663	31.8
17. Oaxaca	71	84.7	118	12,965	79.8
18. Puebla	115	74.1	141	3,597	68.2
19. Queretaro	112	76.5	123	6,953	76.9
20. San Luis Potasi	87	72.5	106	6,143	66.4
21. Sinaloa	244	70.8	87	4,748	52.0
22. Sonora	397	59.2	108	3,022	38.0
23. Tabasco	165	80.6	78	5,656	64.7
24. Tamaulipas	238	55.6	82	1,857	35.3
25. Tlaxcala	93	76.5	150	6,089	59.7
26. Veracruz	172	72.0	83	3,500	64.1
27. Yucatan	305	66.0	118	2,986	50.0
28. Zacatecs	94	77.8	133	16,037	58.9

Source: see text.

X_1, output per agricultural worker (in pesos)
X_2, per cent of labor force in agriculture
X_4, infant deaths per 1,000 live births
X_5, population per physician
X_6, literacy rate

data, which were, however, much less complete in the 1940 census than in 1960. Because of the major changes in Mexican agriculture during these two decades no ready way exists to improve the dependent variable for 1940. After some trial tests with the independent variables (discussed below), analysis was limited to twenty-five states in 1940. All twenty-nine states were used in 1960.*

*In 1940 Coahuila, Nuevo Leon, and Sonora were excluded. In addition the Federal District (where Mexico City is located) was excluded, as were the political subdivisions which came to statehood after 1940 (Baja California, Quintana Reo and the territory south of Baja California).

Table 3: Data for Mexico, 1960

State	X_1	X_2	X_3	X_4	X_5	X_6
1. Aguascalientes	3,612	49.2	16.47	79.0	2,342	29.38
2. Campeche	3,916	54.6	0.33	55.7	1,910	41.96
3. Coahuila	6,049	44.8	45.50	75.6	1,290	24.09
4. Colima	6,255	53.9	25.43	85.5	2,497	25.43
5. Chiapas	3,428	79.7	2.48	65.5	3,858	63.62
6. Chihuahua	8,640	50.0	22.73	84.1	1,878	28.59
7. Durango	7,860	70.3	16.37	63.2	2,489	24.31
8. Guanajuato	2,254	64.5	18.19	99.0	3,201	56.52
9. Guerrero	2,826	81.4	3.40	52.8	3,704	69.18
10. Hidalgo	2,578	71.1	10.44	74.0	3,537	63.50
11. Jalisco	2,916	51.9	16.87	87.2	1,764	41.74
12. Mexico	2,149	61.4	14.69	114.3	4,560	45.30
13. Michoacan	2,167	74.0	20.49	54.3	3,250	51.41
14. Morelos	2,661	60.5	33.13	55.1	1,434	41.29
15. Nayarit	4,584	70.9	2.01	61.8	2,992	37.54
16. Nuevo Leon	4,361	32.2	25.62	58.1	911	27.22
17. Oaxaca	1,749	82.0	14.45	77.2	6,300	62.43
18. Puebla	2,070	67.0	15.48	97.1	2,378	59.53
19. Queretaro	2,242	69.8	14.85	70.5	4,427	64.01
20. San Luis Potosi	2,575	68.7	7.32	67.4	2,669	52.66
21. Sinaloa	5,652	64.6	45.44	49.0	1,624	39.28
22. Sonora	10,867	53.5	84.46	74.2	1,361	30.33
23. Tabasco	3,807	47.6	46.20	61.2	3,166	37.85
24. Tamaulipas	6,936	50.0	0.87	62.1	1,141	27.92
25. Tlaxcala	2,412	68.4	2.32	113.3	4,135	28.64
26. Veracruz	5,980	64.5	1.91	51.6	2,014	54.23
27. Yucatan	6,047	59.0	0.43	70.4	1,155	45.94
28. Zacatecas	3,182	80.0	4.66	66.9	5,357	32.61
29. Baja California	10,430	39.4	65.65	71.5	988	21.81

Source: see text
  X_1, output per agricultural worker (in pesos)
  X_2, per cent of labor force in agriculture
  X_3, per cent of land irrigated
  X_4, infant deaths per 1,000 live births
  X_5, population per physician
  X_6, literacy rate

Data for the following measures were collected for 1940 and 1960:[*]

X_1, output: average production per worker in agriculture (selected crops, 1940)

*As indicated, these data are derived principally from census materials, which also provide information on other agricultural inputs (wooden plows, land in *ejidos*, all from the 1940 material alone) and on other health inputs (hospitalization, attendance at clinics, and the like, for 1960). On the whole, these additional data do not appear comparable from state to state, nor did they reveal any relationship with the dependent variables.

X_2, input, labor: percentage of working population in agriculture

X_3, input, irrigation: percentage of cultivated area in irrigation (1960 only)

X_4, input, health: infant mortality

X_5, input, health: population per physician

X_6, input, education: literacy rate

For 1940, our regression analysis provides the following equation:

$$X_1 = 572 - 1.5X_2 - 1.1X_4 - .0004X_5 - 2.6X_6$$
$$[0.7] \quad [2.7] \quad [1.1] \quad [2.0]$$

For 1960 the relationship is:

$$X_1 = 5842 + 67X_2 + 44X_3 - 6X_4 - 0.9X_5 - 84X_6$$
$$[1.4] \quad [2.4] \quad [0.3] \quad [2.2] \quad [2.7]$$

The two relationships are broadly consistent.* The signs for most coefficients correspond, the sole exception being that for X_2, the percentage of agricultural to total workers. It is not possible to determine which of the signs is more appropriate to the Mexican experience, although the comment earlier in this paper supports a positive coefficient, which is found in all other cases. But a negative relationship for Mexico may reflect its relatively high level of economic development among the world's poor countries. On the other hand, the significance of the coefficients for the labor variable, especially for 1940, is not impressive, nor is the positive figure for 1960 definitely other than zero. Still, as a point of major interest in the present paper, it is noteworthy that some of the health data for Mexico yield the most significant coefficients.

The independent variables "explain" 66 per cent and 63 per cent respectively, of the total variation in agricultural output in 1940 and 1960. Tests were made with such other independent agricultural input measures as could be obtained, notably agricultural equipment; and with additional variables of a less direct economic nature such as the importance of *ejidos* in the states, the percentage of population with piped drinking water, and data on hospital visits. None showed significant variation with the patterns of agricultural output per man in the states. Given the lack of precision in the data and the fact that the states of Mexico are too heterogeneous for an over-all analysis of agricultural output, the level of R^2 appears satisfactory. However, some categorization of regions may permit explicit introduction of additional contributory independent variables, and I am attempting to do this.

---

*Progress and prices increased the value of the output per worker almost 15 times during this twenty-year period.

Table 4: Data for Thailand

Changwad	X_1	X_2	X_3	X_4	X_5	X_6	X_7
1. Chai-Nat	728.9	81.8	59.1	0.24	74	6	15
2. Singh-buri	768.1	76.1	89.5	0.12	82	4	52
3. Lopburi	525.3	70.6	38.5	0.52	77	4	23
4. Sara-buri	499.2	66.8	19.3	0.78	78	12	17
5. Ang-thong	595.9	5.2	81.2	0.37	75	8	26
6. Ayuthya	552.1	53.6	82.3	0.23	81	15	25
7. Nonthaburi	347.6	60.5	77.6	0.04	73	66	2
8. Pathum-thani	746.5	67.0	88.6	0.56	76	65	27
9. Thonburi	58.9	22.9	60.8	0.45	72	37	–
10. Phra-nakhorn	80.1	10.8	87.6	0.67	69	62	2
11. Nakhornayok	686.2	74.0	46.9	0.14	77	20	27
12. Prachinburi	543.0	77.4	35.7	0.55	72	5	5
13. Samutprakan	512.0	54.6	80.1	0.57	76	10	–
14. Cha-choengsao	789.8	68.4	69.9	2.10	78	49	4
15. Cholburi	179.9	60.1	25.5	1.00	70	8	14
16. Rayong	143.9	76.9	7.7	0.53	82	10	23
17. Chant-buri	177.2	76.8	2.0	0.95	73	20	4
18. Trat	207.8	77.1	0.2	0.85	77	9	1
19. Chayaphom	390.5	90.8	38.3	0.64	75	1	1
20. Nakhornratsima	274.4	84.1	19.8	0.93	73	1	2
21. Buriram	328.0	87.8	30.5	0.16	63	0	–
22. Surin	393.3	90.8	18.1	2.50	58	1	–
23. Srisaket	290.9	93.5	14.6	0.28	54	4	–
24. Ubonratthani	316.8	87.6	11.8	0.45	71	7	–
25. Nong-kai	334.8	78.9	11.4	0.90	62	6	3
26. Loei	268.8	89.8	22.1	1.15	55	1	–
27. Udornthani	476.7	85.8	24.5	1.50	70	3	–
28. Sakonnakhorn	397.0	88.5	13.1	0.73	72	4	–
29. Nakhornphanom	275.3	87.0	19.8	0.86	51	2	–

In the observed covariation as measured by these equations, health variables, especially infant mortality, provide an important part (28 to 40 per cent) of the total explained variation in per worker output.*

For Thailand data were obtained for all the provinces (*changwads*) that are primarily rice producers, fifty out of a total of seventy-one. These provinces make up the central plains and the northeast regions of the country. The former is dominated by the reasonably specialized producers of rice as a commercial and export crop; the northeast district does not participate much in export trade and is considered a relatively depressed area. In recent years other crops – kenaf, corn, and cassava – have become more important, especially in the northeast, but they remain secondary by far. Output in our analysis was measured by rice production alone. In the period considered, 94 per cent of all fields cultivated were in rice.

*Basic data appear in Tables 2 and 3.

Table 4 – *continued*

Changwad	X_1	X_2	X_3	X_4	X_5	X_6	X_7
30. Khon-kaen	352.3	85.5	22.7	0.46	71	4	–
31. Mahasarakham	339.5	92.0	13.5	0.50	72	3	–
32. Kalasin	391.9	92.8	15.9	0.55	73	3	–
33. Roi-et	317.1	92.9	19.6	0.47	73	3	–
34. Uttaradit	422.7	86.4	22.9	0.87	73	4	4
35. Tak	247.1	75.0	45.3	1.17	50	–	–
36. Sukhothai	452.5	86.1	38.0	0.36	73	4	9
37. Phitsnulok	549.9	80.7	32.2	1.43	73	4	6
38. Kamphaenghet	614.1	86.4	17.2	0.21	75	20	3
39. Phichit	896.7	80.0	69.8	0.43	77	20	20
40. Phetchbun	537.5	85.2	40.2	0.18	68	1	4
41. Nakhornsawan	590.9	80.0	44.1	0.25	75	6	18
42. Uthai-thani	456.7	83.0	46.2	0.56	77	11	–
43. Kanchanaburi	176.6	83.3	21.9	1.22	64	5	21
44. Suphanburi	592.9	79.0	59.8	0.21	67	9	15
45. Ratburi	197.9	65.7	50.1	0.56	70	12	4
46. Nakhornpathom	462.6	77.1	59.3	0.67	65	31	19
47. Samutsongkhram	20.0	56.1	17.1	1.33	80	14	–
48. Samutsakhorn	317.0	52.3	58.4	0.44	71	32	3
49. Phetburi	353.7	68.0	55.3	0.24	66	1	1
50. Prachrap-khirkhan	50.9	69.7	3.8	0.52	70	3	13

Source: see text

X_1, output: tons of rice produced per capita
X_2, input, labor: percentage of labor force in agriculture
X_3, input, irrigation: percentage of land irrigated
X_4, input, health: percentage improvement in malaria death rate
X_5, input, education: percentage literate in population over age fifteen
X_6, input; percentage of holdings using chemical fertilizer
X_7, input: percentage of land using tractors

Four independent variables were used. The dependent variable could be entered in productivity form, as output per head of rural population. The following specific data were analyzed:

X_1, output: tons of rice produced per capita
X_2, input, labor: percentage of labor force in agriculture
X_3, input, irrigation: percentage of land irrigated
X_4, input, health: percentage of improvement in malaria death rate
X_5, input, education: literacy rate

They yield the relationship:

$$X_1 = -1042 + 7.6X_2 + 6.8X_3 + 31.9X_4 + 8.5X_5$$
$$[3.1] \quad [7.3] \quad [0.76] \quad [3.2]$$

All the coefficients except that of the health variable are statistically significant by the criteria used here. For all the variables the signs of the regressions conform to expectations. In contrast with the previous cases, here the economic factors dominate. Of the 62 per cent of the total variation in productivity accounted for by the four independent variables, almost 85 per cent is associated with labor and irrigation, roughly in equal parts. Literacy accounts for most of the remainder. The malaria index does not yield a quantitatively important contribution.

The Thai material warrants much more study. Of the variation in productivity 38 per cent is not associated with the independent variables in the present study. Moreover, preliminary exploration of statistics on deaths due to malaria raises questions about the malaria index used. Substitution of an estimated for the actual malaria index in nine provinces where irregularities were observed had a marked influence upon the health-productivity relationship for the fifty provinces (the simple correlation coefficient of malaria and output increased from .16 to .48).

On the other hand, Thailand is a major rice-exporting nation in which agriculture, especially in the central areas included in this study, has long been established on a firm commercial basis. Previous analysts have already stressed this more-developed-nation aspect of Thai rice production. There is the possibility that the motivational significance of health is smaller in such a country.* Also, the residuals from the regression analysis suggest a regional pattern which may warrant separate consideration of the central plains and the other provinces. In any event, there are enough additional data and insights to justify continued analysis of the regional statistics in Thailand in order to determine the role of health and other non-economic factors in regional output variations.†

In two states in India, Maharashtra and Uttar Pradesh, research workers have assembled a wide range of data bearing on current modernization trends for twenty development blocks,‡ ten in each state. Combinations of census and field statistics permitted the gathering of data on total value of agricultural output per acre in each block, and also on chemical fertilizers applied, manure pits dug, amount of double cropping, use of new plows, and a range of non-economic data, including numbers of new primary schools, new drinking wells, new latrines, and smallpox vaccinations.

After considerable testing of the data for consistency, regression analysis was based upon these variables:

*This argument may also pertain to the North Pacific area of Mexico.
†See Table 4 for basic data.
‡The "block" is a geographical unit popularized in the community development program. It consists of about a hundred villages and frequently corresponds in size to the *taluka*, a unit below the district.

Table 5: Data for India

Block	X_1	X_2	X_3	X_4	X_5	X_6	X_7	X_8	X_9
1. Deoband	563,389	32.33	568	470	72	2,503	23	215	132
2. Rampur	389,013	42.50	616	568	94	818	28	2,182	215
3. Bulinkheri	220,641	9.26	480	586	92	1,672	24	502	297
4. Bahaddrabad	456,289	61.04	410	324	188	568	28	19	200
5. Muzaffarabad	558,734	24.36	390	548	113	2,070	32	2,036	254
6. Biswan	204,269	3.96	654	818	56	2,014	36	5,046	251
7. Maholi	126,380	13.27	327	222	78	1,438	22	779	113
8. Misrikh	132,485	8.96	216	130	25	155	36	800	130
9. Kasmanda	99,158	27.38	188	260	37	109	30	881	280
10. Alia	115,964	8.73	194	170	41	305	30	292	83
11. Hatkanangle	400,880	1.53	3,416	—	773	51,678	17	245	21
12. Karueer	511,928	2.77	4,169	—	305	99,332	27	526	17
13. Radanagar	336,228	4.04	2,391	—	152	16,007	—	473	78
14. Ajra	163,262	1.14	454	—	97	6,779	15	536	24
15. Vengurla	44,463	3.95	441	—	48	10,538	07	484	16
16. Malwan	90,722	8.00	482	—	39	51,357	—	347	17
17. Deogad	45,291	5.01	923	—	34	30,085	07	596	11
18. Ratnagari	125,417	2.00	260	2	204	53,598	05	1,734	20
19. Guhagar	47,353	1.51	203	—	97	27,021	07	2,345	32
20. Chiplum	199,775	4.19	602	—	128	55,373	30	2,905	12

Source: see text

X_1, output: total value of agriculture output (in rupees)
X_2, input, land: per cent of net sown area used for double cropping
X_3, input, fertilizers: average supply of chemical fertilizers per year (in metric tons)
X_4, input, health: average number of drinking wells constructed per year
X_5, input, health: average number of vaccinations against smallpox per year
X_6, input, health: average number of sanitary latrines constructed per year
X_7, input, education: average number of primary schools opened per year
X_8, input, health: average number of manure pits dug per year
X_9, input, land: average number of plows used per year

X_1, output: total value of agricultural output

X_2, input, land: percentage of net sown area used for double cropping

X_3, input, fertilizers: average supply of chemical fertilizers per year

X_4, input, health: average number of drinking wells constructed per year

X_5, input, health: average number of vaccinations against smallpox per year

X_6, input, health: average number of sanitary latrines constructed per year

X_7, input, education: average number of primary schools opened per year

They yield the following relationship:

$$X_1 = -1878 + 5708X_2 + 93X_3 + 255X_4 + 100X_5 + 0.7X_6 + 382X_7$$
$$[3.0] \quad [2.3] \quad [1.7] \quad [0.44] \quad [0.47] \quad [0.14]$$

Again, there is statistical significance for the agricultural inputs and for an important health variable, new wells, the construction of which was particularly extensive in the Uttar Pradesh development blocks. The regressions for all the variables correspond to our hypotheses on the direction of influence. Together, the independent variables can be associated with 73 per cent of total variation in output, but most of the explained variation is due to fertilizer and double cropping. Drinking wells account for 11.5 per cent of the 73 per cent.*

In the present context there is need to examine other information on Indian development. The community development record is suggestive,[9] but there are no systematic data that would permit comparisons over time or among communities. Conventional health statistics on state or district levels provide measures on personnel, beds, and clinics which are not readily combined, nor has individual analysis yet permitted a statement on the health-output relationship. Although the Indian government does place great reliance upon production gains from certain health programs, the models through which these conclusions emerge are not available, and it is clear that India's health-productivity relationships require much more study.[†]

The table on the opposite page summarizes pertinent results of the cases we have discussed. All show some role in output for health inputs, although

*See Table 5 for basic data.

[†]A nationwide (malaria) control program was launched in 1953 and "resulted in the economic improvement of the farmer. Investigations in certain areas revealed that for every rupee spent on the control programme, a villager had gained 97 rupees" (from a statement by Satya Narain Sinha, Minister for Health, Family Planning and Urban Development, published in *Swasth Hind*, World Health Day Number, March–April 1968, p. 68). I have not yet been able to find the basis for this estimate.

Determinants of Output in Agriculture[a]

Case	Output		Percentage of Covariation Associated with Inputs		
			Economic	Health	Other
Developing nations, 22 countries	Changes in agri-cultural output	(.62)	20	79	1
Mexico	Output per worker in agriculture				
1940		(.66)	1	28	71
1960		(.63)	20	40	40
Thailand, 50 provinces	Output per worker in agriculture	(.62)	85	5	10
India, 20 blocks	Agricultural output	(.73)	85	14	1

[a]Multiple regression coefficients are shown in parentheses.

the relative importance of the role of health varies widely.

The question of the direction of this relationship (health→output vs. output → health) cannot be resolved by statistics alone, particularly by so sparse and irregular a statistical record. Yet the data in each case do suggest that the health observations are not consequences of the output variations. The programs for improved health through malaria control, infant mortality reduction, and better village health facilities seem to have been initiated by the central authorities and on the initiative of a govenment concerned with social welfare. Nor can regional variations have been causally associated with the international health program activities of the World Health Organization, which began in the early 1950s. The population per doctor ratio poses the familiar problem of the urban concentration of medical personnel and facilities. On the whole, where population per physician is important in the observed variation (as in the UN materials and the Mexican data), the internal evidence is consistent with both the importance of the negative regression between density and output and the preponderance of medical personnel in urban areas. Both sets of data show a positive correlation between the population per physician variable and the ratio of agricultural labor to total labor.

Although the results are approximate, a health-output relationship does appear in all the areas studied here. This in itself justifies further research and development of better statistics. On the output side, there is need for more comprehensive crop coverage or agricultural income estimates at state or lower levels. In particular, some estimates of supplementary, perhaps non-farm, income would be useful. There is great need for improved data on health facilities, and especially on new installations that provide drinking water and improved sanitary sewage disposal in poor countries. More data on new nursing and clinical facilities would improve measures of the state of health proper. The existence of a health-output relationship could then be tested on the basis of regional data in societies where labor supply is ample for most agricultural work. More valuable still would be meaningful data for small units, even villages, in poor regions, perhaps for several such units simultaneously. Time series for villages would be still more valuable. Field work, or, at the least, access to systematic records made in the field over a period of years, would be necessary to obtain such data. Perhaps the present type of interregional analysis can be sufficiently refined, with better statistics, to justify such field efforts.

Relationships between health and output were observed in areas where the supply of labor is relatively abundant and where the supply of non-labor productive facilities has not been augmented as a result of malaria control or similar actions. We therefore continue to assume that the health input-production output relations are affected in some measure by motives and attitudes. If man's health can be improved through his actions, he must have the power to affect his life on earth. As this is recognized, passive acceptance can begin to give way to active participation, an essential component of the process of initiating growth in a poor society.

With improved data it may be possible to discover specific parameters for a relationship which is assuming great importance in our understanding of the process of emergence from economic stagnation. Man's health is a basic ingredient of his *quality* as a participant in the economic world, with respect not only to his physical application but also and especially to his attitudinal and motivational drives. As is indicated in the section below, *quality* of factor inputs has a central role in development. Thus, economic growth theory may need the kind of relationships sought in the present paper.

III

Health inputs are properly associated with variations in economic output beyond those which usually are attributed to the inputs of classical economic theory, labor and capital. Given additional data and more refined analysis, the economist is broadening the range of inputs which he can handle explicitly. The health input-economic output relationship can be fitted into this expanded scheme. It is now generally recognized that changes in observed output cannot be adequately explained by changes in the input of labor and capital, when these are measured as quantities of labor and capital without allowance for quality change.

This emerges clearly in a study prepared by the United Nations Economic Commission for Europe for sixteen Western European nations plus the United States and Canada.[10] There the multiple regression equation linking rates of growth of domestic product with rates of fixed capital formation and of growth in the labor force leaves unexplained about one-half of the total variation. The results are essentially the same for manufacturing as for the economy as a whole. Similar investigations for output variations in the United States alone provide comparable results. Thus, from 1869–1878 through 1944–1953 inputs of capital and labor increased in relative terms from 100 to 381; the corresponding relative output was 1325. The unexplained component thus exceeds 70 per cent.[11] And finally, studies for shorter intervals in the United States, for the periods 1909 to 1929 and 1929 to 1957,[12] show an increase in the relative importance of the unexplained residual from 42 to 58 per cent of total output change.

The ECE-type analysis has been extended to thirty-six relatively poor countries in Asia and Latin America.[13] The results confirm the ECE analysis: 69 per cent of the variation in growth rates was unexplained by growth in the labor and capital inputs. Indeed, only in some of the more developed countries is the degree of explanation appreciably higher than 30 per cent. Moreover, this analysis suggests that such covariation as exists between growth of output and the conventional factor inputs is due much more to labor than to capital input.

There is a conceptual inconsistency between the actual record of growth on one side and the unreality of changes in factor inputs, with quality constant, on the other. Technical change is an integral part of the very process of economic growth and may even be embodied in the changing capital base of a growing economy. This changing quality of capital calls for labor of changing quality. Indeed, skills and intellectual command of nature, science, and society are preconditions for the occurrence of technical change. Unless the labor supply has the quality which seeks to innovate and adapt, there can be neither technical progress nor growth. The process of economic expansion must not only take account of changing quality components of capital and labor; it must also recognize the interdependence of the two quality changes.

Considerable effort has been devoted to the measurement of the stock of capital, adjusted for quality change. Usually this has been done by taking into account the average age of capital. It is very difficult to develop measures of capital of constant quality. Efforts at measuring the quality of labor have focused on education and training, but imagination, enthusiasm, motivation, and even entrepreneurial skills may be discernible only through their actual contribution to output. Perhaps advanced nations can introduce monetary rewards for these qualities. These could then serve as weights in the construction of measures of labor input which would take into account these qualities as well as mere growth in numbers. In a poor society, assessment of the contribution of such skills and talents will require the addition of new independent statistical variables. Here, health inputs may provide preliminary beginnings.

Recent formulations of production functions start from:[14]

$$(1) \qquad \frac{\Delta O}{O} = \frac{\Delta A}{A} + b\frac{\Delta L}{L} + (1 - b)\frac{\Delta K}{K}$$

Here the labor and capital terms (L and K) are of constant quality. Total factor productivity (A) is meant to reflect all quality changes in L and K: it is the measure of the "unexplained residuals" above. As explicit adjustments are attempted for qualities embodied in the original capital endowment (age of capital equipment, rates of depreciation), and the original labor endowment (improvement in education, age-sex composition, and numbers of hours of work), the residual total productivity is reduced.[15] Thus:

$$(2) \qquad \frac{\Delta A}{A} = \frac{\Delta A'}{A'} + b\frac{\Delta L'}{L'} + (1 - b)\frac{\Delta K'}{K'}$$

where L' and K' refer to quality dimensions of L and K, respectively. In equation (1) these qualities were presumably "disembodied" and measured as part of the residual, total factor productivity, A. Conceptually, more insight on the factors responsible for A would permit its eventual elimination, as explicit adjustments are made for the real causes of the changes in growth, $\Delta O/O$.*

Such a simple additive sequence of separable items understates the complexity of the process of explaining growth and particularly the interdependence of quality factors. Thus to "separate out" the skills of labor may leave a residual in quality of equipment which could be meaningless without skilled labor. Alternatively, more of one quality might appropriately compensate for less of another; or even more, motivations and drives (labor qualities) may contain the dynamic prerequisites for quality changes in capital. These possibilities are mentioned not only to suggest the dangers of oversimplifying through sequences of sums but also to stress the possibility that labor quality may itself be one of the fundamental ingredients of the growth process. This was suggested by the results of some of the statistical calculations in the paper. Comparable suggestions are made in the ILO and UN studies cited previously.

There will be improvement in the precision of our measures of health-output relations when we have better data, and especially when we can actually derive them on a systematic time series basis. Also, the usefulness of our results in a program for growth may depend on the extent to which interregional comparisons can be used effectively as substitutes for intertem-

*The separation of quality dimensions actually embodied in the original K and L measures means that original approximations to the elasticity of output, b and $(1 - b)$, may need reappraisal as more measures of quality are introduced.

poral changes. Cross-section analysis has often been substituted for time-series analysis in economic research, as in measurements of demand and supply elasticities, but their use always calls for some qualification.

If improved health does contribute to expanded output in poor countries for reasons which are fundamentally different from those that explain the contributions of labor, land, and capital, this insight can help our understanding of the process of development. It may also lead to the restoration of a more positive attitude toward the economic role of health programs in poor nations. From an early tendency to see only the gains from such improvement,[16] "the negative influences [from population growth, reduced savings and a lower productivity of investment] gather strength as time progresses."[17] Inevitably, it is said, the positive gain is offset and replaced by a net loss. This paper moves toward restoring the original position. Health inputs may in fact lead to continued growth of per capita output even though rates of population growth are high.

NOTES

1. See "The Contents and Measurement of Development," in United Nations Research Institute for Social Development, *Research Notes*, no. 1 (Geneva: By the Institute, 1968), pp. 8–23. Of some hundred social and economic indicators in 115 countries, health variables tend to be most highly correlated with all measures of progress (pp. 15–18). See also F. Harbison and C. A. Myers, *Education, Manpower and Economic Growth* (New York: McGraw-Hill, 1964), pp. 23–48.

2. United Nations Research Institute for Social Development, *Research Notes*, p. 13. Important health variables "seem to move more rapidly or less rapidly (after this range) . . . with given increases of per capita national income." The results, however, are tentative. Similarly, D. C. McClelland emphasizes different aspects of the relationship (health and wealth) in different wealth ranges; see "The Relationship of Health and Wealth among Modernizing Nations," a paper prepared in 1964 in connection with a Harvard University research project on economic growth in Tunisia.

3. See Julius S. Prince, "Demonstration and Evaluation Project, Ethiopian Health Center Program: Its Impact on Community Health in Three Towns," *Ethiopian Medical Journal* 5, no. 3 (July 1967).

4. McKim Marriott, "Western Medicine in a Village of Northern India," in *Health, Culture and Community*, ed. B. D. Paul (New York: Russell Sage Foundation, 1955), p. 241: "The facilities of western medicine are largely ignored by the inhabitants of Kishan Garhi, but indigenous folk-medicine, magical, sacred and secular, flourishes in every village of northern India. In terms of numbers of patients, amount of expenditure, and frequency of use, patronage of indigenous medicine surpasses that of western medicine one hundredfold." He goes on to suggest that health programs presented in the western context will not be accepted, and that only when they are modified to conform with the Indian way of life will any benefit be realized. On the other hand, Charlotte V. and William H. Wiser, who had extensive experience in another village of North India, found the people quite willing to receive most medical aid that was offered. In fact, it was through the small dispensary which the Wisers set up that they were able to begin friendships and technical assistance activities with the people (see their *Behind Mud Walls* [Berkeley: University of California Press, 1963]).

5. This statement is based on "Progress Report of the Tufts-Delta Health Center," a mimeographed report issued by its director general, H. Jack Geiger, in October 1968.

(This information subsequently provided the core of a report in the *Wall Street Journal* for January 14, 1969.) The report cited considerable evidence of economic resources underutilized until popular motivation (emanating from the establishment of the Health Center) prompted new economic beginnings.

6. See J. R. Behrman, *Supply Response in Underdeveloped Agriculture: A Case Study of Four Major Annual Crops in Thailand, 1937-1963* (Amsterdam: North-Holland Publishing Co., 1968).

7. United States of Mexico, Department of Industry and Trade, Office of Statistics and Census, *Census of Agriculture, Livestock and "Ejidos," 1960* (Mexico City: United States of Mexico, 1965).

8. A detailed description of the program, its computational system and machine procedure, is provided in W. J. Dixon, ed., *BMD: Biomedical Computer Programs* (Berkeley and Los Angeles: University of California Press, 1967). The best discussion of the method may be found in M. A. Efroymsen, "Multiple Regression Analysis," in *Mathematical Methods for Digital Computers,* ed. A. Ralston and H. S. Wilf (New York: John Wiley & Sons, 1960), pt. 5 (17).

9. See my statement on this subject presented at a 1961 meeting of the Pan American Sanitary Bureau (World Health Organization *Boletin* [January 1962]:46–56).

10. *Some Factors in Economic Growth in Europe during the 1950's: Part 2, Economic Survey of Europe in 1961* (Geneva: Economic Commission for Europe, 1964).

11. Moses Abramovitz, *Resource and Output Trends in the United States since 1870,* National Bureau of Economic Research Occasional Paper No. 52 (New York: By the Bureau, 1956), p. 8.

12. Edward F. Denison, *The Sources of Economic Growth in the United States and the Alternatives before Us,* Supplementary Paper No. 13 (Washington, D.C.: Committee for Economic Development, 1962), Table 19, p. 148.

13. Walter Galenson and Graham Pyatt, *Quality of Labor and Economic Development in Certain Countries* (Geneva: International Labour Office, 1964), pp. 22–38.

14. R. R. Nelson, "Aggregate Production Functions and Medium-Range Growth Projections," *American Economic Review* 54, no. 5 (September 1964):575–606. The additive form of the relationship derives from the convenience offered by the Cobb-Douglas model:

$$O_t = A_t L_t^b K_t^{(1-b)}$$

where O_t, L_t, and K_t are, respectively, total output, labor, and capital in year t, where A_t is an index of total factor productivity in that year, and where b and $(1-b)$ are elasticities of output with respect to labor and capital, respectively. (In a competitive equilibrium position these elasticities indicate the relative shares of the two factors in total output, i.e., in the United States, for example, b would approximate 0.70 and $(1-b)$, 0.30.) The Cobb-Douglas function in logarithmic form converts to a simple equality of rates of change in output and the sum of rates of change of independent variables multiplied by constants b, $(1-b)$.

15. The names most frequently associated with these adjustments are R. M. Solow (especially "Technical Progress, Capital Formation and Economic Growth," *American Economic Review* 52, no. 2 [May 1962]:76–86), and Denison, *Sources of Economic Growth.* The contributions of these studies also are discussed in Nelson, "Aggregate Production Functions."

16. Thus "For economic reasons alone, the effort [of eradicating malaria] would be worthwhile, since the economic results of effective anti-malaria measures are a foregone conclusion" (F. L. Hoffman, *Malaria Problems* [Newark, N.J.: Prudential Press, 1928]).

17. Robin Barlow, "The Economic Effects of Malaria Eradication," *American Economic Review* 57, no. 2 (May 1967):130–48.

Richard Goode
International Monetary Fund

COMMENT

Professor Malenbaum's paper is a most welcome effort to quantify the relationship between health and productivity in less developed countries. He finds an impressive association between health and productivity in a group of twenty-two developing countries and in Mexico (particularly in his equation for 1960), but the results are much less impressive for Thailand and India. I shall return later to a few comments on the possible reasons for the difference in results for Thailand and India on the one hand, and for Mexico and the twenty-two-country group on the other.

Malenbaum enumerates three ways in which improved health may increase output: (a) by increasing the energy potential of workers; (b) by making additional land accessible for use; and (c) by improving the motivation or attitudes of workers. He stresses the last factor as potentially the most important. As I understand it, Malenbaum's reasoning runs as follows. In many — or possibly most — less developed areas there is a surplus of unskilled labor, and its marginal product must be reckoned as zero or close to zero. In these conditions health measures that merely increase the number of unskilled workers or the amount of time that they work will raise output only a little or not at all. An improvement in labor motivation due to better health, however, will constitute an improvement in the quality of labor services, which will be conducive to innovation and technical progress. In short, the marginal product of better motivated workers will be significantly above zero. Another consideration is that the change in attitudes may be associated with a declining birth rate. We may thus escape the Malthusian dilemma that

Interpretations and opinions are my own and do not purport to reflect the official views of the International Monetary Fund.

improvements in health do not raise standards of living or increase per capita productivity because they merely bring with them an increase in population.

Although I find congenial the stress on motivation and attitudes, my interpretation differs in certain respects from that of Malenbaum. The most important source of difference is that I do not assume, as he seems to, that the typical situation in less developed countries is one of underemployment, or disguised unemployment, of labor. This is not the time or place for an extended discussion of this subject. It is a large issue which has become, I sometimes think, almost an ideological question. For whatever it is worth, I will assert that I am highly skeptical of the labor-surplus or disguised-unemployment hypothesis. On this subject, I find persuasive the arguments of T. W. Schultz. Observation suggests that when labor is withdrawn from the agricultural sector without a simultaneous increase in capital investment or improvement in techniques, output suffers. Programs based on the assumption of disguised unemployment have not performed as expected. I believe that increases in the energy potential of workers, even without a change in attitudes, will generally raise output. Also, in many cases public health measures can be expected to increase output by opening up additional natural resources. Nevertheless, I agree with Malenbaum that improved health can facilitate technical progress by changing people's attitudes toward the capacity of men to control their environment and to better their lives. In order to take advantage of the better motivation, however, injections of capital will usually be needed, and often government programs will be required to acquaint people with the better techniques and to prepare them to use these techniques efficiently.

It is interesting to note that in Malenbaum's equations the findings that are most favorable to health are those in which infant mortality is used as a summary measure of health conditions. A reduction in infant mortality may indeed be associated with attitudes toward the external world and the future which are conducive to modernization.

For Thailand and India, where the statistical findings relating to the importance of health are unimpressive, the health variables themselves may be subject to some question. In the case of India, Malenbaum's health variables are in fact inputs of health services rather than output in the form of improved health. The three variables used are the number of drinking wells constructed, the number of vaccinations against smallpox, and the number of sanitary latrines constructed. While it seems clear that these facilities and services may contribute to improved health, they are one stage removed from that result. For Thailand the health variable used is the death rate from malaria. This is a direct measure of health conditions, but it may not be a wholly satisfactory one. It is clear that correct classification of the cause of death puts a greater demand on the keepers of vital statistics than does the mere recording of the fact of death, as in the case of the statistics of infant mortality. As Malenbaum notes, there are some doubts about the reliability of the malaria index used for Thailand. Another question which I raise for possible comment by persons who are acquainted with the facts about malaria, as I am not, is whether the death rate from malaria is closely correlated with the incidence of malaria in debilitating form. Is it possible that malaria deaths, even if accurately recorded, would not show how many people were sick from malaria to a degree that impaired their productivity?

I should also like to stress a question, mentioned by Malenbaum himself, about the suitability of the variable percentage of labor force in agriculture as a measure of labor input. While conceding that the relationship is not unequivocal, Malenbaum posits that a high percentage of the labor force employed in agriculture will be associated with large total agricultural output or large output per capita. Yet in advanced countries rapidly rising agricultural output has been accompanied by rapidly declining proportions of agricultural employment to the total labor force, and it is interesting that for Mexico Malenbaum's findings are not clearly consistent with his hypothesis. It strikes me that *numbers* employed in agriculture, or numbers per unit of cultivated area, would be a more straightforward measure of labor input.

I hope that it is clear that my criticisms are not intended in any way to suggest lack of enthusiasm for this interesting and useful paper. I am sure that many will join me in hoping that Malenbaum will go ahead with his research in this field. Perhaps some of the participants in this conference may be able to help him find additional usable data.

Joseph P. Newhouse
Harvard University

DETERMINANTS OF DAYS LOST FROM WORK DUE TO SICKNESS

INTRODUCTION

One of the most difficult problems in any analytical study of the health of a given area is finding an appropriate criterion to measure health. Previous investigators have concentrated almost entirely upon either over-all or disease-specific mortality or upon infant and maternal mortality.[1] Clearly, such criteria are inadequate measures of the health of a developed country, particularly if one has the World Health Organization's definition of health in mind: "a state of complete physical, mental, and social well-being, and not merely the absence of disease or illness."[2] The lack of a criterion of health more comprehensive than mortality, regrettable as it may be, is not really important until the analyst attempts to appraise the rationality of resource allocation in the area. For that purpose it is crucial to identify a better measure.

The most obvious improvement one might make is to utilize some measure of morbidity (i.e., sickness) in addition to mortality. While this by no means solves the problem (notice that the criterion still violates the World Health Organization definition and does not include the costs of pain or anxiety), it does establish a more useful criterion for policy purposes. Such a criterion is sufficient if other dimensions of health are of negligible relative value or if they are perfectly correlated with an appropriate weighted average of mortality and morbidity.* The intention of this paper is to analyze the determinants of days lost from work because of sickness in order to find a production function for one of the outputs of the medical system, namely, reductions in

*The weights are the relative values assigned to morbidity and mortality.

days lost from work. This paper is based upon a dissertation which attempted to appraise the rationality of present resource allocation in the health area in general by considering the levels of both mortality and morbidity as outputs of the medical care system.[3]

STATISTICAL METHODOLOGY

There is little or no a priori theory to guide one in specifying a model to explain variation in work-loss days. This is primarily because of the data, which are not cause-specific, but, in any event, epidemiological theories are notoriously underdeveloped outside the realm of the classic communicable diseases. The result is that one must use empirical methods; that is, one tries a number of variables to help explain observed work loss, being prepared to discard those which are not helpful. The cost of this methodology is that tests of significance have higher Type I error than they purport to have, though how much higher is, in the present case, difficult to know.[4]

Unfortunately, straightforward application of multiple regression analysis to this problem is undesirable for two reasons. First, there are few observations relative to the number of explanatory variables to be considered; in fact, the number of potential variables exceeds the number of observations in some of our samples. Second, as one might expect with a large number of explanatory variables, several which one would like to use are collinear with each other. In the face of this collinearity, ordinary regression analysis tends to break down.

One may avoid both these difficulties, at least in a statistical sense, by extracting a number of principal components from the set of original explanatory variables and using them as explanatory variables. The first component is the linear combination of the original variables (standardized), which maximizes the proportion of the total variance that is explained by the component.[5] A second component or linear combination of the original variables is then constructed which maximizes the explained portion of the residual variance, subject to the condition that it be orthogonal with the first. The process of extracting components can be continued until there are as many components as there are observations or variables, whichever is fewer (provided no two variables are exactly correlated; the number of components needed to explain all the variance will be reduced by one for every variable exactly correlated with another). Nearly always, however, a few components suffice to explain most of the variation, which is another way of saying that there are really relatively few dimensions of variation in many sets of real-world data.

Two problems are associated with the use of principal components as independent variables. The first is the result of collinearity. Since the components are constructed to be orthogonal to one another, collinearity causes no estimating problem, but, as one might suspect, a conceptual problem remains.

Collinearity manifests itself in the components when two or more variables are highly correlated with one particular component. (If all original variables were orthogonal, each variable would be uniquely associated with a component.) This creates a problem in "identifying" or assigning some meaning to a component. Further clarification of this point, if it is needed, should be provided by the application below.

The second conceptual problem is that one cannot find unambiguous marginal productivities of inputs; that is, principal components allow one to ascertain which variables are related to the dependent variable, but it is not possible to say how much a change in the level of any explanatory variable would change the dependent variable. Unlike the regression coefficients of the set of explanatory variables, which translate straightforwardly into marginal productivities, it is not clear what the coefficients of the components mean. Strictly speaking, the components are like an activity or fixed-proportion bundle of goods. An incremental change in all variables in the component in proportion to their linear weights would change the dependent variable by an amount equal to the estimated coefficient multiplied by the incremental change, but some variables in the components cannot be affected by public policy. It is not clear that a change in one element (or in those elements which are amenable to policy) would lead to a change in the dependent variable. However, it might. This is the dilemma posed for the analyst by the collinear nature of the data.

Because of these disadvantages of regression on components, it is important also to use the original variables in ordinary regression analysis, for only then can one compare the effect upon work loss of one variable with that of another. Regression on the components, however, is a most helpful first step. Inspection of the results of the regressions on the components can yield information on how the independent variable set can be reduced (necessary because of the small number of observations). Also, the components serve as a warning not to ascribe too much meaning to the regression results using the original variables. If only one of several variables correlated with a particular component appears in a regression, it may be acting as a proxy for some or all of the others.

SPECIFICATION OF A MODEL

The dependent variables are work-loss days for all ages and for age groups 17-44 and 45-64, as measured by the National Health Survey.[6] The measure is restricted to the employed population. Disaggregation by age groups is an attempt to control for the age variable. In addition, it is important to know which variables affect which age groups, unless all ages are to be given equal weight in the social welfare function.

There are several explanatory variables to be considered. They can be conveniently grouped in four categories. The first category is demographic: the percentage non-white, the percentage male, the educational status of the population (percentage who finished high school and the percentage with less than five years of education), and the percentage married were considered. The second category is environmental: variables included measures of air pollution (suspended particulate matter, nitrogen dioxide concentration, sulphur dioxide concentration), of climate (average annual number of degree days and days per year with more than 0.01 inches of precipitation), extent of urbanization (percentage of the population urban and percentage living in central cities), and the quality and quantity of housing (percentage of housing units sound and percentage of occupied housing units with more than one person per room). The third category is medical, and it is among these variables that one usually speaks of allocating a health budget. Nevertheless, it cannot be emphasized too strongly that a change in one of the non-medical variables (many of which are clearly amenable to policy) may do more to affect health status than a change in one of the medical variables. We are fortunate that the National Health Survey has gathered data on physician visits and hospital discharges.* Thus, one of the common pitfalls of production function estimation – the need to use capital stock data as a proxy for capital services – could be avoided. In addition, these variables are age-specific (others are not) and are also specific to residents of the units of observation (physician and hospital stock variables generally are not). Two variables which attempt to measure the quality of medicine being practiced were also included, percentage of physicians who are general practitioners and a dummy variable which measures the presence or absence of a medical school. The fourth category is economic. Here a real income variable was included: because it is unlikely that consumption of goods and services which affect health is perfectly correlated with the current year's income, an attempt was made to approximate permanent income by averaging real income for two past years.[7] This procedure also helped to prevent a simultaneous-equation bias in which current income is seen as a function of work days lost. Other economic variables are the percentage of the population with annual income under $3,000 and the percentage with hospital insurance. In the regression analysis using the original variables several additional variables were considered. The most important of these were per capita food expenditure and variables to measure the occupational mix.

The justification for the inclusion of all these variables should be reasonably obvious; I have provided detailed comments upon them as well as data

---

*Number of discharges is not an ideal measure of the flow of hospital services, since one needs data on length of stay as well. This household survey did not collect the latter.

sources elsewhere.[8] The units of observation are twenty-two standard metropolitan statistical areas (SMSAs) during the period July 1963–June 1965.

A valid question can be raised concerning the exogeneity of some of the
explanatory variables, in particular, physician visits, hospital discharges, and
percentage with incomes under $3,000. (Note, however, that since input
levels are not set so as to minimize cost for a given health level, the usual
simultaneity problem of production function estimation is not present.) To
keep the model reasonably tractable, these variables, as a first approximation,
were assumed to be exogenous (the model is currently being revised and that
assumption removed). If the variables are endogenous, the only problem is
the consistency of the parameter estimates, since there can be little doubt
(given the variables included in the equations below) that the number of
excluded exogenous variables would exceed the number of included endogenous variables (so that the equations are overidentified), and with twenty-two
observations one need not be too concerned about consistency.

RESULTS OF THE ESTIMATION PROCEDURE

Observations for three of the twenty-two SMSAs were missing for work
loss in the 17–44 age group, and observations for five were missing in the
45–64 age group. Thus, it was necessary to compute three separate sets of
components, one for each sample. As might be expected, these components
are reasonably similar, and to save space only the correlation matrix between
the components and the original variables for the components used in the
17–44 age group is presented (Table 1). Correlations of under 0.50
have generally been omitted from the table.

Examination of these correlations or loadings indicates the characteristics
of the population which the component is measuring. The first component
seems to be measuring the presence of poverty: it is strongly correlated with
the percentage within the population with income of less than $3,000 and
also has a negative correlation with the income variable and a positive correlation with the percentage with less than five years of education. In addition,
both housing variables load onto this component. The identification of the
second component is not so clear from the loadings, but it seems to be
measuring a well-educated population which sees a physician relatively often.
Also, areas with high values for this component have a warm, dry climate and
relatively little sulphur dioxide pollution. The other two pollutants (nitrogen
dioxide and suspended particulates), as well as hospital discharges, load onto
the third component. Identification of the other components is very tenuous.

The results of regressing work-loss days upon the first six components are
shown in Table 2. The numbers shown are the incremental F-statistics for
each component; the sign preceding each number is the sign of the regression
coefficient of the component. (The coefficients themselves are not presented,

Table 1: Work-Loss Days Correlation Matrix, Ages 17–44

| Variable | Component Number | | | | | | | |
	1	2	3	4	5	6	7	8
Hospital discharges			+.49					−.52
Physician visits		+.64		+.50				
Non-white	+.56							
Dummy medical school		−.58						
Hospital insurance	−.60	−.65						
Income	−.61							
General practitioners	−.57			+.59				
Income under $3,000	+.94							
Less than five years of								
education	+.56	−.56						
High school diploma		+.81						
Suspended particulate matter			−.49	+.56				
No. of degree days	−.60	−.61						
Days with precipitation		−.88						
Urban residents (%)	−.52				+.52	+.40		
Central city residents (%)					+.61			
Sound housing	−.60					−.42		
Occupied housing units with								
more than one person								
per room	+.80							
Married	+.73							
Benzene-soluble suspended								
particulates			−.66			+.49		
Sulphur dioxide concentration		−.60						
Nitrogen dioxide concentration			−.82					
Males				+.70				

since they are not useful.) Comparing the results, one notes that the first component – the presence of poverty – is significant for the older group but not for the younger. This suggests that a poverty variable belongs in the equation to explain work loss in the 45–64 age group, but not in the 17–44 age group. The second and third components are significant in the younger group but not in the older group, suggesting that education, physician visits, air pollution, and hospital discharges may all play a role in the younger group but not in the older group.

These hypotheses are all confirmed by the regression analysis, the results of which are shown in Table 3. Both linear and log-linear forms were tried, with the form that gave the better results being selected. Two results from Table 3 are interesting enough to deserve further comment. The first is that poverty is related to work-loss days in the 45–64 age group but not in the 17–44 age group. A straightforward explanation of this is that age and poverty interact in such a way that health among the poor starts to worsen earlier than among the well-to-do. In other words, the poor age faster, but at relatively young ages their health status is not very different from that of the

Table 2: Work-Loss Days, Incremental F-Statistics, and Signs of Regression Coefficients

Work-Loss Days	Component Number						R^2
	1	2	3	4	5	6	
Identification of components	Poverty	Good education; use of physician	Low air pollution; large use of hospital	N.W.I.	N.W.I.	N.W.I.	
Ages 17–44	Ins.	+25.31**	−17.79**	Ins.	Ins.	−11.84**	0.76
Cumulative percentage of explained variation	26	46	58	69	77	82	
Ages 45–64	+12.67**	Ins.	Ins.	−7.34*	Ins.	Ins.	0.59
Cumulative percentage of explained variation	27	49	65	75	82	87	
All ages	+4.82*	Ins.	−17.73**	Ins.	−12.29**	−5.97*	0.71
Cumulative percentage of explained variation	23	44	58	69	75	80	

*Significant at the .05 level (two-tail test).
**Significant at .01 level (two-tail test).
Ins., insignificant at .05 level (two-tail test).
N.W.I., not well identified.

Table 3: Work-Loss Days, Regressions on Original Variables

Equation No.	Form	Equation
(1)	Log-Linear	Work-loss days per person, ages 17–44 = 2.0073 + 0.4844 physician visits per person, age under 45 (0.1401)**
		+ 0.2195 Nitrogen dioxide concentration + 0.7239 per cent of population completing high school (0.0321)** (0.1494)**
		– 0.9570 Food expenditure per capita – 0.2907 hospital discharges per person, age under 45 (0.2575)** (0.1499)***
		$R^2 = 0.89$
(2)	Linear	Work-loss days per person, ages 45–64 = 10.3458 + 0.2033 per cent of population with income under $3,000 (0.0923)***
		– 0.0532 Hospital discharges per person, age under 45 (0.0187)**
		$R^2 = 0.56$
(3)	Log-Linear	Work-loss days per person, all ages = 4.4364 + 0.4477 physician visits per person, age under 45 (0.1051)**
		– 0.7687 Per cent of population urban + 0.1217 nitrogen dioxide concentration (0.2962)* (0.0269)**
		– 1.1190 Per cent of labor force male – 0.2631 hospital discharges per person, age under 45 (0.4870)* (0.1115)*
		$R^2 = 0.80$

*Significant at the .05 level (two-tail test). **Significant at the .01 level (two-tail test). ***Significant at the .10 level (two-tail test).

well-to-do. After some discussion with physicians, I believed this hypothesis to be reasonable. Among the older poor group, one tends to find a state of chronic morbidity from diseases such as emphysema, chronic bronchitis, disorders of the prostate and urinary tract, hernias, and back injuries, which are not found so frequently among either the younger poor group or among the older, more affluent group. Further testing of this hypothesis seems warranted.

Alternative but less satisfactory explanations are possible because most of the explanatory variables are not restricted to the currently employed population (as is the dependent variable), nor are they generally age group-specific. One possibility is, therefore, that the percentage in the 17–44 age group with income below $3,000 who are unemployed or out of the labor force is high both absolutely and relative to the proportion in the 45–64 age group. In the younger age group the additional poor found in certain SMSAs would tend not to be employed. Hence, poverty would not be associated with work loss in that group. If one could restrict all observations only to those employed, an association would be in evidence for both age groups. Data were not gathered on this point, but somewhat similar results for bed-disability days (which are not restricted to the currently employed population) tend to indicate that this hypothesis is probably incorrect.[9] It is also possible that the younger poor group which is employed tends to be in jobs or industries that are less well covered by sick leave plans than the older poor group. No evidence was available on this point. Another possibility is that the percentage of those aged 45–64 who are poor is high relative to the proportion of the younger group who are poor. Then the poverty component, which is not age group-specific, would primarily reflect variation among the poor aged 45–64. If the proportion of the poor aged 17–44 were not well correlated with the proportion aged 45–64, no significant correlation between poverty and work loss in the younger age group would be observed. This explanation does not seem to be valid. The number of male income recipients aged 20–44 receiving less than $3,000 is about 50 per cent higher than the number aged 45–64 in this income category.*

The second and perhaps even more interesting result in Table 3 revolves around the positive and very significant coefficients in the 17–44 age group of physician visits and the percentage completing high school, contrasted with the insignificance of the same variables in the 45–64 age group. The inference drawn from this is based on the assumption that well-educated people will more readily utilize preventive care when they do not feel well; that is, on their own they will not go to work if they feel ill. This may be because of greater perception of the symptoms of illness, greater knowledge of preven-

---

*Computed from U.S. Bureau of the Census, *Statistical Abstract, 1966* (Washington D.C.: Government Printing Office, 1966), p. 343.

tive techniques, or systematically different risk preferences. Furthermore, if one sees a physician, the physician is likely to follow a conservative course of treatment and recommend that one not go to work. The incentives he faces are in favor of minimizing risk,[10] partly because he does not bear the cost of hedging, partly because he may feel he should do "something" to justify his fee for the office visit.* But at younger ages a conservative course of treatment leads, on balance, to more work-loss days. This does not mean that it is irrational for an individual to follow such a course of treatment: one may rationally accept one day of work loss to avoid a 0.1 chance of ten days of work loss or even a 0.05 chance of ten days of work loss. The decision depends upon one's risk preferences. But the gamble seems to be of the latter variety in the younger age group, where the odds apparently are that an individual who continues to work will get well on his own. Note that there is an inherent bias toward a positive correlation between work loss and physician visits, since a physician visit will often lead to a work-loss day, the day on which the patient sees the physician. This factor cannot be too important, since in the 45-64 age group the physician visits variable (specific to that age group) has a negative (though insignificant) partial correlation with work loss. In the older group the insignificance of the physician visit and percentage completing high school variables makes it appear that preventive care is a statistically fairer gamble. At ages 45-64 there are probably more cases in which the physician can, in fact, prevent serious illness, and these may offset the cases in which the patient would have recovered of his own accord.

A few other results from Table 3 might be commented upon briefly. Hospital discharges under age 45 may have an effect in both the younger and older groups. This variable does not seem to be taking the place of hospital discharges among the 45-64 group in equation (2), since the simple correlation of discharges in the under 45 group with work-loss days in the 45-64 group is - 0.636, while the simple correlation of hospital discharges in the 45-64 group with work loss in the 45-64 group is only + 0.011. The explanation of why nitrogen dioxide concentration and food sales are significant in the younger group but not in the older cannot be explained; however, the explanation of variation in the older group in general is less clear. This ambiguity could be the result of greater sampling variability associated with each observation; also, there are two fewer observations.

The results for all age groups together are an amalgam of the two age groups already considered, with two exceptions. The percentage of males in

---

*Martin Feldstein adduces risk aversion by British National Health Service physicians as one reason why the elasticity of the number of hospital admissions with respect to bed supply should be relatively high, while the elasticity of mean length of stay with respect to bed supply is near zero. Physicians are unwilling to incur the risk of earlier discharge, particularly since they do not bear any of the cost of not admitting a larger number of cases.

the labor force is significant and negative, as expected. Urbanization enters with a negative sign: an explanation of that finding is difficult, since both physician visits and hospital discharges are in the equation; it might be that in a more highly urbanized area a man is more likely to live closer to his work, so that the marginal cost of getting there is less for any given level of sickness. The coefficients of both these variables seem too large, however. The significance of the other variables in equation (3) is reassuring, since the data for all age groups contain more observations and less sampling error in each observation.

POLICY IMPLICATIONS AND CONCLUSIONS

There are several difficulties in drawing policy conclusions from these results. First, they are part of a large number of equations in a study to determine the marginal productivities of various medical care inputs. Hence, any conclusions based solely upon results for work loss would be a case of suboptimization. Desirable reallocations cannot be prescribed until one knows the impact of these and other explanatory variables upon mortality and upon other types of morbidity. (Such knowledge is a necessary but not a sufficient condition for prescribing reallocation.)

Second, of all the explanatory variables, the only one to which a cost can easily be assigned is expenditure upon food. The cost of redistributing income depends upon intangibles, and, as the first component shows, it is not clear whether income alone must be redistributed for the desired result to be achieved. The cost of expanding hospital discharges depends upon whether there is excess capacity, and the cost of reducing length of stay must also be considered. The nitrogen dioxide variable is an index number which takes the values 1 through 5, and the costs of changing it are not easily calculated. The benefits (in terms of reduced work-loss days) from increasing physician visits or high school education are negative and must be deducted from any positive effect those variables have upon other dimensions of health.

We can quantify the benefit and cost of allocating more resources toward food. If we value a work-loss day in the 17–44 age group by using a weighted average of age- and sex-specific earnings, the weights being the proportion of the labor force in each five-year age-sex group (normalized to sum to 1), increasing food expenditures by one dollar per capita would increase earnings approximately thirty cents per capita (figured at the arithmetic mean of the two variables).* In other words, while food expenditures at the margin have investment as well as consumption aspects, the returns (based solely upon work-loss days prevented) are not great enough to warrant the expenditure on

---

*The proportion of the labor force in the 15–20 age group was used as a weight for the 17–20 age group. The resulting error is negligible.

investment grounds; a final conclusion, however, would have to take other outputs into account.

It further appears that resources devoted to reducing poverty might generate additional earnings in the 45–64 age group and so partly pay for themselves. Exactly what reducing poverty means, however, cannot be ascertained from these results. They do not indicate in which age groups poverty must be reduced nor exactly which aspects of poverty must be ameliorated. The answer to the latter question awaits the collection of richer data, since, as the first component points up, several variables related to poverty move together in this sample.

Finally, the results point up the desirability of disaggregating the data by age group. Differences between age groups are apparent, and it is important not to blur parameter estimates through aggregation.

NOTES

1. Edward S. Rogers, *Human Ecology and Health* (New York: Macmillan Co., 1960), p. 129; Harold F. Dorn, "Mortality," in *The Study of Population*, ed. P. Hauser and O. D. Duncan (Chicago: University of Chicago Press, 1959), reprinted in *Chronic Diseases and Public Health*, ed. Abraham M. Lilienfeld and Alice J. Gifford (Baltimore: Johns Hopkins Press, 1966), p. 29.

2. "Constitution, Annex I," *The First Ten Years of the World Health Organization* (Geneva: World Health Organization, 1958).

3. See Joseph P. Newhouse, "Toward a Rational Allocation of Medical Care Resources" (Ph.D. diss., Harvard University, 1968).

4. George E. Klein, "Selection Regression Programs," *Review of Economics and Statistics* 50, no. 2 (May 1968):288–90.

5. M. G. Kendall, *A Course in Multivariate Analysis* (London: Charles Griffin and Co., 1957), chap. 2, a classic reference on components analysis. A short, lucid explanation of the technique is in Gerhard Tintner, *Econometrics* (New York: John Wiley & Sons, 1953), chap. 6.3. A longer but equally lucid explanation is in Harry H. Harman, *Modern Factor Analysis*, 2d ed. (Chicago: University of Chicago Press, 1967), chaps. 1–8, 16.

6. National Center for Health Statistics, *Health Characteristics*, United States Public Health Service Publication no. 1000, ser. 10, no. 36 (Washington, D.C.: Government Printing Office, 1967).

7. Milton Friedman, *A Theory of the Consumption Function* (Princeton: Princeton University Press, 1957).

8. Newhouse, "Toward a Rational Allocation of Medical Care Resources," chap. 5.

9. *Ibid.*, chap. 7.

10. Martin S. Feldstein, "Effects of Differences in Hospital Bed Scarcity on Type of Use," *British Medical Journal* 2 (August 1964):563; Feldstein, "Hospital Bed Scarcity; An Analysis of the Effects of Inter-Regional Differences," *Economica* 32 (November 1965):404.

PART III

DEMAND ANALYSIS

Ronald Andersen and Lee Benham
University of Chicago

FACTORS AFFECTING THE RELATIONSHIP BETWEEN FAMILY INCOME AND MEDICAL CARE CONSUMPTION

The distribution of medical care is receiving increased attention from the government, medical care administrators, researchers, and the general public. There is growing concern that medical care is not "equitably" distributed in terms of quality or quantity.[1] It is asserted that some families receive considerably less care than is warranted, given the general affluence of our society and the potential of the health services system to provide it.[2] Demands for change are based on the ethic that all persons have a right to medical care of reasonably high standards regardless of their means.[3] Most of the recent governmental programs concerning the financing and distribution of health services, including the Hill-Burton Program, the Regional Medical Programs, the Office of Economic Opportunity Medical Care Demonstration Projects, and Medicare and Medicaid, can be viewed as attempts to implement this ethic.[4]

Family income has traditionally served as the prime measure of a family's resources, determining its medical care consumption as well as its demands for more conventional consumer goods and services.[5] The intent of this paper is to measure and assess the importance of some factors which may influence the relationship between family medical care consumption and family income.[6]

Social policies regarding medical care are usually based in part on an assessment of the relationship between income and medical care consumption. Our expectation is that such assessments will vary with the measures of income used. The fundamental hypothesis in the following analysis is that the observed simple relationship between income and medical care expenditures is the result of a complex set of interrelationships among income, illness, and

73

other variables. Specifically, we will consider the following factors which may bias estimates of the association between family income and consumption of physician and dental services: (1) the effects of other variables, including price and quality of medical care, preventive care, and family demographic variables; (2) the substitution of permanent income for observed income as the measure of a family's resources; (3) the expected negative relationship between illness and transitory income; (4) the association between permanent income and illness; and (5) the employment of quantities of service rather than dollar expenditures.

Through the use of regression analysis, we will examine the influence of these factors on observed income elasticities of demand for medical care.[7]

THE DATA

The data used in this paper are from a national survey conducted in 1964 by the Center for Health Administration Studies and the National Opinion Research Center of the University of Chicago. Interviews were conducted with 2,367 families.[8] These families constituted an area probability sample of the civilian non-institutionalized population and contained 7,803 individuals. One or more knowledgeable members of each family provided information regarding use of health services, expenditures for these services, and methods of payment for the calendar year 1963. Information was also collected from hospitals, employers, and insuring organizations about hospitalization and health insurance coverage reported in the family interviews. The latter information served to verify and add additional detail to the family reports.[9]

The family is the unit of analysis for this paper.[10] It has been considered an appropriate unit for studying consumption of many consumer goods and services because it is the primary earning, spending, and consuming unit in our society.[11] It seems particularly important for a study relating illness, family income, and medical care expenditures, since family income is expected to play some part in the determination of medical care expenditures for all family members. Furthermore, the illnesses of family members, particularly those of main wage earners, can reduce family income and the ability of the family to secure medical care for other members. In addition, such general familial characteristics as size, life cycle stage, attitudes toward medical care by the family head or his spouse, and health insurance coverage have all been considered as determinants of the quantity and type of medical care consumed by each family member.[12]

DEPENDENT VARIABLES*

In considering what measures of medical care utilization would be most appropriate for this study, we first examined previous measures used. A num-

*A description of the variables is included in Tables 1 and 2.

ber of studies have shown that the determinants of demand vary considerably from one type of medical care to another.[13] In particular, hospital and hospital-based physician services are found to have a considerably lower correlation with social and economic determinants than dental services.[14] Given the heterogeneity of these medical care components, two types of services were selected for analysis here: physician services, representing a "necessity" component, and dental services, representing a "luxury" component.

Physician services are measured in this paper by dollar expenditures and also by "units" of use. Our first measure consisted of physician charges incurred by the family in 1963, including charges paid by voluntary health insurance programs. This measure, however, does not always adequately reflect the quantity of services families consume because of the variation found in price per unit of service from family to family.[15] The price for a particular service may vary with the ability of the family to pay. Furthermore, free care is available to people with very low incomes or other special characteristics such as old age, disability, or blindness. Finally, costs for various types of services differ according to geographical area and the rural or urban nature of the area in which the family resides.

Table 1: The Dependent Variables

Identification	Mean Value	S.D.	Description
Physician expenditures	$120	$181	Charges incurred by families for physician services during the calendar year 1963: charges incurred for all care provided by physicians except that provided to hospitalized in-patients which are included in the hospital billing are included, as are other hospital in-patient care provided by physicians and physician care provided in hospital out-patient departments and clinics, private offices, and homes. *Includes* charges for which the family was reimbursed by health insurance, but *excludes* health insurance premiums. *Includes* charges incurred by the family which had not been paid at the time of the interview
Physician use	116 units	162 units	Includes the same services as physician expenditures. These services are then weighted by standard prices rather than charges actually incurred by families (see text)
Dental expenditures	$48	$100	Includes charges by dentist for his services and those of his auxiliary personnel and charges for dental appliances incurred during the calendar year 1963. *Includes* charges incurred by the family which had not been paid at the time of the interview

In an attempt to handle these difficulties, our second measure, quantity of services consumed, involved weighting various types of physician services by standard prices. The basic units selected were physician visits and in-hospital surgical procedures. These units were considered to represent, in the main, the services provided by the physician to the patient. The units were weighted according to "relative values" based on fees charged by California physicians in 1960 for various types of visits and surgical procedures,[16] multiplied by a constant (value of 5) to approximate the dollar charges.[17]

Dental services are measured in this paper only by dollar expenditures, as use data were not collected. However, less difference between measures of use and of expenditures is to be expected for dental service consumption than for physician service consumption because less free care is provided for the former. Data from the Social Security Administration indicate that for the calendar year 1963 consumer expenditures accounted for 99 per cent of total expenditures for dental services, as opposed to 93 per cent of total expenditures for physician services.[18] More detailed definitions of our measures of physician expenditures and use and dental expenditures are given in Table 1.*

THE ANALYSIS

Proposition 1: Effects of Other Variables

The simple observed income elasticities for physician and dental expenditures will differ significantly from the corresponding elasticities obtained by holding constant price (p), quality (q), demographic characteristics (d), and preventive care (e). In symbolic notation: $\eta y \neq \eta y \cdot pqde$.

Previous studies indicate that income is only one of several variables that influence the demand for medical care.[19] There is also evidence to suggest that the effects of income are not independent of the effects of these other variables. In order to observe the income elasticity of demand while attempting to hold these other variables constant, we have developed an initial model of the demand for health services. This model asserts that medical care expenditures are a function of family income (y), price (p), quality (q), demographic characteristics (d), and preventive care (e).

Some of the "independent" variables in this model could be considered endogenous variables in a more elaborate model. Our preference in this preliminary effort was to work with a simple model because we believed that at this stage we would be better able to observe basic relationships, even though more subtle associations might be observed in a complex model. Thus EXP = $f(y, p, q, d, e)$. Definitions of the variables representing each of the components of the model are presented in Table 2.

---

*The fact that mean units of physician use per family are slightly less than mean expenditures indicates a conservative bias in the weighting process, particularly since free care is included in the "use" measure.

Table 2: The Independent Variables

Identification	Mean Value	Use[a]	Description
		Family Income (y)	
y	6363	M-P[b]	Reported earned and other income for all family members[c]
		Illness Level (i)	
SYMPTS	4.2	M	Based on a check list of twenty commonly experienced and understood symptoms representative of a fairly wide range of somatic and psychosomatic conditions.[d] The total number of these symptoms experienced during the survey year by all family members as reported in the interview is the family's score
			Series of "health" variables below compared with all family members reported to be in "excellent" health[e]
GOODHE	0.39	M	1 = "good" health, lowest level reported[f]
FAIRHE	0.24	M	1 = "fair" health, lowest level reported
POORHE	0.11	M	1 = one or more family members reported to be in "poor" health
		Price (p)	
INPREM	85.3	M-P	Premium cost of all health insurance paid directly by the family
			Series of health insurance variables below compared with families having no health insurance coverage
EMPCON	0.41	M-P	1 = group health insurance with employer contributing to premium cost
INGRP	0.13	M-P	1 = group health insurance with no employer contribution to premium cost
INNGRP	0.20	M-P	1 = non-group health insurance only
WELFAR	0.05	M	1 = medical care provided to family members at no direct cost or at reduced rates because the family was unable to pay
FREECR	0.03	M	1 = medical care provided for a hospitalization or other major illness at no direct cost or at reduced rates for some reason other than inability to pay (e.g., professional courtesy)

Table 2—*continued*

Identification	Mean Value	Use[a]	Description
			Quality (q)
			Series of "regular source of care" variables below compared with families reporting a specialist (internist, pediatrician, etc.) as regular source of care for at least one family member
GP	0.41	M-P	1 = general practitioner, regular source
CLINIC	0.09	M-P	1 = no specific practitioner mentioned but reference made to clinic or hospital out-patient service
NON-MD	0.01	M-P	1 = some person other than a medical source (e.g., chiropractor)
NONE	0.10	M-P	1 = no regular source of medical care mentioned for any family member
			Preventive Care (e)
EXAMS 5	0.26	M	1 = at least one family member had not had a physical examination within five years
			Demographic Characteristics (d)
			Series of age variables below compared with families headed by persons less than 25 years of age
AGE 25–34	0.19	P	1 = family head 25–34
AGE 35–64	0.57	P	1 = family head 35–64 or "no answer"
AGE 65	0.18	P	1 = family head 65 or over
MARRED	0.75	P	1 = family head married
FEMALE	0.19	M-P	1 = family head female
RETIRE	0.09	P	1 = main earner retired
FAMSIZ	3.4	M-P	number of family members
NWORK	1.3	P	number of wage earners in family (NA coded 1)
			Series of education variables below compared with families headed by persons completing six or fewer years of schooling
ED 7–8	0.19	P	1 = family head has 7–8 yrs schooling
ED 9–11	0.22	P	1 = family head has 9–11 yrs schooling

Table 2—*continued*

Identification	Mean Value	Use[a]	Description
ED 12	0.24	P	1 = family head has 12 yrs schooling
ED 15	0.11	P	1 = family head has 13–15 yrs schooling
ED 16	0.12	P	1 = family head has 16 or more yrs schooling
SOCCLA	4.0	P	Social class ranking according to prestige of last regular occupation of main earner. Ranking developed from responses in a national survey regarding the relative ranking of occupations.[g] Scaled values of original scores used in this paper are: 0–9 = 1, 10–19 = 2; 20–29 = 3, 30–39 = 4; 40–49 = 5, 50–59 = 6, 60–69 = 7, 70–79 = 8, 80–99 = 9 (1 = lowest rank, 9 = highest rank)
NEGRO	0.13	M-P	1 = Negro family; whites, "other," and NA were all coded "O"
			Series of urban-rural variables below compared with families living in the urban area of the ten largest standard metropolitan statistical areas of the country
OMETRO	0.47	M-P	1 = urban "other" metropolitan residence
RURNF	0.22	M-P	1 = rural non-farm residence
FARM	0.08	M-P	1 = rural farm residence
SOUTH	0.32	M-P	1 = residence in southern section of the U.S. according to U.S. census definition

[a]"M" indicates that the variable was used as a predictor of medical care consumption; "P" indicates that the variable was used to predict permanent income; "M-P" indicates that the variable was used for both of the above purposes. See the text for a discussion of the process used to estimate permanent income.

[b]Used as a dependent variable in the permanent income equation.

[c]Unless otherwise stated, all values assuming a time period are for the calendar year 1963.

[d]See Ronald Andersen, *A Behavioral Model of Families' Use of Health Services*, Center for Health Administration Studies Research Series no. 25 (Chicago: By the Center, 1968), pp. 99–100, for exact list.

[e]Here and in the rest of the table, this category was left out of the series of dummy variables to prevent overdetermination in the regression equation.

[f]Here and in the rest of the table this indicates a dummy variable, with all families not specified "1" given a score "0."

[g]O. Duncan, Appendix, in *Occupations and Social Status*, ed. A. Reiss (New York: Free Press of Glencoe, 1961), pp. 263–75.

Price

Economic theory suggests that the quantity of medical care demanded will increase as the price decreases. Proxy measures of price used here include health insurance premiums and method of health insurance enrollment. We assume that the higher the cost of the premiums, the more comprehensive the benefit structure and, consequently, the lower the price per unit of care to the consumer at the time of purchase.* Further, since the return on the premium dollar is higher under group than under non-group enrollment, the actual out-of-pocket cost per unit of service should be lower for families enrolled under group contracts than for those who purchase insurance on an individual basis.[20] Since the measures of medical care expenditures in this study do not exclude health insurance benefits, expenditures as well as use should vary directly with these price surrogates.

The other variables in this price package are receipt of welfare medical care and receipt of substantial medical services free or at reduced rates. It was expected that availability of such services would reduce the relative price per unit of service and thus reduce expenditures but increase use.† These measures of price should have little correlation with dental expenditures, since dental services were not insured and were rarely provided free of charge.

Quality

If price per unit of service were held constant, we might expect quality to be inversely related to expenditures and use. Each unit purchased should be more effective, thus reducing the total number of units purchased. However, there are several problems raised by the introduction of our measure for quality: source of regular medical care. We assume that families who use an internist or other specialist receive higher quality care than do those who use general practitioners or clinics, or who have no regular source. The latter are listed in decreasing order of estimated quality.

Even if this rough measure does indicate quality, there are other reasons to suggest that the sign of the regression coefficients will be negative rather than positive. (A negative coefficient indicates that families using higher quality care also have greater total outlay on medical care.) First, this measure is

---

*Michael Grossman has pointed out that if premiums are actuarially fair, families who have a higher probability of illness will have to pay a larger premium for the same coverage than families with a lower probability of illness. This will introduce a positive bias in the relationship between medical expenditures and insurance premiums, one of the components of "price." For a further discussion of this point, see footnote on p. 87.

†Welfare care and free care are, however, correlated with illness. Families must actually use these medical services to be included in these categories. In a more complete model, eligibility for such services would be estimated.

correlated with price, since specialists tend to charge more per unit of service, and it may also be correlated with illness, since very ill people probably gravitate toward more specialized sources of care. Furthermore, there is little convincing evidence that using higher quality services results in lower over-all utilization rates. In fact, having a regular, specialized source of care may result in greater utilization. It is therefore difficult to predict the regression coefficient for this measure.

Preventive Care

There is some question as to whether preventive care reduces the over-all demand for medical services. We hoped that, by analytically separating families in which at least one member has not had a physical examination within five years from all other families, we would obtain some indication of the importance of past care for the current demand for medical services. If, in fact, preventive care reduces the over-all volume of services consumed, the sign of the coefficient should be positive.

Demographic Variables

If our model of demand for health services were complete, the effects of most sociodemographic variables would be accounted for by other components. In and of themselves, the former do not provide reasons for consumption of medical care. Rather, they serve as proxy measures of other conditions, such as attitudes and values about health and health care, family resources, the availability of health services, and "perceived" and "objective" illness – the most immediate causes of medical care consumption. For example, age and sex are often used in the literature as "substitutes" for illness measures. Differences in consumption patterns accounted for by education are explained in terms of differential information and values. Differences in residence are often related to availability of services.

Given the imperfect operational measures of several of our variables, we decided to add certain sociodemographic variables to the analysis.* Our expectations were that high utilization of medical care would be associated with families living outside the South, in large standard metropolitan statistical areas, white, with a male household head, and with a larger number of members.

Findings

The demand equations in Table 3 show that income elasticities of observed income for both physician and dental expenditures are rather heavily

---

*A family size variable would have been included in any case.

FAMILY INCOME AND MEDICAL CARE CONSUMPTION

influenced by other components of the demand equation.* Proposition 1 is thus supported.

Table 3: Equations for Physician and Dental Expenditures
Using Measured Income

Predictor	Physician Expenditures		Dental Expenditures	
	y	$ypqde$	y	$ypqde$
Income (y)				
Regression coefficient	0.008**	0.004**	0.006**	0.005**
T value	10.0	4.61	14.9	9.46
Elasticity	0.41	0.22	0.83	0.61
Price (p)				
INPREM		0.218**[a]		0.101**[a]
EMPCON		21.1*		-0.083
INGRP		14.7		1.28
INNGRP		18.9		2.84
WELFAR		14.6		-5.51
FREECR		72.2**		-10.08
Quality (q)				
GP		-23.7**		-2.12
CLINIC		-53.5**		1.06
NON-MD		-68.2*		25.7
NONE		-47.7**		-12.0
Preventive care (e)				
EXAMS 5		-22.7**		-10.6*
Demographic (d)				
FEMALE		7.47		-1.87
FAMSIZ		11.4**		4.95**
NEGRO		-31.5**		-22.6**
OMETRO		-14.2		-15.0**
RURNF		-17.3		-29.2**
FARM		-16.7		-19.8*
SOUTH		-0.620		-6.04
CONSTANT	70.7**	60.9**	8.2*	18.0*
R^2	0.041	0.098	0.086	0.124

  [a]Values given are regression coefficients.
  *Significant at .05 level.
  **Significant at .01 level.

---

*It should be noted that the income elasticity for dental expenditures is over twice that for physician expenditures. These findings corroborate those of earlier studies and emphasize the need to investigate the components of medical care separately.

	Physician Expenditures	*Dental Expenditures*
ηy	.41**	.83**
$\eta y \cdot pqde$	.22**	.61**

The introduction of price (p), quality (q), demographic characteristics (d), and preventive care (e) into the equation *reduces* income elasticity for physician expenditures by 46 per cent and that for dental expenditures by 26 per cent.*

Examination of the intermediate steps in these equations[†] suggests that the price component, more than any other, depresses the elasticity for physician expenditures. Quality and demographic characteristics also reduce the elasticity for physician expenditures, but preventive care has little effect.

The most important variables of the price component represent insurance coverage. High-income families had more comprehensive coverage in 1963 than low-income families. According to our model this leads to higher physician care consumption by high-income families because the relative price is lower. Consequently, when the sample is standardized for price, relative differences in consumption between high- and low-income families decrease.

Quality and the demographic components also contribute to the reduction of income elasticity for physician care. As with price, arguments can be made that the variables representing these components provide reasons for higher consumption on the part of high-income families. When the sample is standardized for these variables, the relative differences in consumption according to income decrease. For example, it appears that high-income families spend more for physician services because they make greater use of specialists. They also spend more because they tend to have more family members. When these factors are controlled, the income elasticity for physician services decreases.

The reduction in income elasticity for dental care is accounted for primarily by demographic characteristics. Since price, quality, and preventive care were defined primarily as concerning services provided by or under the direction of a physician, it is not surprising that they show little relationship to dental consumption.

Proposition 2: The Permanent Income Hypothesis

The estimates of elasticity of demand for both physician and dental expenditures will be higher with respect to permanent income than with respect to observed income: $\eta \hat{y} \cdot pqde > \eta y \cdot pqde$, where y is permanent income.

---

*Significance levels for physician and dental expenditures cited in listings in text or in tables are designated as follows: * indicates significance at the .05 level; ** indicates significance at the .01 level; absence of an asterisk indicates the T value was not significant at the .05 level.

†For intermediate steps, see footnote on p. 87.

Evaluating this proposition requires that we be able to measure "permanent" income. Permanent income is a family's "expected regular" income, apart from "unanticipated, transitory" positive or negative components. It can be measured in a number of ways. Individual observations can be pooled on the assumption that within the larger aggregation the positive and negative transitory components of individual observations will tend to cancel each other out.[21] A second approach is to estimate permanent income for each family. We used the latter approach in this study.

To obtain measures of permanent income and permanent income elasticities, we used two-stage instrumental variable analysis.[22] The technique involves first regressing observed income on the instrumental variables. All of the variables described in Table 2 except illness level and preventive care were used as predictors. The results of this regression are shown in Table 4. The resulting estimated value of permanent income $(\hat{y})$ was then substituted into a

Table 4: Estimating Equation for Permanent Income

$\hat{y}$ =   -687.6[a] + 3.89 INPREM + 1338.0 EMPCON + 583.0 INGRP
              (-1.33) (3.96)   (6.19)   (2.00)

+19.61 INNGRP - 1006.0 FEMALE + 56.5 FAMSIZ
    (.08)   (-3.07)   (1.33)

-970.5 NEGRO - 542.6 OMETRO - 968.9 RURNF
  (-3.98)   (-2.77)   (-4.12)

-1341.0 FARM - 301.4 SOUTH - 537.8 GP
   (-4.11)   (-1.73)   (-3.22)

-668.2 CLINIC + 316.0 NON-MD - 412.0 NONE
   (-2.42)   (.49)   (-1.56)

+1298.0 AGE 25-34 + 2803.0 AGE 35-64 + 2124.0 AGE 65
    (3.65)   (8.46)   (5.35)

+1156.0 NWORK + 502.0 ED 7-8 + 977.9 ED 9-11
   (11.28)   (1.81)   (3.51)

+1071.0 ED 12 + 1777.0 ED 15 + 2876.0 ED 16
   (3.68)   (5.15)   (7.85)

+403.1 SOCCLA + 1202.0 MARRED - 1281.0 RETIRE
   (10.19)   (3.83)   (-4.016)

R^2 = .44   DF = 2326

[a]The upper value gives the regression coefficient. The lower value in parentheses gives the T value for that coefficient.

second-stage analysis using the same models as for observed income.* The results of the second-stage analyses are shown in Table 5.†

Table 5: Equations for Physician and Dental Expenditures
Using Estimated Permanent Income

Predictor	Physician Expenditures			Dental Expenditures	
	y	$ypqde$	$ypqdei$	y	$ypqde$
Income (y)					
Regression coefficient	0.012**	0.003	0.006**	0.009**	0.008**
T value	10.2	1.75	3.21	14.7	7.51
Elasticity	0.63	0.17	0.30	1.24	0.99
Price (p)					
INPREM		0.23**[a]	0.20**[a]		0.08**[a]
EMPCON		23.0*	26.6**		-7.18
INGRP		15.7	19.9		-3.02
INNGRP		18.4	16.3		3.39
WELFAR		11.2	-18.4		-5.46
FREECR		72.0**	51.4*		-10.14
Quality (q)					
GP		-24.4**	-19.2*		0.288
CLINIC		-54.4**	-42.9**		4.62
NON-MD		-67.4*	-56.6		25.5
NONE		-48.3**	-19.7		-10.0
Preventive care (e)					
EXAMS 5		-24.9**	-28.7**		-13.0**
Demographic (d)					
FEMALE		5.46	7.49		4.66
FAMSIZ		11.8**	10.7**		4.33**
NEGRO		-32.8**	-28.0*		-18.6**
OMETRO		-14.7	-20.2*		-12.8*
RURNF		-18.3	-24.5*		-25.1**
FARM		-18.4	-28.6		-12.8
SOUTH		-0.75	-5.29		-5.82
Illness level (i)					
SYMPTS			7.7**		
GOODHE			32.2**		
FAIRHE			51.6**		
POORHE			110.9**		
CONSTANT[b]	44.6**	66.2**	-12.5	-11.6**	1.66

[a]Values given are regression coefficients.
[b]R^2 was not computed for the second stage of the two-stage equations.
*Significant at the .05 level.
**Significant at the .01 level.

*The error of measurement (transitory income) should not be correlated with any of the instrumental variables. The set of variables giving condition of health (POORHE, FAIRHE, GOODHE) and the variable giving illness symptoms (SYMPTS) were excluded

The permanent income hypothesis asserts that consumption tends to be a function of the normal or permanent income of families.[23] Measured income is an imperfect indicator of normal or permanent income, since it consists of both permanent and transitory components. These two components are assumed to be uncorrelated. One test of the permanent income hypothesis is to see whether the income elasticity of demand for a commodity is lower for measured than for permanent income.[24]

Findings

Comparisons of the income elasticities from Tables 3 and 5 provide support for the permanent income hypothesis for dental expenditures but not for physician expenditures:

Physician Expenditures	*Dental Expenditures*
$\eta y = .41^{**}$	$\eta y = .83^{**}$
$\eta\hat{y} = .63^{**}$	$\eta\hat{y} = 1.24^{**}$
$\eta y \cdot pqde = .22^{**}$	$\eta y \cdot pqde = .61^{**}$
$\eta\hat{y} \cdot pqde = .17$	$\eta\hat{y} \cdot pqde = .99^{**}$

In the regression equations for physician expenditures where income is the only predictor, the elasticity for permanent income was, as expected, higher

---

because they were associated with a negative transitory income. Preventive care (EXAMS 5) was excluded because it was found unrelated to income in the preliminary analysis. As a group, the families who lost income due to illness in 1963 will probably have a lower permanent income than families who are similar in other respects. An individual who is seriously ill during a particular year, other things being equal, will be more likely to be ill on a permanent basis. By excluding the variables measuring illness, we will overestimate the permanent income of the families who have illness during the survey year. If we are overestimating the permanent incomes of these sick (high-expenditure) families, then there will be a positive bias in our estimates of income elasticity. Margaret Reid has suggested that the number of workers in a family would be correlated with the transitory component of income. We plan to examine this proposition by excluding this variable from the estimating equation in later analyses.

†The predictors of permanent income which were not utilized in the demand equations (age, social class, education) did not make a significant independent contribution to the explanation of either physician or dental expenditures. The lack of significance of age might appear surprising. It should be remembered that the age measure used here is for the family head. If we were studying individuals, the relationship between age and medical expenditures would be more dramatic.

The table presents only our results for the simple linear form of income. We also tested semilog transformations. Stage 1: $\log y = a + \Sigma b_j x_j$; Stage 2: expenditures $= a + b_1 \log \hat{y} + \Sigma b_1 x_1$. The semilog elasticities were somewhat smaller than those obtained from the linear equations.

than the elasticity for observed income. However, when price, quality, demographic variables, and preventive care were taken into account, the permanent income elasticity dropped below that for observed income and was, in fact, *not* significant at the .05 level. This suggests that the apparent increased effect of permanent income on physician expenditures can be largely accounted for by other components of the model. Within the context of the model, with "other things being equal," consumption of physician services is not more closely associated with permanent than with observed income.*

In contrast to the results for physician expenditures, our findings for dental expenditures were quite consistent with the permanent income hypothesis. In both the simple and multiple regression models, permanent income elasticities were considerably higher than observed income elasticities.

Proposition 3: Illness and Transitory Income

Illness simultaneously increases physician expenditures and produces a negative transitory component in family income. Insofar as the effect is important, we will find $\eta\hat{y} \cdot pqde > \eta y \cdot pqde$.

Although the empirical test of this proposition is identical with that for Proposition 2, Proposition 3 suggests that observed income elasticity should be lower than permanent income elasticity for different reasons. The theory of permanent income assumes that consumption of non-durable commodities is uncorrelated with transitory income. But transitory income is likely to be negatively correlated with expenditures on physician care through the intervening variable, illness. Illness is cited by 5.4 per cent of the families in the sample as a cause of negative transitory income. This proposition does not apply to dental care, since illness is not directly associated with dental expenditures.

---

*Michael Grossman argues in the discussion of this paper that the reduction in income elasticity when price and quality are included may be spurious because insurance and quality are themselves highly income-elastic. Examination of the elasticities excluding these components gave the following results:

(1) $\eta y \cdot pde = .23$
(2) $\eta\hat{y} \cdot pde = .24$
(3) $\eta y \cdot p'de = .27$
(4) $\eta\hat{y} \cdot p'de = .37$

where p' is the price component minus the insurance premium (INPREM): $p' = p -$ INPREM.

Equations 1 and 2 exclude the quality components. Equations 3 and 4 exclude the quality components and the insurance premium, INPREM, part of the price package. These results suggest that the exclusion of quality has little effect on our general conclusions. However, equations 3 and 4 suggest that income elasticity resulting from equations excluding INPREM is higher using permanent income than using measured income. Thus our conclusions concerning the permanent income hypothesis must be considered within the context of the particular model employed.

Findings

The results obtained for Proposition 2 for physician expenditures are applicable here, namely:

$$\textit{Physician Expenditures}$$

$$\eta y = .41**$$
$$\eta \hat{y} = .63**$$
$$\eta y \cdot pqde = .22**$$
$$\eta \hat{y} \cdot pqde = .17$$

The same discussion is also relevant. The observed income elasticity for the population as a whole does not appear to be negatively biased by transitory loss of income due to illness.

Proposition 4: Illness and Permanent Income

Permanent income elasticities for physician expenditures will increase when we standardize for family level of illness: $\eta \hat{y} \cdot pqdei > \eta \hat{y} \cdot pqde$, *where i represents illness.*

Our underlying supposition here was that families with low permanent income have poorer health than families with high permanent income because of the chronic incapacity of potential wage earners or the unhealthy environment in which low-income people may live. Poor health in turn leads to increased medical utilization, with the result that income elasticities appear lower than they would if health were taken into account.

Use of a permanent income measure was important because we wanted to distinguish between families who have low incomes *temporarily* because of poor health or some other reason and families who have poor health which is associated with their low *permanent* income. We obtained a measure of the relationship between low permanent income and poor health by introducing a set of variables into our permanent income model to measure illness explicitly.

Our illness variables were "perception of illness" measures based on symptoms reported by the family and on reported general state of health.*

---

*A special problem in developing the illness component concerned time relationships. We wanted to determine the illness levels of each family at the beginning of the period in which medical care consumption was measured. However, only illness levels at the end of the period were reported in the survey. Thus it might be argued that the relationships discovered simply reflected people reporting their health level on the basis of the medical care they consumed over the year. However, to the extent that perception of health is not simply a function of past medical care consumption (and people who are high consumers in one period tend to continue to use large quantities in later periods), relationships found between perceived health levels and medical care consumption will be meaningful.

These variables are defined in Table 2. It may be that some measure of "objective illness," as determined through a physical examination, would be a better predictor of medical care use than is ours. However, the subjective measures used here should also have predictive value, since they are correlated with objective illness. In addition, what people do about illness depends upon their own evaluations as well as upon objective conditions.[25]

Findings

Elasticities taken from Table 5 support the proposition:

Physician Expenditures

$$\eta \hat{y} \cdot pqde = .17$$
$$\eta \hat{y} \cdot pqdei = .30**$$

The permanent income elasticity, which is not significant for the equation that excludes illness, increases and becomes significant at the .01 level when illness is introduced. This evidence suggests that families with lower permanent income do experience more illness and do spend less per "unit" of illness. This result could not have been foretold from the relationship between observed income and illness.

Proposition 5: Quantity versus Expenditure

Income elasticity estimates for physician services will be lowered by the substitution of quantity of services consumed for dollar expenditures in the analysis: $\eta^e \hat{y} \cdot pqdei > \eta^q \hat{y} \cdot pqdei$, *where the superscripts q and e stand for quantity and expenditure, respectively.* *

Expenditures and quantities have both been used as measures of consumption. The measures differ because of care provided at no cost to the consumer and because of price discrimination. We expect income elasticities to be smaller for physician use than for physician expenditure because low-income families use proportionately more services which are not included in the expenditure measure.[†]

Findings

Comparisons of elasticities from Tables 5 and 6 support this final proposition:

---

*We are only considering the proposition for normal goods, i.e., goods where $\eta y \geqslant 0$.

†This result would also be expected if the quality of service for low-income people were lower. The price and quality measures explicitly included in our equations are very imperfect; thus we expect the proposition to hold even where we standardized for price and quality.

	Physician Expenditures	Physician Use
$\eta \hat{y}$	.63**	.31**
$\eta \hat{y} \cdot pqde$	.17	.01
$\eta \hat{y} \cdot pqdei$	.30	.12

Table 6: Equations for Physician Use Using Permanent Income

Predictor	y	$ypqde$	$ypqdei$
Income (y)			
Regression coefficient	0.006**	0.0	0.002
T value	5.25	-.12	1.45
Elasticity	0.31	0.01	0.12
Price (p)			
INPREM		0.130**[a]	0.106*[a]
EMPCON		12.00	16.1
INGRP		13.8	18.3
INNGRP		16.1	14.9
WELFAR		127.8**	99.6**
FREECR		207.6**	187.1**
Quality (q)			
GP		-6.99	-2.24
CLINIC		-35.9**	-25.3*
NON-MD		-27.5	-18.0
NONE		-47.6**	-21.4
Preventive care (e)			
EXAMS 5		-30.4**	-34.4**
Demographic (d)			
FEMALE		-5.24	-3.41
FAMSIZ		12.4**	11.4**
NEGRO		-37.6**	-33.6**
OMETRO		2.53	-2.43
RURNF		7.35	1.33
FARM		-5.37	-15.4
SOUTH		-2.05	-6.77
Illness level (i)			
SYMPTS			6.28**
GOODHE			27.8**
FAIRHE			52.8**
POORHE			111.9**
CONSTANT[b]	80.57	66.44**	-5.57

[a]Values given are regression coefficients.
[b]R^2 was not computed for the second stage of the two-stage equations.
 *Significant at .05 level.
 **Significant at .01 level.

For every equation, from those including only income to those including all components of the model, the elasticities involving physician expenditures exceeded those involving physician use. These data suggest that expenditures significantly underestimate the proportion of all physician services consumed by low-income families.*

SUMMARY

We have examined five propositions concerning family income elasticity and medical care expenditures and use. The central underlying hypothesis is that apparent income elasticities of demand with respect to medical care may be altered significantly when other factors are taken into account. The propositions were tested for physician and dental care consumption using data from a national consumer survey for 1963. The findings supported three propositions unambiguously, supported a fourth for dental but not for physician expenditures, and lent no support to the remaining proposition, as indicated in Table 7.

Table 7: Summary of Results

Proposition	Expectation	Result
1	$\eta y \neq \eta y \cdot pqde$	Supported
2	$\eta \hat{y} \cdot pqde > \eta y \cdot pqde$	Not supported for physician expenditure; supported for dental expenditure
3	$\eta \hat{y} \cdot pqde > \eta y \cdot pqde$ (physician expenditure only)	Not supported
4	$\eta \hat{y} \cdot pqdei > \eta \hat{y} \cdot pqde$	Supported
5	$\eta^e \hat{y} \cdot pqdei > \eta^q \hat{y} \cdot pqdei$	Supported

IMPLICATIONS

1. Our findings corroborate those of other researchers — that the total medical care package includes heterogeneous types of services. They suggest that further research should concentrate on the separate services rather than on the package as a whole because of the considerable difference in determinants from one service to another.

---

*Included in these findings may be the influence on cost to low-income families of low-quality service at low cost, of government subsidies, and of price discrimination.

2. Our results were consistent with the permanent income hypothesis for dental services but not for physician services. The secular increase in the consumption of physician and hospital services would appear to be less closely related to increase in income per se and more closely related to other factors such as the changing methods of financing medical care. The fall in cost to consumers of medical care as a result of federal programs and so forth will have a significant impact upon the level of consumption of medical care. The lower income groups seem particularly sensitive to the method of financing. Insurance coverage for low-income groups apparently results in a dramatic increase in the demand for medical service. This fall in price to the consumer of medical care diminishes the importance of income as a determinant of the consumption of medical care.*

3. Our finding that loss of income due to illness does not seem to reduce measured income elasticities substantially suggests that, although this income loss can be dramatic in individual cases, it is not an important factor in the general association of income and medical care expenditures. Along with point 2, this suggests that the use of measured rather than permanent income to obtain elasticity estimates for physician expenditures may not be as misleading as has often been suggested.

4. Our finding that permanent income elasticity estimates increased when we standardized for amount of illness suggests that families with lower permanent incomes have more illness and spend less per "unit" of illness. Assumptions sometimes made about "random distributions of illness" obscure this issue.

5. Measured differences in consumption patterns by income level are reduced when we substitute quantities for expenditures. Given growing third-party payment for medical care, it appears that in order to investigate the actual distribution of services we will have to rely more and more on units other than consumer dollar expenditures.

---

*This is not to say that income will not continue to be an important determinant of certain categories, such as dental care, for some time. Also, it might be expected to continue to differentiate consumption patterns for amenities or for luxury medical care (e.g., private rooms, extensive preventive care, cosmetic surgery, etc.).

NOTES

1. Anselm Strauss, "Medical Ghettos," *Trans-action* 4 (May 1967):7-15.
2. Charlotte Muller, "Income and the Receipt of Medical Care," *American Journal of Public Health* 55 (April 1965):510-21.
3. As early as 1952 the President's Commission on the Health Needs of the Nation stated: "When the very life of a man, or the lives of his family, may depend upon his

receiving adequate medical services, society must make every effort to provide them. . . . These benefits sometimes can be obtained by the individual's own effort; but when these efforts fail, other means must be found" (*Building America's Health, Findings and Recommendations*, 1:1.) For a review of current issues and research, see "Medical Care for Low Income Families," *Inquiry* 5 (March 1968), entire issue.

4. Victor Fuchs suggests, however, that removal of all variation in use other than that based on some "objective need criteria" may be not only impossible but undesirable; see "The Basic Forces Influencing Costs of Medical Care," his paper presented at the meetings of the National Conference on Medical Care Costs, June 1967.

5. The first national consumer survey to collect detailed data on consumption of and expenditures for medical care was conducted by the Committee on the Costs of Medical Care around 1930 (see I. S. Falk et al., *The Incidence of Illness and the Receipt and Costs of Medical Care among Representative Families: Experiences in Twelve Consecutive Months during 1928-31* [Chicago: University of Chicago Press, 1933]). High positive correlations were found between family income level and both expenditure and use patterns. Such correlations were discovered for all the major components of medical care, including hospital, physician, and dental care.

The next series of social surveys to relate consumption of health services to family income was that conducted by the Center for Health Administration Studies and the National Opinion Research Center of the University of Chicago; see Odin W. Anderson and Jacob J. Feldman, *Family Medical Costs and Voluntary Health Insurance: A Nationwide Survey* (New York: McGraw-Hill Book Co., 1956); Odin W. Anderson et al., *Changes in Family Medical Care Expenditures and Voluntary Health Insurance* (Cambridge, Mass.: Harvard University Press, 1963); Ronald Andersen and Odin W. Anderson, *A Decade of Health Services: Social Survey Trends in Use and Expenditures* (Chicago: University of Chicago Press, 1967). Three studies conducted at five-year intervals from 1953 to 1963 showed that families in the upper income brackets continued to spend more for medical care than those with lower incomes. However, differences in the quantities of services consumed according to income level had largely disappeared for hospital services and were smaller for physician services than they had been in 1930. Only dental care continued to show the large differentiation by income level which had been documented earlier. These national trends are also supported by findings from the National Center for Health Statistics; see *Family Income in Relation to Selected Health Characteristics*, ser. 10, no. 2 (Washington, D.C.: U.S. Department of Health, Education, and Welfare, 1963), and *Medical Care, Health Status and Family Income*, ser. 10, no. 9 (Washington, D.C.: U.S. Department of Health, Education, and Welfare, 1964).

6. Insofar as medical expenditures represent an investment which gives a flow of services over time, the term "consumption" is not appropriate. In this paper "consumption" is used as a generic term to represent both expenditures and quantities consumed at a point in time. See Jerome Rothenberg, "Comment," *Proceedings of the Social Statistics Section of the American Statistical Association* 7 (1964):109.

7. The fundamental definition of income elasticity of demand is:

$$\eta = \frac{\text{relative change in medical care expenditure (quantity)}}{\text{corresponding relative change in income}}$$

This definition leads to a measure which is independent of the units in which the numerator and denominator are quoted. Since the elasticity is an abstract number (having no dimensions), the elasticities for various commodities can be compared; see George Stigler, *The Theory of Price* (New York: Macmillan Company, 1966), p. 329.

8. Since a main component of this study is family income, twelve families with no reported income for the survey year and one family with a reported income of $100,000 were deleted. The units of analysis for this study thus total 2,354.

9. The final report on these data, including details of methodology and a questionnaire, is found in Andersen and Anderson, *A Decade of Health Services*.

10. A family is defined as one person or a group of persons living together and related to each other by blood, marriage, or adoption. However, when two related married couples are found living in a single dwelling unit, each married couple and its unmarried children are a separate family. Any person unrelated to anyone else in the dwelling unit is a separate family.

Alternative units which could have been selected include the individual, as was done by Grover C. Wirick and Robin Barlow ("The Economic and Social Determinants of the Demand for Health Services," in *The Economics of Health and Medical Care*, ed. S. J. Axelrod [Ann Arbor: The University of Michigan, 1964]), or some aggregate geographical unit exemplified by the work of Paul J. Feldstein and Ruth Severson, "The Demand for Medical Care," in American Medical Association, *Report of the Commission on the Cost of Medical Care* (Chicago: By the Association, 1964), 1:57–76, and Gerald D. Rosenthal, *The Demand for General Hospital Facilities*, American Hospital Association Monograph 14 (Chicago: By the Association, 1964). The advantage of using the individual is that the influence of such variables as age, sex, and illness on consumption patterns can be measured more precisely. A chief asset of the geographical unit is that implications concerning regional differences are more easily determined; see J. S. Cramer, "Efficient Grouping, Regression and Correlation in Engle Curve Analysis," *Journal of the American Statistical Association* 59, no. 5 (March 1964).

11. See, for example, Nelson Foote, ed., *Household Decision-Making* (New York: New York University Press, 1961).

12. Ronald Andersen, *A Behavioral Model of Families' Use of Health Services*, Center for Health Administration Studies Research Series no. 25 (Chicago: By the Center, 1968). See pp. 7–8 for literature references relevant to family decision-making with respect to medical care.

13. *Ibid.*; Feldstein and Severson, "Demand for Medical Care"; Grover C. Wirick, "A Multiple Equation Model of Demand," *Health Services Research* 1 (Winter 1966): 301–46.

14. Louis Kriesberg has shown that these patterns are related to secular trends and broader societal change. In 1930, for example, consumption of hospital and physician services, as well as dental services, was highly correlated with family income. He suggests that reduction in these correlations is primarily due to "situational factors" such as the development of health insurance, which allows poorer people to receive care; see "The Relationship between Socio-Economic Rank and Behavior," *Social Problems* 10 (Spring 1963):334–52.

15. Paul J. Feldstein and W. John Carr, "The Effect of Income on Medical Care Spending," *Proceedings of the Social Statistics Section of the American Statistical Association* 7 (1964).

16. California Medical Association, Committee on Fees of the Commission on Medical Service, *Relative Value Studies, 1960* (San Francisco: By the Association, 1960).

17. To illustrate, suppose a person had three office visits to a physician and an appendectomy performed during the survey year. The relative value of the office visit is 1 and the relative value of the appendectomy is 40 (*ibid.*, pp. 5–41). Total physician use units assigned to that person would be calculated as follows: $5[1(3) + 40] = 215$ units. Total family use of physician services was calculated by summing individual physician use for all family members. A comparison of units assigned for a sample of procedures to actual charges for those procedures indicated that 5 would be the appropriate constant; that is, multiplication of the relative value of each procedure by 5 would result in magnitudes approximating "dollar equivalents." A detailed account of this procedure is found in Andersen, "Families' Use of Health Services," pp. 35–53, 181–87. The quantity data were developed in this form for a previous study. The statistical results are unaffected by the multiplication by 5.

18. Derived from Louis S. Reed and Ruth Hanft, "National Health Expenditures," *Social Security Bulletin* 29 (January 1966):3–19.

19. See Feldstein and Severson, "Demand for Medical Care"; Feldstein and Carr, "The Effect of Income on Medical Care Spending"; Rosenthal, *The Demand for General*

Hospital Facilities; Wirick and Barlow, "The Economic and Social Determinants of the Demand for Health Services"; Wirick, "A Multiple Equation Model of Demand"; Hendrick S. Houthakker and Lester Taylor, *Consumer Demand in the United States* (Cambridge, Mass.: Harvard University Press, 1966).

20. In 1964, for example, operating expenses as a percentage of premium income were 12.9 for private insurance group plans and 45.4 for private insurance non-group plans (Louis S. Reed, "Private Health Insurance in the United States: An Overview," *Social Security Bulletin* 28, no. 12 [December 1965]:18).

21. This is the approach used by Feldstein and Severson ("Demand for Medical Care"), Rosenthal (*The Demand for General Hospital Facilities*), and Feldstein and Carr ("The Effect of Income on Medical Care Spending"). We anticipated lower correlation coefficients from the study of individual families used here than for grouped data. When families are grouped (as they were in Feldstein and Severson's study), the variation in group behavior patterns is reduced compared with that of individual families.

22. Henri Theil, *Economic Forecasts and Policy*, 2d rev. ed. (Amsterdam: North-Holland Publishing Co., 1961).

23. Milton Friedman, *A Theory of the Consumption Function*, rev. ed. (Princeton, N.J.: Princeton University Press, 1967).

24. A number of studies have raised the question of the relative effect of permanent and of measured income on expenditure patterns. Musaffer Ahmad investigated this question for life insurance and estimated the income elasticity for life insurance to be approximately 0.4 for measured income and greater than unity for permanent income ("Demand for Life Insurance" [Ph.D. diss., University of Chicago, 1964]). Margaret Reid estimated the income elasticity for housing to be less than unity (approximately 0.35 in 1950) for measured income and between 1.5 and 2.0 for permanent income (*Income and Housing* [Chicago: University of Chicago Press, 1962]). In the area of medical care, Feldstein and Carr obtained an elasticity estimate for total medical expenditures, including insurance, in 1950 of 0.5 for measured income and 1.0 for permanent income ("The Effect of Income on Medical Care Spending").

While all these studies suggest some support for the permanent income hypothesis, a study by Robert C. Jones interjects a note of caution. He investigated the effect of windfall income on the demand for food, housing, and clothing. He concluded that "the propensities to consume [out of transitory income] were stronger than might be expected given the assumptions made under the permanent income hypothesis" ("Transitory Income and Expenditures on Consumption Categories," *American Economic Review* 50 [May 1960]:584-92).

25. For example, farmers who thought that they had heart disease which could not be verified through clinical examination behaved in some respects more like the cardiacs who knew about their disease than did farmers who had clinically verified disease but did not define themselves as cardiacs (Robert L. Eichhorn and Ronald Andersen, "Changes in Personal Adjustment to Perceived and Medically Established Heart Disease: A Panel Study," *Journal of Health and Human Behavior* 3 [Winter 1962]:242-49).

Michael Grossman
National Bureau of Economic Research

COMMENT

In general, I think that Andersen and Benham have selected an interesting and useful technique for obtaining permanent income elasticities. Their paper has many fine aspects, including clear statements of the hypotheses to be tested and a helpful comparison of measured and permanent income elasticities.

I have two types of criticism of their work to offer. In the first place, within the context of their own model of the demand for medical care, I have reservations with regard to certain aspects of their estimating procedure and also with regard to their interpretation of the price, preventive care, and quality variables. In the second place, if one adopts a model in which medical care is an input into the production of a commodity called good health, one has an approach to the demand for health services that is, I feel, more novel and more revealing than the one employed by Andersen and Benham. The rest of my remarks will be limited to these two areas of disagreement.

I am bothered by some of the variables the authors select to predict permanent income. For example, I would exclude age from the estimating equation because the permanent income hypothesis suggests that consumers' decisions are a function of their long-run or average income over the life cycle. What one really wants to measure is permanent wealth, defined as the present value of future income. It is true that income rises with age, but permanent income is fixed over the life cycle.

To take another example, I would think that the dollar value of health insurance premiums should be treated as an endogenous variable, since health insurance has a positive and perhaps a large income elasticity. Of course, this means that the premium variable and the dummies that indicate the presence or absence of insurance should not be used to predict permanent income. If they are used, one ends up estimating an equation with endogenous variables on both sides. This same comment applies to the inclusion of the quality variables that measure the source of regular medical care in the first stage.

My objections to the insurance and quality variables carry over to the estimation of the demand curves for medical care themselves. These variables, as well as preventive care, are functionally dependent on income and should not be held constant in calculating income elasticities. In the second stage, the premium variable is supposed to be a proxy for price. The authors justify this assumption by resorting to the old argument that health insurance creates a differential between the price of medical care and out-of-pocket expenditures per unit of service by consumers. In addition, they aver that this differential is positively correlated with the size of the premium. It should be noted that the positive correlation between premiums and medical outlays is likely to be spurious for the following reason.

Let L_i be the medical outlay against which the ith consumer insures, p_i be the probability of becoming ill, Π_i be the premium for health insurance, K_i be the loading factor, M_i be medical expenditures reported, and O_i be uninsured outlays. Then $M_i = L_i + O_i$ and $\Pi_i = K_i\, p_i\, L_i$. If K_i, P_i, O_i, and L_i are all independent, and if one considers only people who receive insurance benefits,

$$\text{cov}\,(\Pi_i, M_i) = \text{cov}\,(K_i\, p_i\, L_i, L_i + O_i) = \bar{K}\,\bar{p}\,\sigma^2{}_L\,,$$

where cov means covariance, $\bar{K}$ is the mean of K_i, $\bar{p}$ is the mean of p_i, and $\sigma^2{}_L$ is the variance of L_i. Of course, this covariance would be reduced to the extent that L_i equals zero for some of the families in the sample.

The issue I take with the insurance variable is, however, more fundamental than that of the degree of spuriousness it introduces. If consumers purchase health insurance voluntarily, then I deny that its acquisition reduces the price of medical care in any meaningful sense. Premiums are not acquired at zero cost, and the larger the demand for insured services the higher the premium. In viewing insurance, one should realize that it is simply one method of financing the demand for medical care. Presumably, this method is selected by consumers because it reduces uncertainty or increases the stability of their consumption stream. If medical care has a positive income elasticity, an increase in income would increase the demand for it and also the demand for insurance. Put differently, people with more comprehensive health insurance would demand more medical services, not because the relative price of these services is lower but because their income is higher.

I do not deny that certain aspects of insurance influence price. For example, if the government compels people to purchase health insurance and finances it through general taxation, the price of medical care will be reduced. Again, insurance will have price effects if, as the authors suggest, the premium cost of a unit of services is less when purchased under a group plan and if certain consumers are not eligible to buy this type of insurance. But even if the last argument is valid, it is not clear why the premium cost of a unit of services should be negatively correlated with income. If anything, the correlation might be expected to be positive because certain forms of health insurance stipulate that benefit payments are to be lower for higher income claimants.

Andersen and Benham's estimate of the net permanent income elasticity of demand for expenditures on physician services seems to be unreasonably small. Moreover, the permanent and measured income elasticities are roughly the same. The authors report that the gross elasticity is much larger than the net elasticity and that most of this difference is the result of the inclusion of the price variables. But if my remarks are correct, it is difficult to interpret an income elasticity that holds the size of insurance premiums constant. If they excluded the premium variable, they would obtain a much higher and a much more reasonable income elasticity. Besides, because the demand for preventive care and the demand for the quality aspects of physician services are probably income-elastic, the estimated parameter would make more sense if these two variables were omitted.

The reasons for holding quality constant are very puzzling to me, particularly when one considers that Andersen and Benham have separate estimates of expenditure and quantity elasticities for physician services. They argue that the expenditure elasticity exceeds the quantity elasticity because poor people receive care at reduced rates and because physicians engage in price discrimination according to income. I suspect that a more plausible interpretation of their finding is that much of the variation in price reflects quality variation rather than true differences in the price of standard units of service. If price is taken as an index of quality, one has the well-known formula relating the quantity and quality elasticities to the expenditure elasticity: $\eta_M = \eta_Q + \eta_P$. Using the authors' estimates, $\eta_M = .30$, $\eta_Q = .12$, and, therefore, $\eta_P = .18$. While the quality interpretation is mentioned in a footnote, I think it should be stressed more heavily.

The preceding comments have been made in the context of what might be termed Andersen and Benham's conventional approach to the demand for medical care. Stripped to its barest essentials, their model states that demand depends on relative price, permanent income, and tastes. In my opinion, however, the demand for health care can be better understood if it is realized that what people demand when they purchase medical services are not these services per se but rather good health. Medical care and the time of the consumer are inputs into the production of good health, which implies that the shadow price of good health depends on the price of medical care, the value of time, and the efficiency of the production process.

Once the concept of a shadow price of health is introduced, one can illuminate a number of empirical phenomena. Consider the quality income elasticity of medical care, for example. Since the price of time and income are positively correlated, an increase in income would induce consumers to substitute medical care for their own time in the production of health. One way for higher income people to substitute in the direction of medical care would involve the acquisition of higher quality care.

To cite another illustration, consider the explanation of the impact of demographic characteristics like education and age on demand. Andersen and Benham claim that these variables are proxies for tastes or for "attitudes and values about health care," to use their terminology. If this approach is taken, one cannot predict the effects of shifts in these variables; instead one can simply rationalize observed effects in an ad hoc fashion. Suppose it were true, however, that an increase in, say, education did not shift tastes but rather increased the efficiency of the production process by which health is produced. If an increase in education raised productivity, it would lower the relative price of health. Thus, by the fundamental law of the downward-sloping demand curve, more educated people would demand more health. One could easily show that these same consumers would reduce their outlays on medical care unless the price elasticity of demand for health exceeded unity.*[1]

Perhaps the most important implication of the model I have proposed is this: if one accepts the notion that the basic demand is for good health, health status itself becomes an endogenous variable to some extent. It follows that the illness-level variables should be omitted from the demand curve for medical care. Besides, I would challenge the authors' statement that health and permanent income are positively correlated. Several studies done at the National Bureau of Economic Research find that when the appropriate variables are held constant, income and the age-adjusted death rate are positively correlated across the states of this country.[2] I myself have discovered that if the number of sick days is used as an index of the health status of individuals, the relationship between this measure and income is weak but positive.[3]

Let me close my remarks with a warning that is implicit in everything I have said. There is nothing wrong with the assertion that the demand for medical care depends on many other variables in addition to income. But difficulties arise unless one formulates his model of demand with extreme care so that only the exogenous variables are used to estimate the parameters of the system. While Andersen and Benham's estimates of the *net* permanent and measured income elasticities of physician expenditures are approximately equal, the *gross* permanent elasticities of physician and dental expenditures are each 50 per cent higher than the corresponding *gross* measured elasticities.

---

*In reality, consumers produce health and other commodities that enter their utility functions. If education improved efficiency in the production of all these commodities, its impact on the demand for health and on the demand for medical care would reflect income as well as substitution effects.

The magnitude of these gross differences is precisely what one would expect based on a simple model of the demand for medical care, and this finding is potentially the most important one of the study.

NOTES

1. A complete formulation of the model of consumer demand that underlies these remarks has been developed by Gary S. Becker ("A Theory of the Allocation of Time," *Economic Journal* 75, no. 299 [September 1965]).

2. See Victor R. Fuchs, "Some Economic Aspects of Mortality in the United States," mimeographed (New York: National Bureau of Economic Research, 1965); Richard D. Auster, Irving Leveson, and Deborah Sarachek, "The Production of Health: An Exploratory Study," *Journal of Human Resources* 4, no. 4 (Fall 1969):411-36.

3. "The Demand for Health: A Theoretical and Empirical Investigation" (Ph.D. diss., Columbia University, in progress).

Gerald Rosenthal
Brandeis University

PRICE ELASTICITY OF DEMAND FOR SHORT-TERM GENERAL HOSPITAL SERVICES

Although numerous studies have been made of the degree to which various economic factors, especially insurance coverage and income, are associated with the utilization of hospital services, the impact of price has not been of primary interest. A few studies of price elasticity have yielded mixed results. The Feldstein and Severson study showed no price elasticity of demand for hospital services, while my study showed significant price elasticity for general hospital services, primarily in length of stay.[1]

There are a number of reasons why the price elasticity of demand for hospital services is of interest. Much of the discussion about the impact of deductibles in hospital insurance is based on implicit assumptions about the nature of the price elasticity of demand. If there is no price elasticity of demand, then such deductibles are not likely to have any significant effect on the utilization of hospital services. In that case, the deductible itself serves merely as a device to reduce the risk spread over the healthy insured population, while more of the cost is charged to the patient. In effect, the deductible then becomes an additional premium for the user of such services. On the other hand, if there is significant price elasticity of demand, then an understanding of the effect of the deductible on utilization is of great importance.

Two major areas of difficulty are encountered in the development of an effective analysis of price elasticity of demand. One has to do with the nature of the demand for health services itself. Earlier analyses demonstrated that

This research was supported by Grant HM00302, United States Public Health Service. Additional support was provided by Grant No. CH00125-02, Department of Preventive Medicine, Harvard University Medical School. David Yates provided significant programming assistance.

101

the two aspects of the demand for hospital facilities – the admissions rate and the length of stay – were likely to respond very differently to the factors associated with demand.[2] An analysis of the demand for hospital facilities among the states, associated with a number of social, economic, and demographic characteristics, yielded different results for each of these two components of demand. The ability to estimate the admissions rate from these characteristics, as indicated by the multiple correlation coefficient, was much less significant than the estimates of the average length of stay, which implied that factors of importance affecting admissions were left out of the specification of the model. Within the specification of the model, however, differences in the relative importance of the variables were noted.

My earlier study concluded that "the empirical observations support the suggestion that economic constraints and the availability of substitutes . . . affect utilization by affecting the average length of stay. Apparently, the characteristics of the population which reflect physiological requirements for hospitals, (such as age distribution) or perception of the need for care (such as educational level), operate by affecting the admissions rate, and once the admissions rate is set, the other characteristics determine the actual duration of stay within a significant range."[3]

Recent studies of the British experience support the hypothesis that length of stay is highly sensitive to economic characteristics, such as price and insurance, while the admissions rate is far more likely to reflect other differences in the characteristics of the population and the medical care system.[4] In Britain, where insurance coverage can be presumed to be relatively constant, housing is uniformly tight, and the income distribution is far less widely spread than in the United States, the length of stay displays very little sensitivity to differences in supply constraints. Differences in pressures of supply will tend to be reflected in differences in the admissions rate. These observations would support the argument that where the economic characteristics cannot or do not fluctuate or relate differently to different groups, then the length of stay is likely to be considerably more stable than what would otherwise be the case.

The above evidence suggests that the price elasticity of demand is likely to be considerably more relevant in an analysis of length of stay than in an analysis of the admissions rate. If the above evidence leads to the appropriate conclusion, then the price elasticity of demand with respect to the admissions rate is likely to be considerably smaller than the price elasticity with respect to the length of stay. It is this latter aspect of demand which is of interest for this paper.

A second major problem is the difficulty in establishing the appropriate price. For the most part, the stated per diem rates for hospital services are quite independent of the cost incurred by the consumer. Indeed, even within a single institution, considerably different room rates will be encountered for what appear to be essentially similar services. Previous studies have used merely an average price or a most frequently charged price as a surrogate for the price faced by the consumer in making his utilization decisions. There is ample evidence that the price faced by the consumer is affected by a number of other factors. First, the extent to which ancillary services are consumed is likely to differ widely by illness, characteristics of the patient, and the institution rendering hospital services. In addition, the degree to which these services are covered by insurance, a factor which is associated with the individual patient rather than the institution, will have a considerable impact on the out-of-pocket expenses associated with them. There are a number of alternative ways to measure what we will refer to as the price-payment factor.

It might be appropriate to evaluate the degree to which the length of stay is associated with the actual money cost to the patient. This price-payment factor would be measured by the cash outlay incurred by the patient as payment for the services he has consumed. An alternative price-payment factor might be one which reflects the relative money outlay of the consumer. For example, a cash payment which represents a small percentage of the total bill might provide less of a price constraint on consumption than would the same payment as part of a smaller bill. The relative share measured by cash outlay as a percentage of the total bill might prove to be a more relevant price-payment factor in determining the price elasticity of length of stay. A third approach to the determination of the appropriate price might be the marginal price of incremental days to the patient. Since what is of interest here is the length of stay rather than the admissions rate, it may well be that the per diem charge is considerably more indicative of the marginal price of the stay than it is of the average price, since ancillary charges are heavily concentrated in the early days of stay. For individual patient experiences, then, it might be appropriate to use total room charges divided by length of stay, as an indicator of average room charge. It can be argued that average room charge, which represents the consumer's view of the price of an additional day, is the appropriate price for making a determination as to whether or not additional days will be consumed. Each of these price-payment factors will be considered in the ensuing analysis.

Perhaps some insight as to the price elasticity of demand might be derived by a direct comparison of the experience of paying with non-paying patients. It is obvious that such a dichotomous comparison may tend to obscure a number of attributes which are relevant for a length-of-stay analysis. There are considerable differences in the degree to which patients covered by third-party insurance are required to pay part of their bills out-of-pocket. In addition, there may be considerable differences between the two populations with regard to age, sex, and various diagnostic characteristics. There may also be an association with certain other characteristics of the population and the likelihood that they are covered through welfare or through some other third-party mechanism for payment for hospital services.

The object of the analysis presented here is to examine the degree to which the length of stay is associated with various price-payment factors for groups of patients with considerably more homogeneous characteristics than a broad-scale analysis will allow. The presentation really amounts to a number of separate analyses of length of stay as a function of the price-payment factors and some other characteristics which have been suggested as significant for determining the length of stay. The data used in each analysis are based on a significant number of patients of similar age, sex, and diagnostic characteristics. In this manner, it is hoped that the differences in length of stay will be more likely to reflect the effects of differences in the price-payment factors.

THE DATA

Essential to this study was the effort to develop such homogeneous groups. The analyses presented here are based on the results of an investigation of admissions in the year 1962 to New England hospitals. Data are drawn from a sample of medical records and financial information derived from 68 individual institutions. The sample was chosen from the universe of non-federal, short-term general and special hospitals in the states of Maine, New Hampshire, Vermont, Massachusetts, and Rhode Island. There were, in 1962, a total of 218 non-teaching, short-term general hospitals in this universe. Separate samples of teaching and special hospitals were also taken. The sample was stratified by size in an effort to examine the institutions themselves as well as individual patient experiences. In each case, the hospitals in the sample represent at least 25 per cent of each size group in the five-state region. In the year 1962 this population represented 1,112,058 admissions. Within each hospital a random sample of admissions was taken in an effort to obtain at least 1 per cent of the admissions for that year in that size group of hospitals.

The original sample was made up of 71 hospitals, of which 3 refused to participate. The total number of admissions expected in the sample was 17,994. The loss, as a result of non-participation, was 880 cases, somewhere under 5 per cent of the sample.

The abstracting of clinical records was undertaken on the basis that no hospital was completed until at least 95 per cent of the records within the sample had been found. The over-all response for clinical records was above 98 per cent. The financial records, however, presented considerably greater problems, and it was often difficult to link them with the clinical records. However, the over-all group of admissions for which both records were present and related was approximately 90 per cent. The resulting final sample consisted of 15,685 admissions, a loss of 12.83 per cent. It is a matter of interest that, with the exception of the hospitals that refused to participate in the sample, the larger the hospital, the higher the percentage of non-usable observations.

These data provide considerable opportunity for illuminating studies. In the course of accumulating this information, factors such as the day of admission, the number of days prior to surgery for surgical admissions, the distance of the patient's home location from the institution, and other information believed to be useful was obtained.[5]

Of primary interest for this paper was the opportunity to do initial analysis of the price elasticity of the length of stay. As a first step, all of the data were distributed by diagnostic category, using the ICDA categorization, age, and sex. All of the data, including charges, payment sources, hospital size, and medical records data, are presently organized in this form. For this analysis 28 cells defined by age, sex, and diagnosis, with large numbers of observations, were pulled out and subjected to a separate analysis.* (Certain diagnostic categories, such as "other diseases of the circulatory system" and "other diseases of the central nervous system," were not included because the presumption of homogeneity was unrealistic.)

As a first step, the distribution of lengths of stay within each of these cells was obtained in an effort to determine whether variation in the length of stay significant enough for meaningful analysis was likely to be encountered. The length of stay distributions by medical categories are presented in Table 1, and by surgical category in Table 2.† It will be evident from a quick examination that considerable differences in the distributions can be found among these groups. In some cases there is a tight distribution with significant clustering around a few values. In other cases the distribution is bimodal, and in some cases there is no apparent systematic distribution. Of even more significance, there is a considerable range of length of stay within even these so-called homogeneous groups. They provide the basis for the analysis that follows.

THE ANALYSIS

There are two aspects of the analysis that are of interest. First, the basic hypothesis being tested is that the length of stay is a function of some

---

*The 28 groups selected represent the largest cells in the sample. The choice of the number 28 is primarily a function of the ability of the computer program to deal with no more than 28 separate sets of data simultaneously.

†The surgical categories represent subsets of the medical diagnoses. For example, the surgical group "tonsillectomy and adenoidectomy" represents approximately two-thirds of the observations in the medical categories "hypertrophy of tonsils and adenoids."

Table 1: Length of Stay Distribution by Medical Category

Length of Stay[a]	Medical Category[b]																			
	1	2	3	4	5	6	7	8	9	10	11	12	13	14	15	16	17	18	19	20
0	1	4	0	0	0	1	1	0	7	2	5	14	1	2	0	0	0	0	0	0
1	5	12	26	0	5	5	1	6	64	40	101	115	6	12	4	1	5	4	1	5
2	29	19	40	6	0	3	1	7	55	47	135	136	70	34	4	1	5	4	0	6
3	32	15	29	2	2	4	6	14	2	1	4	12	3	12	2	1	3	6	3	6
4	13	5	11	7	4	7	6	15	4	1	0	0	0	5	7	2	1	4	5	5
5	11	2	4	6	2	7	5	4	1	0	—	2	1	2	11	6	1	5	3	3
6	11	3	2	6	6	1	9	2	0	1	—	2	0	2	15	7	1	3	0	5
7	11	2	2	4	1	10	5	4	—	1	—	1	—	1	11	8	4	7	4	1
8	24	13	1	6	5	5	5	3	—	0	—	0	—	2	14	12	9	5	5	3
9	26	10	1	2	2	7	5	2	—	0	—	—	—	0	13	7	7	8	6	3
10	14	8	0	1	0	4	8	0	—	2	—	—	—	0	3	9	6	8	5	1
11	11	6	0	4	0	4	4	2	—	0	0	—	—	1	4	2	6	7	3	3
12	7	10	0	2	1	2	5	2	—	—	1	—	—	0	3	0	5	5	5	3
13	7	5	1	0	2	0	5	0	—	—	0	—	—	—	1	1	4	5	8	2
14	3	2	1	4	5	8	7	2	—	—	—	—	—	—	2	2	5	4	2	2
15	4	2	0	0	2	4	4	0	—	—	—	—	—	—	2	2	0	1	1	2
16	1	0	0	2	2	2	7	—	—	—	—	—	—	—	0	1	1	1	0	1
17	0	2	0	0	1	3	3	—	—	—	—	—	—	—	—	0	1	1	1	2
18	0	0	0	6	3	1	2	—	—	—	—	—	0	—	—	1	1	2	2	1
19	0	2	2	3	3	1	0	—	—	—	—	—	1	—	—	0	0	1	3	0
20	0	0	0	1	0	4	5	—	—	—	—	—	0	—	—	1	—	0	1	0
21	1	—	0	11	1	2	2	—	—	—	—	—	—	—	—	1	—	0	3	2
22	0	—	0	5	3	3	0	0	—	—	—	—	—	—	—	0	—	2	1	3
23	1	—	0	6	1	3	3	1	—	—	—	—	—	—	—	—	—	0	0	2
24	1	—	1	4	0	3	0	0	—	—	—	—	—	—	—	—	—	0	0	2
25	0	—	0	6	1	3	1	—	—	—	—	—	—	—	—	—	—	1	0	0
26	—	—	1	3	2	3	1	—	—	—	—	—	—	—	—	—	—	—	0	3

	1	2	3	4	5	6	7	8	9	10	11	12	13	14	15	16	17	18	19	20
27	—	—	—	0	3	2	2	0	—	—	—	—	—	—	—	1	—	1	1	2
28	—	—	—	0	4	3	2	0	—	—	—	—	—	—	—	0	0	1	0	2
29	—	—	—	0	2	1	0	0	—	—	—	—	—	—	0	0	1	1	1	1
30	—	—	1	1	0	2	0	—	—	—	—	—	—	—	1	1	1	0	0	—
31–40	—	—	0	0	5	5	4	5	—	—	—	—	—	—	1	1	0	2	2	6
41–50	—	—	1	—	1	0	1	2	—	—	—	—	—	—	0	0	1	0	1	1
Over 50	0	0	0	1	1	1	3	0	0	0	0	0	0	0	0	0	0	0	1	5
Total	213	122	123	122	66	108	111	64	133	95	246	282	82	73	99	70	68	87	68	80
Median	6.4	6.5	1.9	16.8	13.8	10.0	11.0	3.3	1.0	1.0	1.1	1.1	2.0	1.8	6.8	8.0	8.6	8.8	10.7	12.0

[a] Zero indicates less than one day.

[b] Medical category code:

1. Female, 25–44, benign neoplasms and neoplasms of unspecified nature
2. Female, 45–64, benign neoplasms and neoplasms of unspecified nature
3. Female, 25–44, psychoses
4. Male, 45–64, arteriosclerotic and degenerative heart disease
5. Female, 45–64, arteriosclerotic and degenerative heart disease
6. Male, over 64, arteriosclerotic and degenerative heart disease
7. Female, over 64, arteriosclerotic and degenerative heart disease
8. Male, 0–4, acute upper respiratory infection
9. Male, 0–4, hypertrophy of tonsils and adenoids
10. Female, 0–4, hypertrophy of tonsils and adenoids
11. Male, 5–14, hypertrophy of tonsils and adenoids
12. Female, 5–14, hypertrophy of tonsils and adenoids
13. Female, 25–44, diseases of teeth and supporting structures
14. Male, 0–4, intestinal obstructions and hernias
15. Male, 45–64, intestinal obstructions and hernias
16. Male, over 64, intestinal obstructions and hernias
17. Female, 25–44, cholthiasis and cholecystitis
18. Female, 45–64, cholthiasis and cholecystitis
19. Female, over 64, cholthiasis and cholecystitis
20. Female, over 64, accidental poisoning

Table 2: Length of Stay Distribution by Surgical Category

Length of Stay[a]	Surgical Category[b]							
	1	2	3	4	5	6	7	8
0	7	3	5	13	0	0	1	0
1	59	39	92	99	1	16	28	5
2	33	44	125	124	0	25	77	24
3	2	1	4	9	0	17	69	10
4	3	0	0	0	0	9	22	7
5	0	0	–	2	1	3	8	3
6	–	1	–	1	4	3	5	1
7	–	1	–	1	8	5	6	3
8	–	0	–	0	16	2	5	3
9	–	1	–	0	15	2	2	1
10	–	1	–	0	13	0	1	2
11	0	0	–	0	10	1	3	1
12	1	–	–	1	6	0	0	2
13	0	–	0	0	3	–	0	2
14	–	–	1	–	4	–	1	0
15	–	–	0	–	3	–	0	–
16	–	–	–	–	1	–	2	–
17	–	–	–	–	1	–	0	–
18	–	–	–	–	1	–	1	–
19	–	–	–	–	0	–	2	–
20	–	–	–	–	0	–	0	–
21	–	–	–	–	2	–	–	–
22	–	–	–	–	0	–	–	–
23	–	–	–	–	0	–	–	–
24	–	–	–	–	1	–	–	–
25	–	–	–	–	0	–	–	–
26	–	–	–	–	–	–	–	–
27	–	–	–	–	–	–	–	–
28	–	–	–	–	–	–	–	–
29	–	–	–	–	–	–	–	–
30	–	–	–	–	–	–	–	–
31–40	–	–	–	–	–	–	–	–
41–50	–	–	–	–	–	–	–	–
Over 50	0	0	0	0	0	0	0	0
Total	125	91	227	250	90	83	233	64
Median	1.0	2.0	1.1	1.2	9.0	2.0	2.2	3.0

[a]Zero indicates less than one day.
[b]Surgical category code:
    1. Male, 0-4, tonsillectomy and adenoidectomy
    2. Female, 0-4, tonsillectomy and adenoidectomy
    3. Male, 5-14, tonsillectomy and adenoidectomy
    4. Female, 5-14, tonsillectomy and adenoidectomy
    5. Female, 25-44, hysterectomy
    6. Female, 15-24, curettage of uterus
    7. Female, 25-44, curettage of uterus
    8. Female, 45-64, curettage of uterus

price-payment measure. Two specific price-payment measures are examined: cash outlay as a percentage of the total bill and average daily room charge. These price-payment factors are roughly indicative of the relative charge and the marginal price as stated in the billing. In each case, length of stay will be stated as a function of each of these price-payment factors for each of the groups being examined. For the surgical categories, the analysis employs as the dependent variable both length of total stay and postoperative length of stay.

There is a second analysis implicit in this exercise, however, which reflects the hypothesis that certain diagnostic categories will be more likely to show a high price elasticity of length of stay than others. It can be posited that certain diagnostic categories have a length of stay which is far more technically determined than others. In the former case, the length of stay should be considerably more insensitive to differences in the price-payment factor than those other categories where the actual length of stay is less a technological requirement than a matter of patient preference.

One can speculate in advance about a number of aspects of the diagnosis which ought to show up in the price elasticity analysis. First, one can hypothesize that the more serious the illness, the less likely it is that the price elasticity of length of stay will be significant. However, the counter-hypothesis can be proposed that for diagnostic categories with a longer average length of stay, the potential for technically required marginal days is reduced. The difficulty raised by these two hypotheses is that they lead to opposite expectations. If longer average lengths of stay for a diagnostic category are associated with more serious illnesses, then such illnesses should show a smaller price elasticity of demand. However, if longer lengths of stay are associated with a diminishing technical requirement for marginal days, those illnesses should have a higher price elasticity of demand. A comparison will be made among the groups being examined in this paper in an effort to see whether some light can be shed on this associated hypothesis about the nature of the length of stay.

The analysis consisted of two regressions for each group in the following form:

1. $Y = aX_1{}^{b_1}$ $[\log Y = a + b_1 \log X_1]$

2. $Y = aX_2{}^{b_2}$ $[\log y = a + b_2 \log X_2]$

where Y represents length of stay, X_1 represents cash payment as percentage of total bill, and X_2 represents average room charge.

The bs represent elasticities of length of stay with respect to each price variable. These data are presented in Table 3 for the medical categories and

Table 3: Medical Regression Equations Coefficients
(Dependent Variable = Length of Stay)

Medical Category[a]	Constant	Cash / Total Bill	Average Daily Room Charge	R^2
1	0.76	0.0118		.0399
	1.09	(0.58)[b]		
			-.2536	.1314
			(-1.93)	
2	0.6280	-0.0384		.0958
		(-1.05)		
	0.4315		.1872	.2668
			(3.03)	
3	0.4113	0.0064		.0232
		(0.25)		
	0.8841		-.3479	.2258
			(-2.55)	
4	1.09	0.0085		.0227
		(0.25)		
	1.54		-.3336	.1504
			(-1.67)	
5	1.07	0.0091		.0247
		(0.20)		
	2.01		-.7037	.3814
			(-3.30)	
6	1.09	0.0793		.2335
		(2.47)		
	1.36		-.2778	.2004
			(-2.11)	
7	0.96	-0.0618		.2257
		(-2.42)		
	1.35		-.2392	.1406
			(-1.48)	
8	0.50	-0.0646		.2532
		(-2.06)		
	1.47		-.6689	.2209
			(-1.78)	
9	0.11	-0.0190		.1106
		(-1.27)		
	0.87		-.5515	.4069
			(-5.10)	
10	0.19	-0.0024		.0119
		(-0.11)		
	1.03		-.6411	.3342
			(-3.42)	
11	0.15	-0.0103		.0687
		(-1.08)		
	0.57		-.3012	.3728
			(-6.28)	
12	0.17	0.0031		.0173
		(0.29)		
	0.51		-.2567	.2672
			(-4.64)	

Table 3—*continued*

Medical Category[a]	Constant	Cash / Total Bill	Average Daily Room Charge	R^2
13	0.26	-0.0311 (-2.02)		.2204
	1.05		-.5527 (-6.03)	.5590
14	0.35	-0.0041 (-0.15)		.0178
	0.42		-.0564 (-0.95)	.1118
15	0.80	-0.0168 (-0.77)		.0781
	0.63		.1456 (0.69)	.0694
16	0.91	-0.0199 (-0.89)		.1072
	1.00		-.0504 (-0.48)	.0580
17	0.93	0.0374 (1.08)		.1315
	1.01		-.0966 (-0.37)	.0455
18	0.94	0.0283 (0.80)		.0864
	0.78		.0919 (0.45)	.0491
19	1.00	-0.0296 (-0.91)		.1121
	0.43		.4404 (1.33)	.1632
20	1.06	0.0458 (1.07)		.1208
	1.13		-.0867 (-0.16)	.0177

[a]See note to Table 1 for medical category code.
[b]Figures in parentheses represent *t* values, coefficient divided by its standard error.

Table 4 for the surgical categories. Table 5 presents the results for the surgical categories using postoperative length of stay as the dependent variable.

The results of the analysis provide evidence of significant price elasticity of demand. It is evident that the "persuasive" price is the average daily room charge, which, in almost every case, shows greater elasticity and is considerably more "explanatory" of the length of stay than relative out-of-pocket cost. The degree to which length of stay can be accounted for by the price variable is, in many cases, small. Nevertheless, for well over half the categories, the elasticity is over 0.2 and is significant at the 5 per cent level. In all but a few cases cash as a percentage of total bill showed a very low elasticity.

Table 4: Surgical Regression Equations Coefficients
(Dependent Variable = Length of Stay)

Surgical Category[a]	Constant	Cash / Total Bill	Average Daily Room Charge	R^2
1	0.11	-.0210 (-1.30)[b]		.1165
	0.93		-.5920 (-5.04)	.4134
2	0.18	-.0007 (-0.03)		.0035
	1.04		-.6536 (-3.33)	.3333
3	0.15	-.0128 (-1.27)		.0846
	0.58		-.3016 (-6.13)	.3785
4	0.18	.0047 (0.41)		.0257
	0.48		-.2349 (-3.90)	.2403
5	0.99	.0009 (0.07)		.0076
	1.14		-.1114 (-1.17)	.1235
6	0.42	-.0008 (-0.03)		.0037
	0.72		-.2208 (-0.78)	.0865
7	0.41	-.0242 (-1.48)		.0970
	0.76		-.2353 (-2.59)	.1678
8	0.55	.0163 (0.41)		.0524
	1.00		-.3353 (-0.96)	.1206

[a]See note to Table 2 for surgical category code.
[b]Figures in parentheses represent t values, coefficient divided by its standard error.

For some categories interesting price elasticities were observed: for arteriosclerotic and degenerative heart diseases, the price elasticity (based on average daily charge) of length of stay was considerably higher for the group aged 45–64 than for the group over 64. This suggests an association between the seriousness of the episode of illness (presumably greater for the older group) and the ability of price to affect the length of stay. Among the pediatric surgical categories the price elasticities are higher for younger children than for teenagers, and in the adult surgical categories they are higher for older adults than for younger. For the surgical categories the price elasticity of

Table 5: Surgical Regression Equations Coefficients
(Dependent Variable = Postoperative Length of Stay)

Surgical Category[a]	Constant	Cash / Total Bill	Average Daily Room Charge	R^2
1	-0.34	-.0601 (-2.18)[b]		.1929
	0.56		-.6001 (-2.77)	.2420
2	-0.7	-.0014 (-0.05)		.0054
	1.11		-.9726 (-3.77)	.3712
3	-0.17	-.0091 (-0.61)		.0403
	0.35		-.3747 (-4.96)	.3141
4	-0.15	.0234 (1.29)		.0819
	0.29		-.3539 (-3.74)	.2309
5	0.93	.0041 (0.30)		.0323
	1.08		-.1156 (-1.15)	.1212
6	0.14	.0025 (0.06)		.0070
	0.71		-.4264 (-0.94)	.1039
7	0.16	-.0348 (-1.65)		.1081
	0.62		-.3001 (-2.56)	.1660
8	0.34	.0644 (1.03)		.1300
	1.62		-.9689 (-1.77)	.2192

[a]See note to Table 2 for surgical category code.
[b]Figures in parentheses represent t values, coefficient divided by its standard error.

length of stay was considerably higher when postoperative length of stay was used as the dependent variable. The economic preferences of consumers are not likely to be felt until after the surgical input.*

The analysis could be summarized as evidence of significant price elasticity of length of stay when the price variable is the average daily room charge. This particular price variable is most likely to be known by the patient, since

*In almost all cases the explanation provided by the regressions done in the logs was considerably greater than that obtained in an earlier run of strictly linear regressions.

it conforms quite closely to the stated daily room charge posted by the institution. It is interesting that far less price elasticity of demand is demonstrated with respect to relative cash outlay, although the actual cash outlay would be expected to influence the utilization of the facility by the patient. It is likely that the actual cash outlay and the cash outlay relative to the total bill is not known by the patient until the moment of discharge from the institution and is therefore not likely to motivate him to reduce the length of his stay. On the other hand, the fifty- or sixty-dollar daily rate is well known to the patient and is likely to be quite influential in determining his behavior. The evidence here is wholly consistent with this observation.

The analysis also sheds some light on the association between the median length of stay and price elasticity of demand. The results suggest that for shorter lengths of stay there is likely to be less price elasticity. A Spearman Rank Correlation Coefficient calculated by using length of stay and the average daily room charge for the price variable indicates a negative association. When the lengths of stay were ranked from longest to shortest and the price elasticities of length of stay, using average daily room charge as the price variable, were ranked from most negative to most positive, the coefficient had a value of -.2926. It should be noted that only the first twelve most negative price elasticity estimates were significant, while the others ranked on the continuum were, with one exception, not significantly different from zero.

In the surgical categories it is interesting that the tonsillectomies and adenoidectomies, with their extremely short lengths of stay, tended to have the highest price elasticities. This finding may reflect the fact that these patients are all pediatric cases, in which decisions on stay are made by parents who are much more responsive to direct price constraints. The loss of a day's work or the need to bring in someone to care for the child does not have the same effect on the utilization decision as in the case of adult admissions.

While this analysis was primarily directed at evaluating the degree to which the price-payment variables are associated with variation in the length of stay, there are a number of other factors which are likely to have some influence. A more intensive analysis on some of these factors is in process. One attempt was made to examine the impact of marital status on length of stay for the adult surgical categories (5, 6, 7, and 8). There is considerable evidence that marital status is highly associated with length of stay: widowed, single, and divorced persons stay longer on the average than married persons, both in England and in the United States. The presumption is that married persons are more likely to have alternatives to continued stay in the hospital. In an effort to examine the degree to which the factor is likely to affect the price-payment associations, the analysis was also run with a dummy variable with a value of 0 for married persons and 1 for single persons. This particular analysis was undertaken only on the adult surgical groups. Each of these four groups (surgical categories 5-8) consists of females for whom, at least in part, marriage is likely to represent an increased demand for their presence at home. Home might, therefore, represent an environment which is less conducive to recuperation than the hospital, particularly since all of the females with the exception of number 8 are of child-bearing age and are likely to have child-care responsibilities at home.

The results of this analysis are shown in Table 6 and present rather an interesting set of observations.* For those in age group 25-44 who were hospitalized for hysterectomies, and for the other category in this age group (category 7), the coefficients on the marital status variable tended to be more significant than for the younger and older groups. In the other two categories, both of which (like category 7) were curettage of the uterus in age groups 15-24 and 45-64, the addition of the marital status variable in the regression made little difference. Of perhaps more importance, however, is the fact that for the very serious operation hysterectomy, marital status coefficients all were negative, suggesting that being married was associated with longer length of stay, while for the category curettage of the uterus there were no negative coefficients. This leads to the interesting hypothesis that perhaps, in the case

Table 6: Length of Stay as Function of Price-Payment Marital Status, Adult Surgical Category

Surgical Category[a]	Constant	Cash / Total Bill	Average Daily Room Charge	Marital Status	R^2
5	10.36	.6555 (0.47)[b]		-1.4593 (-1.42)	.1545
	12.11		-.0701 (-1.08)	-1.3885 (-1.37)	.1859
6	3.42	-.7714 (-1.07)		.1700 (0.28)	.1252
	4.03		-.0355 (-0.85)	.1456 (0.24)	.1015
7	3.59	-1.2689 (-1.84)		1.0009 (1.53)	.1503
	3.41		-.0026 (-1.08)	.8842 (1.35)	.1151
8	4.40	-.5963 (-0.72)		.8320 (0.75)	.1171
	5.08		-.0320 (-0.65)	.5776 (0.54)	.1107

[a]See note to Table 2 for surgical category code.
[b]Figures in parentheses represent t values, coefficient divided by its standard error.

*These regressions are linear and were not calculated in logs.

of more serious illness, females with children in the house are more likely to stay longer in the hospital than are males with the same illness in the same age bracket. (A further analysis is being undertaken at the current time of the twenty medical categories and the twenty-eight next largest categories in an effort to carry some of these observations further.)

The results of this analysis, while indicating considerable price elasticity of demand in a number of the diagnostic categories, also suggest that the categories are less homogeneous than might be desired. As noted earlier, a direct examination of the distribution of length of stay in some categories reveals well-defined bimodal distributions, suggesting that within some age, sex, and diagnostic categories there are two separate types of experience which should be analyzed separately. Efforts are being made, particularly for the surgical categories, to develop a number of severity measures which should permit specific analysis, with the severity of the diagnosis for each individual patient included as a separate variable. As an approximation to this method, it might be possible to use two other types of information which are available within the study. An effort is now being made to evaluate the price elasticity of length of stay using only observations without recorded secondary diagnoses. This procedure would eliminate from the sample the length of stay response that reflects multiple illness. In addition, because there is information on distance traveled, it might be possible to evaluate and distribute these data according to the distance traveled to given institutions, particularly to the larger institutions. This finding may be correlated with the severity of illness and might provide some way of differentiating the more serious diagnoses from the less serious ones.

It is also possible to narrow the age range of each of the cells. Nevertheless, it is evident from the analysis here that even without such "purification" there is considerable price elasticity of demand in terms of length of stay even in the cells described. Each of these adjustments represents a refinement which is unlikely to reduce the price elasticity observed here.

In the beginning of this paper it was suggested that much of the discussion about deductibles and co-insurance was based on implicit assumptions about the nature of the price elasticity of demand. The analysis indicates that co-insurance, since it represents a requirement for an additional cash outlay each day, might result in some reduction of the length of stay, although the significance of this influence does not appear to be very great. On the other hand, the relative impact of the deductible on the total bill tends to diminish over time. Neither deductibles nor co-insurance are likely to have any impact on the average room service charge. While the possibility still exists that such financial devices may influence the admissions rate, this analysis has not provided any insight into this question.

SUMMARY

Some of the initial results of an extensive analysis of factors affecting the length of stay in a sample of short-term general hospitals in New England in the year 1962 have been described. Specifically, an attempt was made to ascertain the degree to which length of stay is associated with a number of price-payment factors for twenty-eight groups of patients within specific age, sex, and diagnostic categories. The results suggest that, for most categories, while the price-payment variable does not provide a significant degree of explanation for the variations observed in length of stay, there is significant price elasticity with respect to the average room charge. Additional analysis of the influence of marital status on the adult surgical category suggests that the influence of this factor may be associated with the relative seriousness of the diagnosis.

Some light is shed on the potential significance of the price elasticity of demand in terms of length of stay. While not determinate, the results nevertheless suggest that many of the assumptions implicit in the discussion of deductibles and co-insurance merit further study. It is hoped that further analysis of the data presented here may yield additional insight.

NOTES

1. Paul J. Feldstein and Ruth Severson, "The Demand for Medical Care," in American Medical Association, *Report of the Commission on the Cost of Medical Care* (Chicago: By the Association, 1964); Gerald Rosenthal, *The Demand for Medical Care Facilities* (Chicago: American Hospital Association, 1964).

2. Gerald D. Rosenthal, Progress Report, 1964, Grant HM00302, United States Public Health Service.

3. Rosenthal, *The Demand for Medical Care Facilities*, pp. 44–45.

4. Martin S. Feldstein, *Economic Analysis for Health Service Efficiency* (Amsterdam: North-Holland Publishing Co., 1968).

5. For a more complete description of the sampling procedure and the data, see report on Contract PH108-66-188, Bureau of Public Health Economics.

Victor R. Fuchs

National Bureau of Economic Research and The City University of New York

COMMENT

The title of this paper is misleading. It is described as a study of the price elasticity of demand for short-term general hospital services. In fact, the analysis is limited to only one dimension of demand — length of stay — and the empirical portion does not properly identify a price elasticity.

The author states that it is important to know the effect of price on the quantity of services demanded in order to predict the impact of deductibles and co-insurance on hospital utilization. He also states that price is much more likely to affect length of stay than to affect the admission rate. However, deductibles are much more likely to influence the admission rate than the length of stay. Once the deductible amount has been used up (usually in the first day or two of hospitalization), it has no effect on length of stay. Furthermore, the author implicitly assumes that the amount of insurance an individual carries is independent of the price of hospital services and other demand factors. There may be some instances of completely involuntary insurance, but most often the amount and type of insurance coverage have to be explained in a study of the demand for hospital services.

A true study of price elasticity would have quantity as the dependent variable and price and other relevant factors as the independent variables. The regressions run in Rosenthal's study depart from this standard in several important respects.

First, the dependent variable is length of stay, not quantity of hospital services. The latter consists of patient days plus services such as X-rays and the like. Patient days depend upon admission rates and length of stay. Use of length of stay as a measure of quantity might be acceptable if it were not correlated with admission rate and if the number of services per day were independent of length of stay; but neither assumption is plausible. The elasticities observed in the paper, therefore, are presumably biased estimates of the true quantity-price elasticities.

Second, the so-called price variables in the first two sets of regressions do not measure price or anything even resembling price, as the author admits. How, then, can their coefficients be regarded as price elasticities? The second set of regressions does make a start toward answering the question of whether the length of stay depends upon the payment status of the patient. K. K. Ro has been investigating this question through a multivariate analysis of some nine thousand discharges from short-term general hospitals in Pittsburgh,* and he does find a significant difference in length of stay depending upon payment status. Patients who pay their own bills tend to have appreciably shorter stays than do those patients whose bills are paid for by government, *ceteris paribus.* I have reworked some of Ro's data for hernia cases, and the table below shows the relation between several variables, including payment status and length of stay. Color and age are significant, in addition to payment status. The importance of multiple diagnoses relative to a single diagnosis should also be noted.

The price variable in the paper's third set of regressions, the average price of a room, is calculated by dividing the total room charge by length of stay. The appearance of the dependent variable as a denominator in the independent variable does introduce the possibility of some negative regression bias.

Regression Analysis of Length of Stay for Hernia Surgery,
Pittsburgh Short-Term Hospitals, 1963 (N = 239)

Independent Variable	Simple Regression Coefficient	(t value)	Partial Regression Coefficient	(t value)
Occupancy rate	8.8	(1.7)	4.1	(0.9)
Residency program	0.4	(0.2)	1.6	(1.2)
Female	3.2	(3.4)	1.4	(1.5)
Non-white	-2.8	(-2.3)	-2.5	(-2.0)
20–44[a]	4.3	(3.3)	3.7	(2.9)
45 and over[a]	6.6	(6.5)	6.7	(6.3)
Blue Cross and other insurance[b]	-0.5	(-0.3)	-0.5	(-0.2)
Government and unpaid[b]	0.6	(0.3)	3.7	(1.7)
Multiple diagnoses	3.6	(3.9)	3.1	(3.6)

[a]Compared with 0–19 age group.
[b]Compared with patient as primary source of payment.

---

*See K. K. Ro, "Hospital Characteristics, Patient Characteristics, and Hospital Use," *Medical Care* 48, no. 4 (July–August 1969).

A more serious problem is the omission of other relevant variables that may be correlated with average room charge and length of stay. These include the availability of home care programs, outpatient clinics, and other hospital-related characteristics. Also omitted are such standard economic variables as the patient's income and education. Moreover, neither the quantity nor the price variables have been adjusted for differences in quality such as type of room and other amenities. To the extent that the price variable is affected by the quality of the room, the observed coefficient is an underestimate of the true price elasticity.

Although the author presents his tentative conclusions with commendable caution, the above remarks should serve as an additional warning concerning the theoretical and empirical difficulties which surround this problem.

Morris Silver
City College of New York and the
National Bureau of Economic Research

AN ECONOMIC ANALYSIS OF VARIATIONS IN MEDICAL EXPENSES AND WORK-LOSS RATES

I. OBJECTIVES AND ORGANIZATION

This paper employs a number of the standard tools of economic analysis to explore unpublished data on the medical expenses and work-loss days due to illness or injury of currently employed persons. Section II deals with the data, statistical techniques, and variables employed in the study. The primary objective of Section III is to estimate elasticities of demand for medical care (totally and by type) with respect to family income. Knowledge of these elasticities should contribute to more accurate forecasts of the demand for medical care and aid in the formulation of policy-related judgments concerning the equity of the current distribution of medical services.

Like earlier studies of the demand for medical care[1] which have utilized other bodies of data, the present study utilizes data on medical expenses to measure the amount of care received. Expense data are useful because, unlike the available physical measures, they reflect not only the quantity but the quality of medical care. On the other hand, the use of expense data creates a number of problems (e.g., free care) which are given detailed consideration in Section III.

This research was carried out at the National Bureau of Economic Research and was supported in part by grants from the Commonwealth Fund and by the National Center for Health Services Research and Development Grant 1P01CH00374-01. I am indebted to Richard Auster, Gary Becker, Michael Grossman, Irving Leveson, Jacob Mincer, Kong Kyun Ro, and, most of all, to Victor R. Fuchs for many helpful comments. Special thanks are due Mrs. Geraldine A. Gleeson, Chief, Analysis and Reports Branch, Division of Health Interview Statistics, National Center for Health Statistics, United States Public Health Service, for providing me with the work-loss and medical expense data.

Unlike many previous studies, this study makes use of grouped or "ecological" data. The use of average incomes to estimate income elasticities which describe individual behavior can be justified in two ways. First, grouped data should minimize "simultaneous-equation bias." The individual correlation between income and medical care will reflect not only the effect of income on the amount of medical care demanded but also the effect of health on income. This problem would be more severe for individual than for grouped data because individual health is affected not only by differences in "erratic" factors among groups but by intra-group variations in such factors. Second, measurement errors (including transitory influences) in individual incomes would lead to underestimates of regression coefficients even if these errors were not correlated with the true (or long-run) individual incomes.[2] Errors of this type often cancel out in grouped data.

One of the important innovations of Section III is the inclusion of the earnings rate with family income in the regressions. This allows empirically for the previously ignored possibility that higher income individuals may need more medical care or use less patient-time–intensive methods of dealing with their medical problems.

The mortality rate has been the most widely used measure of health for many years, but the recent growth of quantitative interest in the determinants of health status has sharply increased the demand for more flexible measures. One of the most promising alternative measures of health is the work-loss rate due to illness or injury. Section IV attempts to test the validity of using the work-loss rate as a measure of health by ascertaining whether variations in work-loss rates reflect differences in the degree to which individuals can afford to lose income or in the amounts that would be lost, and, if so, the extent to which they do so. The principal findings of the study are summarized in Section V.

II. DATA, VARIABLES, AND STATISTICAL TECHNIQUES

The medical expense and work-loss data analyzed are drawn from the National Health Survey of the National Center for Health Statistics. These data, which are restricted to currently employed persons, are in the form of averages for each of twenty-four regions (Northeast, North Central, South, and West) by age group (17–44, 45–64, and 65 and over) and by sex.

The information was obtained through household health interviews and mail-in questionnaires left after completion of the interviews. The averages for medical expenses are based on a sample of about 71,000 persons from 22,000 households and include all medical bills paid, or to be paid, by the ill person, his family or friends, and any part paid by insurance. The average work-loss rates are based upon a sample of 134,000 persons from 42,000 households. The expense data refer to the twelve months prior to the inter-

view period of July 1, 1962–December 31, 1962, while the work-loss data
refer to the interview period July 1962–June 1963.[3]

The primary data utilized in the paper are shown in Table 1. The data for
the quantitative independent variables are, of necessity, also in the form of
averages for each of the twenty-four region-age-sex cells and refer to employed persons at work. However, those averages which refer to 1959 or 1960
are derived from a different sample than the medical expenses and work-loss
rates, the 1-in-1,000 sample of the census of 1960.[4]

Table 1: Selected Data on Medical Expenses and
Days Lost from Work, by Age Group and Sex

Region	Age Group	Sex	Average Total Medical Expenses per Currently Employed Person per Year (July–December 1962)	Average Days Lost from Work due to Illness or Injury per Currently Employed Person per Year (July 1962–June 1963)
NE	17–44	M	$106.99	3.5
NE	45–64	M	175.12	7.1
NE	65 and over	M	228.89	8.2
NE	17–44	F	154.47	6.5
NE	45–64	F	193.81	8.7
NE	65 and over	F	269.79	6.4
NC	17–44	M	90.30	3.9
NC	45–64	M	161.00	6.9
NC	65 and over	M	190.45	10.6
NC	17–44	F	129.83	5.5
NC	45–64	F	181.17	6.7
NC	65 and over	F	163.53	5.4
S	17–44	M	95.50	5.4
S	45–64	M	156.92	9.8
S	65 and over	M	175.12	13.8
S	17–44	F	140.95	6.5
S	45–64	F	168.23	6.3
S	65 and over	F	142.09	7.1
W	17–44	M	114.59	4.8
W	45–64	M	192.37	6.2
W	65 and over	M	203.94	9.8
W	17–44	F	216.81	6.6
W	45–64	F	249.30	6.0
W	65 and over	F	183.05	7.5

The more important variables employed in the multiple regressions of Sections III and IV are listed below and discussed when appropriate.

Dependent Variables

Y_1, total medical expense per currently employed person per year

Y_2, hospital expense per currently employed person per year

Y_3, medicine expense per currently employed person per year

Y_4, doctor expense per currently employed person per year

Y_5, dentist expense per currently employed person per year

Y_6, days lost from work due to illness or injury per currently employed person per year

*Independent Variables**

X_1, adjusted mean total family income for employed persons at work who are in families.

Average weekly earnings are obtained by dividing mean total earnings for a given cell by its mean number of weeks worked. Earnings per day are estimated by dividing the above quotient by 5; the resulting dollar figure is multipled by mean work-loss days in the cell to obtain the value of lost time, which was then added to X_{1u}.

X_{1u}, unadjusted mean total family income for employed persons at work who are in families

X_{1d}, 0 if adjusted mean total family income for employed persons at work in families (X_1) is below its median value; the actual value of X_1 when it is above its median

X_2, sex: 0 for female, 1 for male

X_3, region: 0 for non-South, 1 for South

X_4, age: 0 for 17–44, 1 for 45–46, 2 for 65 and over

X_3 and X_4 are the primary measures of region and age utilized in the study. The forms of these variables are derived from a priori considerations and from a desire to conserve degrees of freedom, to limit multicollinearity problems, and to avoid exhausting the sample space. The age variable is the most controversial, but it is important to note that the possibility that its use biases the coefficients of the economic variables upon which our interest centers is lessened by the use of a variety of regression forms. However, as an additional precaution key results are checked by replacing X_3 with:

X_5, age: 1 if age 17–44, 0 otherwise

and

*The following midpoints were assumed for open-ended classes: total family income of employed persons at work in families (Item 60, Code X), $60,000; total earnings of employed persons at work (Item 39, Code X), $40,000; highest grade of school completed by employed persons at work (Item 26, Code X), 17.5 years.

X_6, age: 1 if age 45–64, 0 otherwise

X_7, mean highest grade of school completed by employed persons at work

X_8, percentage of employed persons at work residing in rural areas

X_9, percentage of employed persons at work residing outside SMSAs

X_{10}, percentage of employed persons at work who are married with spouse present

X_{11}, percentage of employed persons at work who are Negro

X_{12}, earnings per week worked of employed persons at work (estimated by dividing mean total earnings in 1959 for those with earnings by the mean number of weeks worked in 1959 by those who worked)

Since the relevant bodies of theory do not specify functional forms, both natural values and a logarithmic transformation are employed. Further, the regressions are run in both unweighted and weighted form in which the weights are the number of persons in each of the twenty-four region-age-sex cells. The use of weights is designed to achieve homoscedasticity and reduce the chances of errors in regression coefficients caused by large random errors in a small cell. However, unweighted regressions are run also because relevant information might be lost by the assignment of low weights to small but extreme cells (e.g., those for the 65 and over age group).

III. REGRESSION ANALYSES OF MEDICAL EXPENSES

The primary objective of this section is to estimate elasticities of demand for medical care with respect to command over goods and services. Amounts of medical services received are measured by the mean medical expenses of currently employed persons in a region-age-sex cell ($Y_1 - Y_5$), while command over goods and services is measured by a cell's adjusted mean total family income for employed persons at work who are in families (X_1).

An important advantage of expense data is that they reflect both the quantity and quality of medical care, whereas the available physical measures (e.g., physician visits) reflect only the quantity. However, as in previous studies, the use of expenses gives rise to a number of difficulties. First there is the (probably minor) problem of "free" care which is received by some currently employed persons with very low incomes but is not included in the expense data. Second, medical care prices may be positively correlated with income because physicians charge the more affluent higher prices for given services or because the more affluent are more likely to have health insurance and those covered by insurance are charged higher prices.[5] Third, and most important, when more affluent individuals are ill or undergoing preventive care, they attempt to maintain their customary living standards by purchasing amenities and complements to medical care such as private hospital rooms and "Park Avenue doctors." As a result, the medical expenses of the more affluent overstate the amount of medical care they have received.

The available data do not permit dealing with the last two problems. However, the purchase of amenities is probably most important in the case of hospital expense, and the data do permit the estimation of separate income elasticities for the various components of medical care.

As has been pointed out in Section I, the use of mean incomes helps to minimize bias due to errors of measurement and simultaneous-equation problems. However, if variables not included in the statistical model reduced health in certain of our region-age-sex cells and resulted in higher medical expenses and lower family income, income elasticities still would be biased. In order to deal with this possibility, data for each region-age-sex cell on average earnings rates and work-loss days due to illness or injury were used to estimate the value of working time lost due to poor health. These estimates were added to the mean family income figure for each of the cells to secure "adjusted" mean total family income (X_1), which was utilized in the regressions.

Since higher income individuals can afford to purchase more and better medical care and are unlikely to prefer purchases of other types of consumer goods when they are ill, and since it seems unlikely that most consumers regard the services provided by preventive medical care as lower quality members of some broader family of services (as is margarine in the family of table fats), there is reason to expect the income elasticity to be positive. On the other hand, given appropriate assumptions about time preferences, it is possible that those with higher incomes might purchase more preventive care, resulting in lower average current expenses.[6] In the opinion of this writer the arguments suggesting a positive relationship are far stronger than those supporting a negative one, but in the final analysis the issue must be resolved by the data.

Previous empirical studies indicate that the income elasticity is positive and somewhat below unity. The latter magnitude is a useful benchmark because of the "necessity" character of much, if not most, medical expenditure. If we continue to think in terms of the "degree of necessity," it seems reasonable to expect the income elasticity of dentist expense to be relatively high and that of hospital expense to be relatively low. This hypothesis receives support from the findings of Feldstein and Severson[7] and is reexamined in the present study.

Because of their intrinsic interest and to avoid biased estimation of the income elasticity, a number of additional independent variables are included in the regressions. Dummy variables measuring age, sex, and region are utilized because they may reflect differences in physiological or psychological needs for medical care,[8] or perhaps in its cost. Later in the analysis, the percentage rural, the percentage living outside SMSAs, the percentage Negro, and measures of marital status and education are included in the regressions.

In the final phase the earnings rate is introduced. The studies cited above suggest that being younger and better educated lowers expenses, while being female raises them. The results of the regressions are presented in Table 2.

Regressions 1-4 show that whatever the form employed, the coefficient of income is positive and statistically significant at conventional levels.* The estimated income elasticities of demand for medical services, which range from 1.4 to 2.0, are quite high in comparison with those observed in previous studies.

The inclusion of bills paid by insurance in the expense data, taken together with a positive correlation between family income and the amount of health insurance (whether directly paid for by the family or by third parties), may help to explain the above discrepancy. Along the same lines, some studies include insurance coverage as an independent variable which causes income elasticities to be underestimated since, to a large extent, insurance coverage is a positive function of income. Unfortunately, the data at my disposal do not permit quantitative statements of the role of these factors. Another possibility which is difficult to test is that preventive care, which is probably more income-elastic than care of the curative variety, comprises a larger fraction of total medical expenses for the currently employed population than for the population as a whole.

Since the LW form showed the strongest results, sole reliance was now placed upon it. The next step taken was to replace X_4 by the less demanding age variables X_5 and X_6 (see regression 5).† Since the coefficients of these variables were found to be statistically significant, to increase the unadjusted coefficient of determination slightly, and to raise the estimated income elasticity from 2.0 to 2.5, it was decided to retain them in the succeeding regressions. Regressions 6-9 are for the separate components of medical expense and show the relative magnitudes of the income elasticities to be consistent with a priori considerations and previous empirical work — i.e., the income elasticities range from 1.8 for hospital expense to 3.2 for dentist expense.

The results for the other independent variables utilized in regressions 1-9 may be summarized as follows: other things being equal, the proxy for the quantity of medical services is higher for females, southerners, and older

---

*X_{1d} was introduced into the regressions in order to ascertain whether the effect of income varies with its level. It was found that the coefficient of this variable, which measures the difference in the effect of income in the range below its median from that in the range above its median, fluctuates in sign and is statistically insignificant.

In practice, the use of "adjusted" income did not matter very much; when regression 4 was rerun utilizing unadjusted income (X_{1u}), the income elasticity was 2.04 and its computed T value was 5.44, while the adjusted coefficient of determination was .89.

†The coefficients of X_5 and X_6 show how much the level of the entire equation must be adjusted for the influence of the corresponding age groups; the influence of the age group 65 and over is reflected in the constant term of the equation.

Table 2: Regressions of Medical Expenses per Currently Employed Person per Year on Various Independent Variables for Twenty-Four Region-Age-Sex Cells[a]

Regression No.	Form of Regression[b] and Dependent Variable	Regression Coefficient and Computed T Value (in Parentheses)[c]						Biased Coefficient of Determination and Unbiased Coefficient of Determination (in Parentheses)
		Income (X_1)	Sex (X_2)	Region (X_3)	Age (X_4) or Age (X_5)	Age (X_6)	$X_7 - X_{12}$	
(1)	(2)	(3)	(4)	(5)	(6)	(7)	(8)	(9)
1	NU_W Tot. exp. (Y_1)	0.03 (3.42)**	-34.90 (-3.01)**	33.50 (1.45)	37.19 (5.27)**			.70 (.63)
2	NW Tot. exp. (Y_1)	0.03 (4.32)**	-43.95 (-6.15)**	47.33 (2.92)**	36.10 (5.38)**			.88 (.85)
3	LU_W Tot. exp. (Y_1)	1.55 (4.01)**	-0.10 (-3.61)**	0.12 (2.04)	0.11 (6.24)**			.75 (.70)
4	LW Tot. exp. (Y_1)	2.02 (5.61)**	-0.14 (-7.64)**	0.18 (4.16)**	0.11 (6.40)**			.91 (.90)
5	LW Tot. exp. (Y_1)	2.53 (5.38)**	-0.14 (-8.10)**	0.24 (4.35)**	-0.26 (-6.34)**	-0.18 (-3.79)**		.92 (.90)
6	LW Hos. exp. (Y_2)	1.82 (1.74)	-0.14 (-3.69)**	0.17 (1.43)	-0.32 (-3.56)**	-0.19 (-1.77)		.74 (.67)
7	LW Med. exp. (Y_3)	2.23 (5.62)**	-0.15 (-10.52)**	0.29 (6.16)**	-0.34 (-10.05)**	-0.20 (-4.93)**		.96 (.95)
8	LW Dr. exp. (Y_4)	2.88 (4.56)**	-0.15 (-6.42)**	0.29 (3.94)**	-0.21 (-4.04)**	-0.18 (-2.78)*		.86 (.82)

	Dep. var.							R^2
9	LW Den. exp. (Y_5)	3.19 (3.55)**	-0.13 (-3.75)**	0.22 (2.08)	0.04 (0.47)	-0.04 (-0.44)		.71 (.62)
10	LW Tot. exp. (Y_1)	2.61 (5.47)**	-0.13 (-5.70)**	0.28 (4.11)**	-0.34 (-3.81)**	-0.22 (-3.58)**	Ed. X_7 0.74 (1.01)	.93 (.90)
11	LW Tot. exp. (Y_1)	2.39 (4.12)**	-0.13 (-5.24)**	0.24 (4.17)**	-0.26 (-6.19)**	-0.17 (-3.35)**	% rural X_8 -0.05 (-0.43)	.92 (.90)
12	LW Tot. exp. (Y_1)	2.38 (4.16)**	-0.14 (-7.34)**	0.23 (4.08)**	-0.25 (-6.21)**	-0.18 (-3.50)**	% out. SMSA X_9 -0.04 (-0.47)	.93 (.90)
13	LW Tot. exp. (Y_1)	2.35 (5.30)**	-0.20 (-6.32)**	0.21 (4.08)**	-0.29 (-7.11)**	-0.22 (-4.59)**	% married X_{10} 0.35 (2.06)	.94 (.92)
14	LW Tot. exp. (Y_1)	2.29 (4.70)**	-0.16 (-8.09)**	0.27 (4.69)**	-0.24 (-5.77)**	-0.16 (-3.37)**	% Negro X_{11} -0.11 (-1.45)	.93 (.91)
15	LW Hos. exp. (Y_2)	1.56 (1.51)	-0.19 (-3.87)**	0.05 (0.34)	-0.08 (-0.41)	-0.07 (-0.51)	Ed. X_7 -2.26 (-1.44)	.77 (.69)
16	LW Med. exp. (Y_3)	2.37 (6.54)**	-0.13 (-7.71)**	0.36 (6.87)**	-0.48 (-7.15)**	-0.27 (-5.69)**	1.26 (2.28)*	.97 (.96)
17	LW Dr. exp. (Y_4)	3.06 (5.02)**	-0.12 (-4.21)**	0.38 (4.35)**	-0.39 (-3.47)**	-0.26 (-3.35)**	1.59 (1.71)	.88 (.84)
18	LW Den. exp. (Y_5)	3.20 (3.41)**	-0.12 (-2.80)*	0.22 (1.67)	0.02 (0.15)	-0.04 (-0.38)	0.10 (0.07)	.71 (.60)
19	LW Hos. exp. (Y_2)	1.28 (1.44)	-0.31 (-4.84)**	0.10 (0.93)	-0.42 (-5.12)**	-0.31 (-3.15)**	% married X_{10} 1.03 (2.97)**	.83 (.77)

Table 2–continued

Regression No.	Form of Regression[b] and Dependent Variable	Regression Coefficient and Computed T Value (in Parentheses)[c]						Biased Coefficient of Determination and Unbiased Coefficient of Determination (in parentheses)
		Income (X_1)	Sex (X_2)	Region (X_3)	Age (X_4) or Age (X_5)	Age (X_6)	X_7–X_{12}	
(1)	(2)	(3)	(4)	(5)	(6)	(7)	(8)	(9)
20	LW Med. exp. (Y_3)	2.23 (5.34)**	-0.16 (-5.35)**	0.28 (5.79)**	-0.34 (-8.88)**	-0.20 (-4.41)**	0.01 (0.05)	.96 (.95)
21	LW Dr. exp. (Y_4)	2.57 (4.67)**	-0.25 (-6.30)**	0.25 (3.80)**	-0.28 (-5.48)**	-0.25 (-4.11)**	0.60 (2.79)*	.91 (.87)
22	LW Den. exp. (Y_5)	3.33 (3.60)**	-0.08 (-1.26)	0.24 (2.18)*	0.06 (0.74)	-0.01 (-0.09)	-0.28 (-0.77)	.72 (.62)
23	LW Hos. exp. (Y_2)	2.04 (1.81)	-0.13 (-2.97)**	0.14 (1.05)	-0.34 (-3.50)**	-0.21 (-1.83)	% Negro X_{11} 0.10 (0.58)	.75 (.66)
24	LW Med. exp. (Y_3)	2.08 (4.93)**	-0.16 (-9.89)**	0.31 (6.09)**	-0.33 (-9.27)**	-0.19 (-4.48)**	-0.07 (-1.06)	.96 (.95)
25	LW Dr. exp. (Y_4)	2.35 (4.02)**	-0.18 (-7.79)**	0.36 (5.21)**	-0.18 (-3.62)**	-0.14 (-2.38)*	-0.24 (-2.63)*	.90 (.87)
26	LW Den. exp. (Y_5)	3.22 (3.28)**	-0.12 (-3.20)**	0.21 (1.81)	0.03 (0.40)	-0.04 (-0.43)	0.01 (0.10)	.71 (.60)
27	LW Tot. exp. (Y_1)	1.20 (2.30)*	-0.69 (-4.50)**	0.28 (6.34)**	-0.37 (-8.22)**	-0.32 (-5.94)**	Earn. rate X_{12} 2.07 (3.58)**	.96 (.94)

28	LW Hos. exp. (Y_2)	1.20 (0.79)	-0.40 (-0.89)	0.19 (1.50)	-0.25 (-1.61)	0.96 (0.57)	.75 (.66)
29	LW Med. exp. (Y_3)	1.46 (2.81)*	-0.47 (-3.12)**	0.31 (7.03)**	-0.28 (-5.21)**	1.20 (2.10)*	.97 (.96)
30	LW Dr. exp. (Y_4)	0.85 (1.38)	-0.99 (-5.43)**	0.35 (6.74)**	-0.40 (-6.13)**	3.15 (4.60)**	.94 (.92)
31	LW Den. exp. (Y_5)	2.39 (1.85)	-0.45 (-1.20)	0.24 (2.22)*	-0.12 (-0.93)	1.24 (0.87)	.72 (.62)

[a]For detailed definitions of the variables employed in the regressions, see Section II.
[b]Natural unweighted, NU_W; natural weighted, NW; logarithmic unweighted, LU_W; logarithmic weighted, LW. The weights are as follows:

Region	Age	Sex	No. of Persons	Region	Age	Sex	No. of Persons
NE	17–44	M	6,338	S	17–44	M	7,103
NE	45–64	M	3,980	S	45–64	M	3,820
NE	65 and over	M	525	S	65 and over	M	495
NE	17–44	F	3,031	S	17–44	F	3,460
NE	45–64	F	2,036	S	45–64	F	1,833
NE	65 and over	F	190	S	65 and over	F	181
NC	17–44	M	7,372	W	17–44	M	3,977
NC	45–64	M	4,236	W	45–64	M	2,205
NC	65 and over	M	589	W	65 and over	M	300
NC	17–44	F	3,181	W	17–44	F	1,800
NC	45–64	F	1,939	W	45–64	F	1,062
NC	65 and over	F	248	W	65 and over	F	102

[c]The estimated income elasticities at points of means for the natural regressions are 1.44 (regression 1) and 1.83 (regression 2).
*Statistically significant at the .05 level on a one-tail test for the earnings rate (X_{12}) and on a two-tail test for all other variables.
**Statistically significant at the .01 level on a one-tail test for the earnings rate (X_{12}) and on a two-tail test for all other variables.

persons (with the exception of dental care) than for males, non-southerners, and younger persons.* Some possible interpretations are (1) that younger persons and non-southerners require less medical care because they are healthier than older persons and southerners, and (2) that for physiological and/or psychological reasons females purchase more and/or more expensive medical care than males.

In regressions 10–14 some new independent variables are introduced one at a time into regressions for total expenses. The coefficients of the percentage rural (X_8) and the percentage outside SMSAs (X_9) are found to be insignificant, and it is wisest to ignore them. The computed T value for the education variable (X_7) is more respectable but is statistically insignificant. However, in view of the wide interest in the role of this variable, it is worth noting that its sign is positive, which might be interpreted to mean that education leads individuals to take better care of their health. The coefficient of the percentage Negro (X_{11}) is negative, which might mean that, other things equal, Negroes are healthier than whites and therefore require less medical care but is more likely to mean that cultural and other factors result in Negroes' receiving less medical care for a given problem. However, these speculations should not be emphasized, since the coefficient of X_{11} is not statistically significant. Finally, the coefficient of the marital status variable (X_{10}) is positive and is in the range of statistical significance. In order to obtain further information on the role of the last three independent variables, they were included in regressions for each of the four types of medical expense, with the results shown in regressions 15–26.

The results for the education variable (regressions 15–18) are quite interesting: the coefficient of X_7 is negative for hospital expenses, positive for medicine and physician expense, and positive but of negligible magnitude for dentist expense. A possible interpretation is that education results in emphasis being placed on preventive care, which leads to relatively low hospital and dentist expense and relatively high medicine and physician expense.[†]

The coefficient of the marital status variable is found to be positive and statistically significant for hospital and physician expense, positive but insignificant for medicine expense, and negative but insignificant for dentist expense (regressions 19–22). These results probably mean that the positive correlation between X_{10} and total expenses is a reflection of the fact that being married with a spouse present is associated with child-bearing expenses

---

*When X_4 is used in regressions 6–9 instead of X_5 and X_6, the ordering of income elasticities remains the same while the coefficients of X_4 are 0.15, 0.16, 0.08, and -0.04, respectively. The corresponding computed T values are 4.20, 11.67, 3.73, and -1.25, respectively.

[†] Caution is justified here, as the computed T values of the education variable are not very large, and there is evidence of harmful multicollinearity in regression 15.

for females; child-bearing raises hospital and physician expenses but does not greatly affect dentist and medicine expenses.

It is found that the inverse relationship between the percentage Negro and total expenses is derived from a strong negative relationship for physician expense and a somewhat weaker negative effect on medicine expense (regressions 24 and 25). The basis for the observed differences in the results for the various components is not apparent to the present writer.*

To the extent that analysts have been willing to take a position on this issue, they have tended to interpret positive relationships between income and medical expenses to mean that higher income permits individuals and groups to receive the benefits flowing from more and better medical care. At the same time, policy-related judgments concerning the equity of the current distribution of medical services are in part based upon the magnitude of the income elasticity. However, aside from the problems that arise in using expenses as a measure of the amount of medical care, such interpretations and judgments are spurious to the extent that (1) activities raising money incomes simultaneously depress health status and consequently increase the demand for medical services, and (2) individuals or groups with higher income use less patient-time–intensive methods (more medical-goods-and-services–intensive methods) of dealing with their medical problems.

Both of these conditions that give rise to upward-biased income elasticities might occur because of a positive correlation between income and the earnings rate.† A higher earnings rate may reduce health status while raising income by inducing individuals to "work harder," to go to work instead of staying at home when they are ill, to take more sedentary jobs, or to take more dangerous jobs. Further, it seems reasonable to believe that an increase in the earnings rate, and hence in income, will lead patients or their physicians to substitute medical goods and services for the patient's time in dealing with a given medical problem. In recognition of these possible sources of biased income elasticities, the earnings rate (X_{12}) is included in regression 27. It is found that the coefficient of the earnings rate has the expected positive sign and is statistically significant, while its inclusion lowers the income elas-

---

*Charlotte Muller suggests that these differences may be explained by the fact that in the Negro subculture (and in other subcultures of poverty) there exists a tendency to substitute medicine for the services of physicians (self-medication) and to substitute home remedies for market purchase of medicines.

†Actually, the bias could be downward if (1) an increase in the volume of medical services needed to produce a given level of health resulted in a *decline* in medical expenditures (i.e., the price elasticity of demand for health was numerically greater than 1), and (2) health were relatively time-intensive and substitution in consumption outweighed substitution in production. These possibilities were called to my attention by Michael Grossman.

ticity of total expenses from 2.5 (regression 5) to 1.2 and raises the adjusted coefficient of determination from .90 to .94.

In interpreting the results of the above regression it should be noted that the correlation coefficient between the earnings rate and sex variables is in the range of .9.* Intercorrelations of this magnitude often produce highly unstable parameter estimates. A check on the stability of the conclusions suggested by regression 27 is provided by regressions 28–31, which are for the separate components of medical expense. Although multicollinearity problems are evident in each of the regressions, the results are consistent with expectations: in every case the coefficient of the earnings rate is positive, and its inclusion in the regression causes a perceptible decline in the estimated income elasticity. The explanatory value of the earnings rate is greatest for physician expense (the adjusted coefficient of determination rises from .82 to .92) and weakest for hospital and dentist expense (virtually no change occurs in the adjusted coefficient of determination). The statistically insignificant result for dentist expense seems reasonable, since it is unlikely that higher earnings rates lead individuals to substitute money income for dental health or to use higher ratios of dental services to their own time in the production of dental health. A factor which may help to explain the exceptional showing of the earnings rate for physician expense is that in the absence of information about income doctors may discriminate in their charges on the basis of occupation, which is more highly correlated with the earnings rate than with income.

With the inclusion of the earnings rate in the regressions, the legitimacy of interpreting the estimated coefficients of income as "income elasticities" is increased. Using expected values, it is found that the elasticity for medical care as a whole is 1.2, while the elasticities for its components range from a low of .85 for physician expense to a high of 2.4 or 3.2[†] for dentist expense.[‡]

These results demonstrate that, even when proper account is taken of the earnings rate, command over goods and services as measured by family income exerts a strong positive influence upon the amount of medical care received by individuals.[§]

*The correlation between the income and sex variables is only .05, while that between the earnings rate and income is .41.

[†] The latter value results when the statistically insignificant earnings rate is dropped from the regression.

[‡] Medical care is produced by the market goods analyzed above together with *the patient's time.* The best available measure of the latter input is days lost from work due to illness or injury per currently employed person (Y_6), which in Section IV is found to have an income elasticity of about 2 – i.e., intermediate between medicine and dentist expense.

[§] The reader is reminded that since some free care is available to persons with very low incomes, the income elasticities in the text, which apply to the relatively affluent,

IV. REGRESSION ANALYSIS OF WORK-LOSS RATES

The primary objective of this section is to obtain information on the question of whether the work-loss rate due to illness or injury is a worthwhile addition to the currently scant stock of quantitative health measures. This purpose is accomplished by testing two hypotheses suggesting that variations in the work-loss rate reflect differences in economic variables (health status remaining constant), rather than in the objective state of health. The primary hypothesis is that the higher the earnings rate in a region-age-sex cell, the lower its rate of work loss. The secondary hypothesis is that the higher the adjusted mean total family income in a cell, the higher its work-loss rate.

The prediction concerning the earnings rate flows from both consumption and production considerations. The consumption argument runs as follows: (1) it is more pleasant to recover from an illness while resting at home than while working; (2) the earnings rate can be considered the price of the consumption good "recovery at home" or "rest"; (3) the "law of demand" predicts an inverse relationship between price and quantity. The production argument is based upon the belief that individuals with higher earnings rates (or their physicians) substitute medical goods and services for their own time in dealing with a given medical problem. Since the patient's time input is, at least in part, reflected in the work-loss rate, the above substitution results in a negative correlation between the earnings rate and the work-loss rate.

The predicted relationship between family income and the work-loss rate rests upon a consumption argument and a mixed consumption-production argument. Stated briefly, the consumption argument is that "recovery at home" or "rest" is a superior consumption good. The mixed argument is based on the assumption that health or "recovery" is a superior consumption good produced according to a production function which is homogeneous of degree one (or of any other form which excludes the possibility of "inferior" factors of production). If these assumptions hold, an increase in family income would increase the demand for health, and hence the demand for all the relevant factors of production, including the patient's own time. An increase in the patient's time input would be reflected in an increased work-loss rate.

In order to avoid biasing the results and to increase their reliability, dummy variables representing region, age, and sex were included in the regressions shown in Table 3.

Negative regression coefficients for the earnings rate and positive ones for family income* are observed in three of the four forms utilized in regressions 1-4. In the fourth case (regression 3) the signs of family income, the earnings

---

currently employed segment of the population, overestimate to an unknown degree the differential benefits received by the more affluent members of our society.

*It is worth noting that the simple correlations between family income and work-loss days are small and negative.

Table 3: Regressions of Days Lost from Work due to Illness or Injury per Currently Employed Person per Year (Y_6) on Various Independent Variables[a]

Regression No.	Form of Regression[b] and No. of Observations	Regression Coefficient and Partial Correlation Coefficient (Computed T Value in Parentheses)						Biased Coefficient of Determination and Unbiased Coefficient of Determination (in Parentheses)
		Income[c] (X_1)	Sex (X_2)	Region (X_3)	Age (X_4) or Age (X_5)	Age (X_6)	Earnings Rate[c] (X_7)	
(1)	(2)	(3)	(4)	(5)	(6)	(7)	(8)	(9)
1	NU$_W$ 24	0.001 0.22 (0.94)	3.55 0.26 (1.14)	2.07 0.31 (1.39)	1.42 0.53 (2.65*)		-0.05 -0.21 (-0.90)	.52 (.38)
2	NW 24	0.002 0.43 (2.04*)	3.27 0.26 (1.13)	3.23 0.56 (2.85**)	1.85 0.67 (3.88**)		-0.08 -0.32 (-1.44)	.74 (.67)
3	LU$_W$ 24	-0.05 -0.01 (-0.06)	-0.21 -0.23 (-1.02)	0.15 0.38 (1.73)	0.13 0.67 (3.86**)		0.83 0.25 (1.11)	.54 (.41)
4	LW 24	1.96 0.35 (1.61)	0.02 0.02 (0.10)	0.28 0.63 (3.44**)	0.12 0.66 (3.69**)		-0.42 -0.10 (-0.42)	.77 (.71)
5	NW 24	0.001 0.39 (1.85*)	0.52 (2.66*)	2.96	2.02 0.71 (4.39**)		-0.02 -0.40 (-1.92*)	.73 (.67)
6	LW 24	1.86 0.55 (2.91**)	0.64 (3.64**)	0.27	0.12 0.70 (4.23**)		-0.33 -0.53 (-2.76**)	.77 (.72)
7	LW 24	2.28 0.53 (2.64**)	0.61 (3.24**)	0.32	-0.28 -0.67 (-3.83**)	-0.18 -0.45 (-2.13)	-0.33 -0.54 (-2.76**)	.78 (.72)

8	LW Males 12	0.24	-0.86			.82
		0.90	-0.56			(.78)
		(6.39**)	(-2.04*)			
9	LW Females 12	0.03	0.24			.18
		0.37	0.24			(-.00)
		(1.20)	(0.73)			

[a]For detailed definitions of the variables employed in the regressions, see Section II.
[b]See n. b to Table 2.
[c]The estimated income elasticities at points of means for the natural regressions are 0.79 (regression 1), 2.38 (regression 2), and 1.32 (regression 5). The corresponding values for the earnings rate are -0.66 (regression 1), -1.29 (regression 2), and -0.29 (regression 5).
*Statistically significant at the .05 level on a one-tail test for income and the earnings rate and on a two-tail test for all other variables.
**Statistically significant at the .01 level on a one-tail test for income and the earnings rate and on a two-tail test for all other variables.

rate, and the sex variable (positive in the other three cases) are reversed. While none of the computed T values are impressive, the strongest results are obtained in regression 2, in which the positive coefficient of income is statistically significant while the negative one for the earnings rate is insignificant but respectable.

It is well known that high intercorrelations between independent variables often result in unstable parameter estimates and small computed T values. In the present analysis the previously noted deviant results for regression 3 and generally small computed T values may be symptoms of harmful multicollinearity (primarily) between the earnings rate and sex variables whose coefficient of correlation is in the range of .9. One method for dealing with this type of problem is to narrow the scope of the model by removing the less theoretically interesting variable, which in this case is the dummy for sex. This is done in regressions 5 and 6 for the weighted forms, which earlier yielded higher multiple correlation coefficients than the unweighted forms. It is found that the coefficients of family income and the earnings rate maintain the predicted signs and, especially in the case of the LW form, are statistically significant. The results are not greatly affected by the use of the less restrictive age variables X_5 and X_6 (see regression 7).

Of course, the danger inherent in the above procedure is that the price of avoiding harmful multicollinearity may be biased parameter estimates. Little can be done to deal with this possibility beyond running separate regressions for the twelve observations on each sex. This is done in regressions 8 and 9, which exclude the family income and region variables because they are now highly correlated with the earnings rate.* The results are ambiguous: while the coefficient of the male earnings rate is negative and statistically significant, the coefficient for females is positive and unreliable.

Obviously, the results are far from conclusive, but in my opinion they lend some support to the economic arguments presented above. The observed signs of the income and earnings rate variables, together with their relatively high partial correlation coefficients, suggest that differences in work-loss days may be unreliable measures of health status.† To the extent that the magnitudes of the regression coefficients can be taken seriously, it appears that the elas-

---

*Taking all twenty-four observations together, the simple correlations between the earnings rate and the family income and regional variables are .41 and -.31, respectively, while for males the corresponding values are .97 and -.83 and for females .89 and -.79. The correlation between the earnings rate and age is .06 for all the observations, .21 for males, and close to 0 for females.

†There are alternative, but in my opinion less plausible, interpretations according to which the empirical results are consistent with the view that the work-loss rate is a pure measure of health. First, the earnings rate might be negatively correlated with the work-

ticity of the work-loss rate with respect to family income is surprisingly high, while that with respect to the earnings rate is low.

Turning to the other independent variables, it is found that, other things being equal, work-loss rates are higher for males, southerners, and older persons than for females, non-southerners, and younger persons. Like the findings for medical expenses (see Section III) the results are consistent with the view that non-southerners and younger persons enjoy better health than southerners and older persons. The generally positive signs for sex are subject to a variety of interpretations, including the notion that females enjoy better health than males.

V. SUMMARY OF MAJOR FINDINGS

The empirical analysis in Section III reveals an income elasticity of demand of 1.2 for medical care as a whole, while the elasticities for its components range from 0.85 for physician expense to 3.2 for dentist expense. The ordering of the income elasticities is not unreasonable, and the magnitudes suggest that family income exerts a strong influence upon the amount of medical care received by individuals. However, an important question for future research is why the income elasticities reported in the present study are so high relative to those estimated from other bodies of data. The elasticity of total expenses with respect to the earnings rate is positive and statistically significant and is not negligible in magnitude — its value is 2.1.

In Section IV it is seen that work-loss days due to illness or injury are usually positively related to family income and inversely related to the earnings rate, which suggests the tentative conclusion that differences in unadjusted work-loss days may be unreliable measures of variations in health status.

---

loss rate because the former is an "efficiency variable"; that is, market skills might be positively correlated with skill in the production of health. Second, even after adjusting for differences in the earnings rate it might be the case that groups with higher incomes have poorer health.

A crude check of the alternative explanations presented above were obtained by running LW regressions utilizing a less ambiguous measure of health, the mortality rate, Y_M, as the dependent variable. (The mortality data utilized include deaths of persons who were not employed during the relevant period; the data were taken from the 1962 and 1963 volumes of *Vital Statistics of the United States*, from National Center for Health Statistics, *Health Insurance Coverage, United States: July 1962-June 1963*, Table 13, and from the *1960 Census of Population*, vol. 1, Pt. 1, Table 52.) The regressions offered little if any support for the alternative interpretations: (1) when the sex variable is included, the coefficient of income is positive but far from statistical significance, while the coefficient of the earnings rate is positive and insignificant; (2) when sex is dropped from the regression in order to avoid multicollinearity problems, the coefficient of income becomes *negative* and insignificant, while the coefficient of the earnings rate is positive and highly significant.

NOTES

1. Paul J. Feldstein and Ruth Severson, "The Demand for Medical Care," in American Medical Association, *Report of the Commission on the Cost of Medical Care* (Chicago: By the Association, 1964), 1:57–76; Grover Wirick and Robin Barlow, "The Economic and Social Determinants of the Demand for Health Services," in *The Economics of Health and Medical Care*, ed. S. J. Axelrod (Ann Arbor: The University of Michigan, 1964), pp. 95–125; Paul J. Feldstein and W. John Carr, "The Effect of Income on Medical Care Spending," *Proceedings of the Social Statistics Section of the American Statistical Association* 7 (1964):93–105; R. Auster, I. Leveson, and D. Sarachek, "The Production of Health, an Exploratory Study," *Journal of Human Resources* 4, no. 4 (Fall 1969):411–36. For useful summaries, references to the literature, and discussions of many of the relevant issues in the theory and empirical application of the demand for medical services, see Herbert E. Klarman, *The Economics of Health* (New York: Columbia University Press, 1965), chap. 2; Paul J. Feldstein, "Research on the Demand for Health Services," *Milbank Memorial Fund Quarterly* 44, no. 3 (July 1966), Pt. 2, pp. 128–62; and Jerome Rothenberg, "Comment," *Proceedings of the Social Statistics Section of the American Statistical Association* 7 (1964):109–10.

2. J. Johnston, *Econometric Methods* (New York: McGraw-Hill Book Co., 1963), pp. 148–50.

3. For more detailed discussions of the work-loss and expense data, see U.S., Department of Health, Education, and Welfare, Public Health Service, National Center for Health Statistics, *Personal Health Expenses Per Capita Annual Expenses United States: July–December 1962*, Vital and Health Statistics, ser. 10, no. 27 (Washington, D.C.: U.S. Government Printing Office, 1966), and *Disability Days in the United States: July 1963–June 1964*, Vital and Health Statistics, ser. 10, no. 24 (Washington, D.C.: U.S. Government Printing Office, 1965).

4. U.S. Department of Commerce, Bureau of the Census, Census of Population and Housing, *1/1,000 and 1/10,000: Two National Samples of the Population of the United States* (Washington, D.C.: By the Bureau, 1960).

5. These possibilities are mentioned by Victor R. Fuchs in his Comment in *The Economics of Health and Medical Care*, p. 126. It should be noted that the direction of the bias caused by a sliding scale of fees depends upon the elasticity of demand for medical care with respect to its price. If, as is generally assumed, demand is inelastic, a positive correlation between medical care prices and income would lead to overestimation of income elasticities.

6. Wirick and Barlow, "The Economic and Social Determinants of the Demand for Health Services," p. 107.

7. "The Demand for Medical Care."

8. Wirick and Barlow, "The Economic and Social Determinants of the Demand for Health Services," pp. 101, 104.

Rashi Fein
Harvard University

COMMENT

In the last sentence of his original paper, subsequently deleted, Morris Silver states, "The present paper adds to a growing body of research suggesting that economists armed with traditional tools such as demand and production functions can contribute to an understanding of behavior and to the formulation of policy in the 'health industry.' "

There is little doubt in my mind that economists can do and are doing what Silver says. Thus far much of this contribution — indeed, most — has been based upon an economic formulation of issues, arguments, and criteria, upon what to the economist has seemed relatively simple economics and statistical techniques. In part this is the case because the economic sophistication of those who make decisions for (or involving) the industry has been such that the provision of a framework of thought and of criteria, the raising of economic issues and questions, the explicit confronting of the problem of "choice," the presentation of some rough data — in other words, addressing the applied area in language considered too elementary for the *American Economic Review* — has been a significant contribution. In part this is the case because the data available were so limited in quantity and quality that if one were to contribute to policy, one often had to rely on "expert opinion" and "intuition," and the economist's chief contribution was to force people to consider the questions which they should ask of the experts and the issues that the experts should be forced to consider.

In many ways this conference may represent a watershed. The papers are, it seems to me, rather different in style from those presented in Ann Arbor some six years ago (though I cannot refrain from noting that if some of those papers were short on numbers, some of these are short on words). These empirically oriented papers represent attempts to answer some questions (not just to ask them), attempts to get quantitative estimates of the importance of different variables (not just directions of change). In a word, they are written for economists, for the *AER* (though perhaps not for policymakers – but more on that later).

The Silver paper is representative of the newer research (newer not only in time but in style) in the field. It adds to our body of knowledge, as Silver says. In no way do I want to minimize the importance of this research and of this paper. The careful and imaginative examination of data is important. Ultimately, such efforts will provide some of the answers we seek. Indeed, as the economic sophistication of the decisionmakers and practitioners increases, they will turn to the economist for numbers to plug into the economic framework that has been provided. We economists had better be prepared. I submit that Silver's paper, because it assembles and examines data and attempts to come to grips with measurement, helps in that preparation.

But having noted the importance of Silver's contribution, I think we should also be clear on what the paper does not do. I do not believe that it significantly assists in policy formulation, a claim which was made in Silver's original version. There may be those who would agree with me, but for the wrong reasons. I reject the argument that because the paper is replete with tables (and complex ones at that) the policymaker will not understand and use it. That argument, of course, *is* true, but it is irrelevant. Not every author should feel compelled to provide a translation of his work for the outside world. There are many hands to assume different tasks. If some researchers prefer to let others cull the journals and report their findings to the decisionmakers, that is certainly appropriate. It should, of course, be noted that there are risks in such a procedure, and we should be aware of them. One risk is that there will, in fact, be no communication of new findings because some unimaginative translator may feel that they have little relevance. Another risk is that of mistranslation. The researcher, after all, is more familiar with his work than is his reader and may see implications that escape others.

I have emphasized this because it seems to me that it is real. Indeed, if Silver argues that my subsequent comments, which question the usefulness of his findings – though not the importance of the effort – are incorrect, if he draws inferences from his work that have escaped me, my apprehensions about the risks of having the reader rather than the author do the translating would only be reinforced.

Why, then, do I feel that the paper does not assist in a significant way in the formulation of policy? The answer requires consideration of Silver's findings. In Section III of the paper, he attempts to estimate the income elasticity of the demand for medical services. In this section he does a first-rate job of taking account of a number of variables (though, regrettably, the data do not permit a quantitative assessment of the role of health insurance). Silver finds a high income elasticity. If we accept this result, it has important and obvious implications. One need only to turn to the Gorham report on medical care prices* to see the uses to which the estimate of income elasticity can be put. There the long-run projection of demand hinged very heavily on just that estimate. Furthermore, if one projects ahead for a period of a decade or more, the growth in income is sufficiently large to make even "reasonable" differences in the estimate create significant differences in the projection of demand, with important implications for public policy.

If, therefore, the income elasticity is as high as Silver estimates, we had better take account of that. However, the validity of Silver's result is, it seems to me, quite questionable. He himself is, of course, aware of the problem of using expenditures as a proxy for services. Price discrimination, free care, and the insurance component purchased *are* significant: I believe that they are so significant and that the income elasticity is therefore reduced so much that for policy purposes the numbers presented may be very misleading. Using the roughest of data, and not taking account of differences in patterns of care by physicians, I calculate that the average price of a physician visit may vary between about $8.65 and $11.30 as a function of income. Of even greater relevance, of course, are the Andersen and Benham data. They too suggest the radical difference between the elasticity computed using visits and that computed using expenditure data. I would question whether we dare use the Silver estimate at all for policy purposes, except, perhaps, with so many caveats as to reduce its usefulness substantially.

There may be those who believe that in dwelling thus upon the policy criterion, I have set up a straw man. Silver, after all, set forth that criterion in his last sentence, perhaps as an afterthought. Nonetheless, I do feel that it is relevant. Economics does have something to say, and economists do seem to be held in some regard among policymakers. If our empirical results are to be used, then it is incumbent upon us to refine them. Perhaps today we do have more confidence in measuring the direction of change than we do in measuring magnitudes. If so, we had better be about the job of refining our estimates of magnitudes. Silver has contributed to that refinement both by starting the task and showing us how much further we have to go.

In Section IV, Silver examines the extent to which variations in work-loss days reflect differences in economic variables rather than in the objective state of health. I found this section provocative and stimulating, even though the results, as Silver himself says, are "far from being conclusive." The eco-

*William Gorham, Assistant Secretary, Department of Health, Education, and Welfare, *A Report to the President on Medical Care Prices* (Washington, D.C.: Department of Health, Education, and Welfare, 1967).

nomic arguments do have a certain appeal. I am somewhat puzzled about the seriousness with which to treat the regression results, given sick leave compensation, difficulty of defining work-loss days, correlation between income and earnings, and patterns of work loss as a function of the type of job held (and of self-employment). Clearly, my reservations relate to the usefulness of work-loss days as a measure of health status: on this point Silver and I are in agreement. Correction of work-loss days as a proxy for health is valuable, and Silver has taken a first step, but at this stage the results do not have the definitiveness that would make them useful. Silver's paper, then, makes a contribution. With the exception of the estimate of income elasticity, the size of which is important for policy analysis, the fact that the other statistics are not firm may not be too troublesome, for I confess that while interesting for our understanding of behavior, they do not seem to me to be vital for policy. I find the ideas far more interesting than the numbers, and since the ideas make economic sense, I accept them as right.

George N. Monsma, Jr.
Amherst College

MARGINAL REVENUE AND THE DEMAND FOR PHYSICIANS' SERVICES

I. INTRODUCTION

It is not usually assumed that the amount of a good demanded by a person is a function, *ceteris paribus*, of the marginal revenue his purchase yields to the supplier of the good; that is, if the price (and marginal cost to the consumer) of a good is, say, ten dollars, it is implicitly assumed that the same amount will be demanded regardless of the marginal return to the supplier. There are, however, some cases in which this assumption (that quantity demanded is independent of marginal revenue to the supplier) does not conform to reality.

This study shows that conditions necessary for this assumption to be valid are not present in the case of the demand for physicians' services. It also suggests ways in which, given the prevailing institutional arrangements, the demand for physicians' services would be expected to vary in response to the marginal return to the physician, and examines the available empirical evidence to see whether, in fact, the demand for physicians' services is influenced by the marginal revenue physicians receive in the manner suggested by the theory.

The analysis which follows neither implies nor assumes that most physicians are slaves of mammon or that their primary goal in their practices is financial gain. It does imply that monetary considerations play a part in

This paper is based on a chapter in my Ph.D. dissertation, "The Supply of and Demand for Physicians' Services," submitted to the Department of Economics of Princeton University. I would like to thank the members of my dissertation committee, Professors Frederick Harbison and Charles Berry, for their many helpful comments, and the members of the Seminar on Research in Progress of the Department of Economics of Princeton, where this paper was first given in December 1966, for their criticism.

physicians' decisions in medical practice, and that in at least some cases such considerations are a decisive factor in the recommendation of treatment; that is, the effect of the monetary factor is not so weak as always to be insignificant.

II. CONDITIONS IN THE MARKET FOR PHYSICIANS' SERVICES

If the market for physicians' services met the conditions of the model for pure and perfect competition, this problem would not arise. Consumers would determine the quantities purchased on the basis of their evaluation of the relative marginal values (utilities) and costs of physicians' services and other goods. The marginal return to the producer would make no difference to the consumer except as it influenced his marginal cost. The same would be true under a monopoly or oligopoly model: given the marginal costs of goods to the consumer, he would make his consumption decisions independently of the marginal returns to the supplier; the consumer would equate ratios of marginal cost and marginal utility for all goods* (income is assumed to be given, of course). However, many of the conditions assumed in the standard models are not present in the market for physicians' services. One such departure is especially relevant to the question at hand. Consumers have little knowledge about the goods (services) available in the market.[†][1]

Consumer Ignorance

Many, probably most, consumers cannot judge the quality of physicians or the relative merits of one course of treatment of a disease over another. Illnesses are often non-recurring. Thus when treatment is needed, consumers have little or no personal experience to guide them. Even if they have had experience, it is usually difficult for them to judge the quality of the treatment they received because they do not know what the optimal course of treatment for their illness would have been.

This lack of knowledge is compounded by the fact that once a physician has passed a licensure examination he is generally deemed competent for the rest of his life. His competence is not questioned unless he very clearly shows himself to be grossly incompetent. The "ethics" of the medical profession, enforced by the medical societies, prohibit advertising or other attempts by a

---

*Consumers do not explicitly determine these ratios for all goods, but they do implicitly equalize them if they maximize their utility from a given income.

[†]Kenneth Arrow has discussed this fact and has pointed out that, in the face of this lack of knowledge, consumers rely on physicians themselves for advice concerning the purchase of physicians' services. However, he does not mention the fact, shown in this study, that in this situation the magnitude of the marginal revenue to the physician may influence his recommendation of treatment and thus the treatment demanded by the patient.

physician to publicize his merits, and individual physicians and medical societies are extremely reluctant to critize the ability of their fellows. While there are some indicators of physician quality, such as specialty board certification, specialty society membership, and hospital affiliation, these are by no means infallible guides and are probably not utilized by the majority of the public.

It is not surprising, then, that studies have shown that consumers do not choose their physicians on the basis of quality. The classic study of the quality of physicians is the one undertaken by Dr. Osler L. Peterson and his colleagues at the University of North Carolina. They found a wide variation in the skill of the general practitioners studied, from those who "performed at a level that would have been acceptable in the outpatient clinic of a university hospital" to those whose "practice would have been unsatisfactory in a senior medical student." In addition, they found that "a doctor's success, as measured by the number of patients he saw during the week, bore no relation to his knowledge and skill."[2]

Other studies have also shown a variation in the quality of treatment rendered by physicians. Virgil Slee of the Commission on Professional and Hospital Activities examined the records of fifteen hospitals and found that the percentage of diagnoses of appendicitis that were confirmed (by the finding of disease in the excised appendix by the hospital pathology laboratory) ranged from 70 per cent in one hospital to 20 per cent in another.[3] The fact that a hospital can exhibit such a low percentage of correct diagnoses suggests strongly that a considerable number of persons can judge neither the quality of a physician nor the quality of his recommendations for treatment (in this case, the recommendation of appendectomy).

In a study of care given to families of members of the Teamsters Union in New York City who had been hospitalized for certain types of disease, it was judged that the care given was "excellent" or "good" in only 57 per cent of the cases, "fair" in 20 per cent, and "poor" in 23 per cent. One-third of the hysterectomies performed were judged unnecessary, and another 10 per cent were questionable. The surveyors also seriously questioned the necessity of over half of the Caesarean sections performed.[4] Again, the evidence indicates that the average consumer is a good judge neither of the quality of his physician nor of a given course of treatment once he has chosen a physician (of course, the two are closely connected because the basic criterion for the quality of a physician is the quality of the treatment he provides).

Reliance on Physicians' Advice

Lack of knowledge alone, however, is not sufficient by itself to cause the marginal revenue to physicians to influence the amount of their services demanded. There is an additional factor present here. Owing to his ignorance, the consumer relies on the advice of his physician concerning the course of treatment to follow. He may presume that the physician's advice is based solely on his judgment of what is best for his patient; however, since the physician often has a financial interest in the treatment, the patient's interest may not be the only factor affecting his advice.

Medical practice is subject to error and uncertainty: diagnoses may be mistaken, and, in many instances, the optimal course of treatment for a specific illness is somewhat uncertain. In order for financial considerations to play a part in a physician's choice of which treatment to recommend, he need not recommend a treatment which he is absolutely sure is not optimal; the point is that in cases of some uncertainty the fact that he will gain financially from a given treatment will, consciously or unconsciously, affect his judgment, so that he will recommend this treatment more often than he would if he received no marginal revenue from it. The recent Senate Antitrust Subcommittee hearings into the ownership of drug companies and drugstores and the dispensing of eyeglasses by physicians produced evidence that financial considerations can affect the recommendations of at least some physicians in such a manner that optimal care at the lowest cost is not always provided to the patient. The hearings also made it clear that organized medicine is not willing to take the steps necessary to eliminate the conflict of interest in these areas.[5] It is interesting to note that the American Medical Association, in its recent study of the economics of medical care,[6] portrayed the physician in a dual role as a "manager," "businessman," or "agent for the patient," who determines the inputs of goods and services into the total process of patient care, and as a "practitioner," that is, the supplier of one of the inputs – physicians' services. The AMA did not, however, mention the potential conflict between these two roles; that is, a physician's actions as "agent" for the consumer (patient) may be influenced by the fact that he is also a supplier of one of the inputs with a financial interest in the matter.

We would expect, then, that the demand for a physician's services would be higher, *ceteris paribus*, the higher his marginal revenue for the performance of the service.* In order to make the *ceteris paribus* assumption more realis-

---

*The correct concept here is marginal revenue net of the marginal costs to the physician of providing the service (including both opportunity costs and direct payments; e.g., the marginal cost to the physician would include the value of the time spent in performing the procedure and the cost of any drugs or supplies used). Since data are not available which would permit measuring the difference in marginal cost among physicians receiving different marginal revenues for similar services, it will be assumed that the difference in marginal cost to the physician is less than the difference in the marginal revenue he receives, so that if one physician receives a higher fee for a service than does another, his "net marginal revenue" (marginal profit) for this service is also higher. This is probably true in the cases where the marginal revenue for the group of physicians with the lower marginal revenue is zero, for it would hold whenever the marginal cost to the other group of physicians was lower than their revenue (i.e., when-

tic, a distinction must be made between different types of physicians' services. First of all, they must be categorized according to the degree to which the patient relies on the advice of the physician in deciding whether or not to have a service performed. There are some obvious variations here. In the case of home and office visits, the decision for the first visit in any illness is (generally) independent of the advice of a physician, and further ones are based on the patient's conception of the progress he is making as well as on the advice the physician may give. These are also cases where the consumer is likely to have some past experience to use as a guide (however unreliable). On the other hand, in the case of surgery (or any procedure that requires hospitalization) a physician's recommendation is mandatory. Such a patient is less likely to have any comparable experience on which to base an independent decision. The illness is likely to be more serious and the patient more hesitant to disregard a physician's recommendation. Thus, since the degree to which the return to the physician influences the demand should be correlated with the degree to which the patient relies on the recommendation of a physician, *ceteris paribus,* it would be expected that the amount of surgery demanded would be more highly influenced by the return to the physician than would the number of home and office calls.

Second, the marginal revenue to the physician is only one of the factors determining *his* decision as to which treatment to recommend. It seems reasonable to assume that the greater the likelihood that a questionable treatment will cause serious damage to the patient (as opposed to its being of little or no positive value to him) and the more strongly he feels that it is unnecessary, the less likely he will be to recommend it.* Thus in an activity such as surgery, the influence of financial considerations will probably be greatest when the surgery is not likely to impair the future functioning of the patient and can at least be rationalized as potentially beneficial.

Thus the hypotheses to be tested are first, that, *ceteris paribus,* the higher the marginal revenue to the physician for performing a given service, the greater the demand for it will be; second, that this increased demand will be greater for surgical procedures (and other procedures that require hospitalization) than for home and office visits; and third, that the increased demand for

---

ever they made any positive marginal profit) and, in some cases, it would hold even if the marginal profit to the physicians receiving a fee for each service was negative.

*This certainty of knowledge is itself in many cases a function of the procedure followed by the physician – for example, the number of tests he has performed before deciding on a course of action. Thus the system of payment for surgery may influence the choice between the "when in doubt, cut it out" and the "when in doubt, make more tests" philosophies. Each individual decision to recommend a certain treatment may not be consciously influenced by the financial incentive; instead, these decisions may be affected indirectly through the influence of this incentive on the general attitude a physician takes toward the practice of medicine.

surgery will be concentrated among those procedures which involve the removal of organs the absence of which will not greatly impair the functioning of the individual and for which the need for the procedure is subject to some doubt (for example, tonsillectomies, appendectomies, and hysterectomies).

III. THE EMPIRICAL EVIDENCE

Under different institutional arrangements for the payment for physicians' services, the marginal revenue to the physician is not a single-valued function of the marginal cost to the consumer. In other words, under various arrangements the marginal cost to the patient for a given procedure may be the same while the marginal revenue to the physician is considerably different. A few studies of utilization under such situations have been performed, and their results can be used to test the hypotheses. These studies were focused on other questions, including determination of the percentage of costs paid for by various insurance plans and of how the use of hospitals differs under different plans, but some of the data are also relevant here. In general, all three of our hypotheses are supported by these data.

Some of the most useful data were collected in a survey by the National Opinion Research Center, undertaken for the Health Information Foundation, reported by Odin Anderson and Paul Sheatsley.[7] This survey of families covered by two comprehensive health insurance plans in New York City, the Health Insurance Plan of Greater New York (HIP) and Group Health Insurance, Inc. (GHI), included slightly more than four hundred families (including single individuals) in each plan. The samples from the two plans were closely matched in age, sex, and family size and quite closely matched in education and family income. The subscribers to the two plans were also found to be similar in the way in which they perceived the health status of their families (excellent, good, etc.) and in their attitudes toward health care.[8]

The benefit structures of the two plans can be described briefly. Basically, GHI provides free home, office, and hospital calls by physicians and free surgery if the service is performed by a participating physician (a participating physician is any licensed physician in New York City who has agreed to accept the fee GHI pays as full compensation for the service he performs for a subscriber; a majority of the physicians in New York City are in this category). If a patient goes to a non-participating physician, the physician will be paid the GHI fee but is free to make an additional charge to the patient, and apparently often does so (specialists called in for consultation may also charge more than the GHI fee). HIP provides free home, office, and hospital calls (including specialist consultations) and free surgery if it is rendered by an HIP physician. A patient using a non-HIP physician must pay the total cost himself. Subscribers to both plans have identical Blue Cross hospitalization insurance.[9]

Although the marginal costs of physicians' services under the two plans are similar (zero in most instances), the marginal revenue to the physician is very different in the two plans because of the difference in the method of payment. GHI pays a fee for each service performed, as is customary in the United States, specified in a fee schedule, which participating physicians agree to accept. HIP does not pay a fee for each service performed; instead, it contracts with groups of physicians, who agree to provide care to its enrollees in return for payment on an annual capitation basis. At the time of the survey HIP had contracts with thirty-one groups; a subscriber chooses to receive his care from one of these groups, and the group is paid an amount determined by the number of enrollees who choose it.[10] Thus there is a positive marginal revenue associated with physicians' services under GHI and a zero marginal revenue under HIP.

As Table 1 shows, the survey showed no significant difference between the mean number of non-surgical, non-obstetrical physician visits; the rate was 5.88 per person per year for GHI, slightly higher than the 5.55 for HIP, but the standard error of the difference in the means was larger than the difference itself. However, this is not true for surgical care. GHI enrollees had an average of 7.18 hospitalized surgical procedures per hundred persons per year, but the rate for HIP enrollees was only 4.38. The difference, 2.80 procedures per hundred persons per year, is significant at a .95 confidence level and is almost two-thirds as large as the rate for HIP. Rates for surgery performed out of hospital are not given, but it is stated that they are also higher for GHI.[11]

These data, then, support the hypotheses that a higher marginal revenue to physicians is associated with a higher demand for services, *ceteris paribus*, and that this effect is greater for surgical than for non-surgical visits. The data shed no light on possible differences between different types of surgery.

There are, however, some differences between the two groups which result from the institutional arrangements for providing care, and these should be examined for their possible effect on the findings. First, while in theory subscribers could receive almost all physician care at a zero marginal cost under either plan, 40 per cent of the actual cost of hospital surgery and 44 per cent of the cost of physicians' services other than surgical and obstetrical services for GHI subscribers was *not* paid for by GHI (because some participating physicians charged more than the GHI fee schedule in spite of their agreements and/or because subscribers used non-participating physicians). The comparable figures for HIP are 7 per cent and 23 per cent, respectively (these figures must reflect the use of non-HIP physicians).[12] Thus the average marginal cost of physicians' services was higher for GHI subscribers than for HIP subscribers. This finding does not change the conclusions to be drawn from the utilization data; if anything, it reinforces them: the demand on the part of GHI subscribers is higher even though they pay a higher marginal cost.

Table 1: Utilization of Physicians' Services by Groups under
Fee-for-Service Plans and Plans Using Physicians on
Salary or Capitation

Study and Population Group	Non-Surgical, Non-Obstetrical Visits	Surgical Procedures in Hospital	Annual Utilization Rate			
			Surgical Admissions	Appendectomies	Tonsillectomies	"Female Surgery"[a]
	(per person)	(per 100 persons)	(per 100 persons)	(per 1,000 persons)		
Anderson-Sheatsley						
HIP[b]	5.55	4.38[c]				
GHI[d]	5.88	7.18[c]				
Densen-A						
Adult males						
HIP			4.61			
GHI			4.86			
Adult females						
HIP			4.97[c]			
GHI			6.56[c]			
Densen-B						
HIP			4.11[c]	e	e	
Blue Shield[d]			5.02[c]	e	e	
United Steelworkers						
Kaiser[b]		3.3[f]				
Blue Cross-Blue Shield[d]		6.9[f]				
Commercial insurance[d]		6.3[f]				
Perrott-Federal Employees						
Group plans[b]		3.9[f]		1.4[f]	4.0[f]	5.4[f]

| Blue Cross-Blue Shield | 7.0[f] | 2.6[f] | 10.6[f] | 8.2[f] |

Note: Rates in any one survey are not comparable with rates in other surveys because age and sex distributions and other characteristics are apt to differ between surveys.

[a] "Female surgery" includes mastectomy, hysterectomy, and dilation and curettage (non-maternal). Most of the difference between the two groups is due to higher mastectomy and hysterectomy rates for Blue Cross-Blue Shield subscribers.

[b] Under these plans physicians *do not* receive a fee for each service performed.

[c] Significant at the .95 level.

[d] Under these plans physicians *do* receive a fee for each service performed.

[e] The actual rates for tonsillectomies and appendectomies were not given, but the report states that rates for both were significantly higher for the Blue Shield group than for the HIP group.

[f] In these studies tests of statistical significance were not reported, nor was data reported from which such tests could be made. In addition, the age and sex distributions were not reported, so that it is not possible to tell whether these affected the differences. Thus these figures must be viewed with caution.

A second relevant consideration is the fact that care is provided by HIP through physicians working in group practice, where preventive care and the subscriber's health education are emphasized. It might be argued that because of this fact HIP subscribers actually need less surgery: even if financial considerations played no part in the decision process and physicians all used the same decision criteria, the surgery rates for HIP subscribers would be lower than those for GHI. This hypothesis may be true to some extent; at present no data are available to test it. However, the variant of this proposition, which states that HIP patients need less surgery because they get more non-surgical care rather than because the care they get is in some sense better, would not hold in this case, as the amount of non-surgical care provided was the same in the two samples. In any case, it is implausible to explain such a large difference in rates in this manner.* Furthermore, it will be shown below that the more frequent recourse to surgery under the fee-for-service system reported in other surveys is, for the most part, concentrated in procedures such as tonsillectomies and appendectomies. It is unlikely that the effects of better care through group practice would be associated so specifically with these procedures.

Thus, in spite of these complicating factors, the evidence supports the hypothesis that the marginal revenue to the physician influences the demand for physicians' services. It does not in itself indicate whether there is over-utilization by the GHI subscribers or underutilization by the HIP group. This issue will be considered below after the data from other surveys are examined.

Other Surveys

Another comparison of subscribers to GHI and HIP was made by Paul Densen and his associates at HIP.[13] This study is primarily concerned with hospitalization, not physicians' services, but it also provides some data on surgical admissions, which are a good proxy for surgical procedures. The samples comprised some forty thousand members of three locals of the International Ladies' Garment Workers' Union; since their dependents were not included, the sample contains only adults. They found no significant difference in the surgical admission rates for males (4.61 per hundred per year for HIP, 4.86 for GHI) but did find a significantly higher rate for females in GHI (4.97 for HIP, 6.56 for GHI).†[14] The data for adult females support the

---

*If it could be so explained, it would be a strong argument for encouraging a HIP-type system, even if a fee-for-service system did not result in overutilization.

†These rates have been adjusted to take account of the fact that the GHI and HIP populations varied in age and proportion belonging to the various locals. Rates between surveys should not be compared with each other because age, sex, and other characteristics are apt to differ.

hypothesis of a higher incidence of surgery under fee-for-service practice, but the data for males do not. The data are classified by diagnostic categories, but the categories are generally too broad to be useful in distinguishing frequency differences among specific surgical procedures.

In a second study Densen and his associates compared the hospitalization experience of a sample of over fifty thousand HIP subscribers with a sample of over fifty thousand persons having Blue Shield coverage. The Blue Shield insurance covered only in-hospital physician services (for some only surgery was covered); it is not so desirable a comparison for testing the hypotheses because the consumer may have some incentive to substitute surgery (which is covered) for other care (which is not). This substitution is not likely to be too great, however. Both groups had Blue Cross hospitalization insurance. The difference in surgical admissions between the two samples was significant at a .95 level; the HIP rate per hundred persons per year was 4.11, and the Blue Shield rate was 5.02. The differences were significant for both the males alone and the females alone, and they were also significant whether obstetrical care was included or excluded. The rates are unfortunately not adjusted for the varying age composition of the two samples, but in this case such an adjustment would probably increase rather than decrease the differences. The data also indicate that the difference is greatest for those under 15 years of age; here the rate was 3.37 for HIP and 5.28 for Blue Shield. For the age group 15–44 the differences are only significant for the males; however, the two populations differed considerably in this age group. The Blue Shield sample had relatively more persons in the 15–24 age category and relatively fewer in the 35–44 age category. The data as published do not allow an adjustment for this variation, but other data from the survey tend to indicate that if such an adjustment were possible the difference for the females might also be significant because the 15–24 age group had considerably less total hospitalization than the 35–44 age group. In the 45 and over age group the difference was significant for the total group and for the males, but not for the females.[15]

Some information on admissions by diagnostic category is also available from this study. The tonsillectomy rate was twice as high for the Blue Shield group as for the HIP group, and this accounted for the higher surgical admission rate for children in the Blue Shield sample. The data also show that the admission rates for appendicitis, hemorrhoids, and diseases of the prostate were significantly higher for the Blue Shield sample.[16] These are the only cases in which hospitalization for a disease category which could be associated fairly specifically with a certain operation showed a significantly higher rate for one group. Unfortunately, the rates for most operations cannot be determined because the disease categories are too broad. The data from this survey support the hypotheses that more surgery is performed under the fee-for-service system and that the increase is concentrated in certain procedures such as tonsillectomies and appendectomies.

A third study by Densen compared the experience of some forty thousand members of the retail, wholesale and department store unions under HIP and under a union-administered fee-for-service plan.[17] The hospitalization rates for all admissions were almost the same for the two plans (the difference would not be significant). In view of this finding, it is possible that the over-all surgical admission rates were also similar. Densen hypothesized that the low hospitalization rate under the union plan could be ascribed to the union's "continuous educational effort directed primarily at the union member but also reaching the participating physician" which was "designed to promote necessary but conservative use of the health benefits available."[18] In spite of the low over-all hospitalization rates, the admission rate for tonsillectomies appeared to be about 50 per cent higher for the fee-for-service group than for the HIP group, and the appendectomy rate was over twice as high for the fee-for-service group as for the HIP group.[19]

Lower rates for surgery under non-fee-for-service practice have also been found in other studies. The United Steelworkers of America under various negotiated health insurance plans had an average rate of hospitalized surgery of 3.3 per hundred persons per year for members covered by the Kaiser Foundation Health Plans (a prepaid system using salaried physicians), as compared with a rate of 6.9 for those covered by Blue Cross-Blue Shield and 6.3 for those covered by commercial insurance. The figures for surgery performed out of hospital are 6.3 for Kaiser, 8.2 for Blue Cross-Blue Shield, and 3.9 for the commercial insurance group.[20] Once again, these figures (with the exception of the out-of-hospital commercial insurance figure) tend to support the hypothesis that there is more demand under a fee-for-service system, but they must be viewed with caution because the age and sex composition of the populations are not given and the populations are taken from different geographical regions.

A study by George S. Perrott of experience under the Federal Employees Health Benefits Program between November 1, 1961, and October 31, 1962, showed that those covered by Blue Shield had an in-hospital, non-maternity surgical procedure rate of 7.0 per hundred persons per year, while those covered by group plans belonging to the Group Health Association of America (in which there is no fee-for-service payment) had a rate of only 3.9 per hundred persons per year. Approximately one-third of this difference represented higher rates for tonsillectomy and adenoidectomy, appendectomy, and "female surgery" for those covered by the Blue Shield plan. The appendectomy rate was only about half as great for those covered by the group plans as it was for those covered by Blue Shield, and the rate for tonsillectomies was two and one-half times as high for those covered by Blue

Shield as it was for those covered by the group practice plans. The rate for "female surgery" was over 50 per cent higher for those covered by Blue Shield. "Female surgery" includes mastectomy, hysterectomy, and non-maternal dilation and curettage. Most of the difference between the two groups is due to higher mastectomy and hysterectomy rates for Blue Shield subscribers.[21] These data also support the hypotheses, but again they are not adjusted for age and sex and thus must be viewed with caution.

A comparison of persons covered by the United Mine Workers of America programs of medical care showed that the number of surgical operations was 37 per cent lower for those served by salaried physicians than for those served by fee-for-service physicians, and that the rate for appendectomies was 59 per cent lower.[22]

IV. IMPLICATIONS OF THE EVIDENCE

Taken as a whole, the data from these surveys support the hypotheses stated above; that is, they indicate (1) that institutional arrangements for the purchase of physicians' services which include a positive marginal revenue to the physician result in a higher demand for physicians' services than do arrangements which include a zero marginal revenue; (2) that this effect is more pronounced in surgery than in home and office visits; and (3) that it is most pronouned in certain types of surgery, such as tonsillectomies and appendectomies, which involve the removal of "useless" parts of the body.

The data also indicate that this effect is not uniform over all groups, thus supporting the hypothesis that financial considerations are only one of a number of factors influencing the decision of a physician to recommend a given procedure. The experience of the store workers' unions indicates that other pressures may be brought on the physician which may offset financial incentives to some extent. The variation among hospitals in the percentage of appendectomies involving normal tissue, mentioned above, and the experience of the Teamsters sample in New York, where half of the hysterectomies performed in proprietary hospitals were questionable, as compared with only one-fourth of those performed in voluntary hospitals,[23] indicate that a hospital can reduce the number of unnecessary operations performed. One way in which this can be done is to set up an active tissue committee, which examines compilations of the pathology reports of all operations performed in the hospital, has power to take action against physicians who excise normal tissue too often, and is willing to use this power. (One action that can be taken is to withdraw operating privileges at the hospital after a warning.) For such an arrangement to be really effective for an entire community, however, such committees have to be operative in all or most of the hospitals in the area; otherwise, such questionable surgery can be shifted to the hospitals with the laxest controls (the Teamsters experience may be an indication of such a shift). While these pressures on physicians may plausibly be expected to counterbalance the financial incentives, little is known about how physicians make decisions, and a full explanation of the variations in the data from the several surveys is not possible.

If more surgery does take place under a fee-for-service system of practice, the question arises as to whether it is resorted to excessively under this system or whether it is underutilized under a salaried or capitation system. A categorical answer to this question cannot be given. There are no data comparing mortality and morbidity experience of similar groups under the two types of care. However, certain of the available facts suggest that there is overutilization of surgery under the fee-for-service system, rather than underutilization under the alternative system. When the Commission on Medical Care Plans of the American Medical Association studied prepaid, salaried group practice plans, a study which included visits to the major plans (including HIP), it concluded that "good medical care is being provided, within the scope of services offered, by the units (of the plans) visited" and that "medical care for many persons in the low income groups now covered by these plans has improved. Some of these people live under conditions which would make it difficult for them to obtain adequate care through the usual available sources."[24]

One study of the health of two groups, one of which was operating under a fee-for-service arrangement, is also available.[25] This is a study of the perinatal mortality rate* among groups cared for by HIP physicians and by private physicians in New York City. A significantly lower rate was found in the HIP group.† This evidence, though not by any means conclusive, tends to contradict the hypothesis of underutilization in the salaried, group practice situation. The evidence of unnecessary surgery, and of concentration of the "excess" surgery under fee-for-service arrangements in procedures such as appendectomies, which has been mentioned, supports the hypothesis of overutilization in the latter situation.‡

---

*Infant deaths under seven days plus fetal deaths of at least twenty weeks' gestation are divided by live births plus fetal deaths of at least twenty weeks' gestation to arrive at the perinatal mortality rate.

†The difference remained after adjustment for differences in age, ethnic group, and hospital used. While the data could not be directly adjusted for possible differences in family income, the fact that the non-HIP members who did not receive the care of a private physician (i.e., who were general-service ward patients) were excluded from this comparison means that most non-HIP members with low incomes were excluded. Also, the HIP rate was lower than the rates for two groups of health areas in the city with high median incomes.

‡This conclusion does not imply that salaried practice never leads to underutilization.

V. SUMMARY

This study suggests that because consumers rely on the advice of physicians in an attempt to remedy their ignorance about the utility of physicians' services, the higher the marginal revenue received by physicians for certain services, the more they will be used. The available data were examined, and they support the hypothesis. They also indicate that the marginal revenue, while significant, was not so dominant that other influences had no discernible role. Finally, it was concluded that the differences in rates of recourse to surgery seem to represent overutilization in the insured, fee-for-service situation rather than underutilization in the salaried, group practice situation. Thus there is a possibility of better resource allocation if this overutilization can be reduced by changing either financial or institutional conditions in the market.

NOTES

1. Kenneth Arrow, "Uncertainty and the Welfare Economics of Medical Care," *American Economic Review* 53, no. 5 (December 1963):941-73.
2. Osler L. Peterson, "Medical Care in the U.S.," *Scientific American* 209, no. 2 (August 1963):20, 21.
3. *Ibid.*, p. 22.
4. Columbia University School of Public Health and Administrative Medicine, *The Quantity, Quality and Costs of Medical and Hospital Care Secured by a Sample of Teamster Families in the New York Area* (New York: Teamsters Joint Council No. 16 and Management Hospitalization Trust Fund, 1962), pp. 3, 15.
5. Morton Mintz, "Doctors Assail 'Greed' of Some Eye Specialists," *Washington Post*, August 9, 1965, p. A6.
6. American Medical Association, *Report of the Commission on the Cost of Medical Care* (Chicago: By the Association, 1964), 1:9-21.
7. Odin W. Anderson and Paul B. Sheatsley, *Comprehensive Medical Insurance*, Health Information Foundation Research Series no. 9 (New York: Health Information Foundation, 1959).
8. *Ibid.*, pp. 44, 45, 94, 95.
9. *Ibid.*, pp. 24-31.
10. *Ibid.*, p. 11.
11. *Ibid.*, pp. 37, 38, 90.
12. *Ibid.*, p. 31.
13. Paul Densen et al., "Prepaid Medical Care and Hospital Utilization in a Dual Choice Situation," *American Journal of Public Health* 50, no. 11 (November 1960):1710-26.
14. *Ibid.*, pp. 1715, 1717.
15. Paul Densen et al., *Prepaid Medical Care and Hospital Utilization*, Hospital Monograph Series no. 3 (Chicago: American Hospital Association, 1958), pp. 14, 17.
16. *Ibid.*, p. 24.
17. Paul Densen et al., "Comparison of a Group Practice and a Self-Insurance Situation," *Hospitals* 36, no. 22 (November 1962):63-68, 138.
18. *Ibid.*, p. 67.
19. *Ibid.*, p. 66.

20. United Steelworkers of America, *Special Study on the Medical Care Program for Steelworkers and Their Families* (Pittsburgh, Pa.: United Steelworkers of America, 1960), p. 89.

21. George S. Perrott, "Utilization of Hospital Services," *American Journal of Public Health* 56, no. 1 (January 1966):62, 63.

22. Milton I. Roemer, "On Paying the Doctor and the Implications of Different Methods," *Journal of Health and Human Behavior* 3, no. 1 (Spring 1962):10.

23. Columbia University School of Public Health and Administrative Medicine, *Medical and Hospital Care Secured by Teamster Families*, p. 30.

24. American Medical Association Commission on Medical Care Plans, "Report," *Journal of the American Medical Association*, spec. ed., January 17, 1959, Pt. 1, p. 49.

25. Sam Shapiro et al., "Comparison of Prematurity and Perinatal Mortality in a General Population and in the Population of a Prepaid Group Practice, Medical Care Plan," *American Journal of Public Health* 48, no. 2 (February 1958):170–87.

CONTRIBUTED COMMENTS ON
DEMAND ANALYSIS PAPERS

Eli Ginzberg
Columbia University

THE LIMITS OF FORMAL ANALYSIS

The papers presented in this section of the Second Conference on Health Economics sought to clarify such basic questions as whether, and to what extent, the demand for medical care is price- and income-elastic. The analysts sought to incorporate into their hypotheses recent refinements in the theory of consumption by considering both time and income as limited resources the use of which the consumer seeks to maximize. An effort was made to explore the potentialities of applying linear programming to alternative measures that might be used in a developing country to reduce the incidence and prevalence of tuberculosis.

While each of the papers provided some interesting new data and suggested how more sophisticated econometric techniques might be employed to study the demand for medical care, they were not able to surmount intractable conceptual difficulties. For instance, is the expressed demand for additional days of hospital care a reflection of the preferences of consumers for spending more time in the hospital, or does it reflect professional and hospital practices?

In comparing the demand for medical care among the poor with that among the non-poor, how does one deal with the fact that ill health is likely to be more common among the poor and that therefore they will need more services? The analysis of gross differences will be significantly affected by whether the health status of consumers is regarded as an endogenous or exogenous variable.

Without an objective determination of health status, what meaning attaches to a finding that different income groups spend differing numbers of

161

days away from work because of sickness? Unless the analysis goes beyond income and expenditures and takes account of such factors as paid sick leave, manual versus white-collar occupations, family conditions, group attitudes toward illness, etc., the meaning of the regressions presented at the conference must be questioned.

Whether or not linear programming for health planning in developing or developed countries offers significant promise depends, of course, not on a static model but on a model that has been dynamized to take account of the reactions of both parties – the purveyors of health service as well as the consumers – to the earlier stages of the programming. But a dynamic model has not yet been developed. Even at this early date it may be suggested that the accumulation of the relevant data may be so horrendous a task as to make the outcome highly problematic.

The past three years, after the introduction of Medicare and Medicaid, have witnessed significant changes in the dollar terms of the medical trade. As a result, all contemporary data are likely to be criticized when used to illustrate changes in the demand for medical care during the past decade. The large changes in dollar expenditures for medical care in 1967–68 compared with 1963–64 may obscure the fact that little change has taken place in the quantity or quality of the services provided, especially to low-income families.

Given these and other conceptual and statistical problems, the question must be raised concerning the value of developing elaborate econometric models for the study of the demand for medical care. Such studies may contribute to a refinement of methodology, but it is doubtful whether they provide much hard new knowledge about the industry or many leads for public policy.

A serious economist will want more control over the facets of demand, but he might profit from rereading the relevant section in Alfred Marshall's *Principles*, which warns of the difficulties of such a task. The following catena lists the many institutional considerations that are likely to doom such an effort, no matter how elegant the analytic structure and no matter how complete the statistical data.

THE MANY FACETS OF DEMAND

1. The demand for medical care is a combined demand for diagnosis, therapy, reassurance, and specific types of consumption – i.e., massage, round-the-clock nursing services, a private room, etc.

2. The demand for medical care is – or should be – a demand for health, but the relation of the former to the latter is often indirect.

3. The demand for health clearly varies according to consumers' knowledge and preferences as well as their incomes, although all these factors are

interrelated. However, within the same income class, among people with the same general health status, the demand varies considerably.

4. Since the demand for medical care services is generally local, the availability of the supply is a major determinant of whether latent demand becomes manifest or effective.

5. As with the demand for other goods and services, there is a big element of "fashion" in the demand for medical services, which is usually a result of professional attitudes and behavior but is also influenced by the preferences of the public. The decline in tonsillectomies and the apparently waning interest in classical psychoanalytic therapy are examples.

6. In most instances the individual patient initiates the demand for medical care, but the physician has a major influence on the total number and range of services provided during the course of an illness. It is regrettable but true that his decisions are influenced not only by his professional judgment of the patient's condition but also by such factors as the patient's ability to pay, occupation, and the practices followed by the physician's colleagues.

7. To assume that from the patient's point of view more services are preferable to fewer services is an error, since no intervention is often the preferred therapy. However, the physician does not get paid for services that he does not provide, hence the tendency to "overdoctor."

8. There is a widespread assumption that more preventive services will tend to reduce the demand for therapeutic services. Aside from basic immunization procedures in childhood and a limited number of diagnostic procedures in adulthood, there is no hard evidence to support this belief, which has been translated, in turn, into a potentially large unmet demand for preventive services.

9. The demand for many services which is initiated by the patient or the physician or both is often determined more by the arrangements governing hospitalization and financing than by purely professional considerations.

10. The behavior of the American people with regard to eating, drinking, smoking, drugs, driving, recreation, and illness itself underscores the willingness of many to run considerable risks with their health in favor of other needs and desires. One conclusion is unequivocal. The demand for medical care cannot be disentangled easily from the demand for health, which in turn is linked in many different ways to the totality of an individual's value structure.

SOME TENTATIVE CONCLUSIONS

It is commendable that economists have belatedly become interested in matters of health and medicine. An industry that spends approximately $56 billion annually and provides employment for almost four million persons is worthy of their attention. But the difficult question remains: how can economists best contribute to new knowledge and improved policy in this field?

The basic model with which most economists work is one that describes a competitive situation under static conditions. But this model is not apposite for the medical care industry, which is neither competitive nor static. Economists should therefore be modest about the transferability of their tools and techniques.

If the gap between the conventional model and reality is wide, and if economists seek to be relevant and constructive, it is necessary that they achieve substantial mastery of the structure of the industry. They must learn how the system actually operates. This is not easy, if they are to select problems the solution of which will add to knowledge and improve policy. Moreover, they must allow the problems they select to determine the methods they will employ. There is evidence that in this instance economists have been operating in a vacuum. Many have become interested in health because of the accretion of large bodies of data that lend themselves to manipulation by econometric and other sophisticated techniques. These techniques lead to more scholarly papers, but not necessarily to a better understanding of the medical care industry or of health policy.

Irving Leveson
The RAND Corporation

The papers presented in this section attempt to consider specific types of medical care rather than all medical care, and in doing so add to our body of knowledge. Rosenthal deals with length of stay in non-federal, short-term general and special hospitals in the New England states. Andersen and Benham examine expenditures for physicians' and dentists' services and a measure of physician use in a nationwide sample of families. Silver considers variation in total, hospital, drug, physician and dental expense per person per year among means of region-age-sex cells. He also examines the relationship of work-loss days to family income and wage rates and investigates substitution between medical care and the patient's time. On the whole, the authors maintain the classification of demand determinants into price, income, and tastes, focusing on price and income variables. Rosenthal emphasizes the price effects of insurance, Anderson and Benham stress income and include insurance variables, and Silver deals with both income and the price of time. In addition to the traditional emphases there are, in portions of the work of both authors and discussants, beginnings in the direction of considering health as an explicit determinant of the demand for medical care. I submit that explicit treatment of health as an independent variable is essential in demand analysis and that its study leads to a fundamental mechanism for explaining the interrelationships among demands for different types of medical care.

The most explicit treatment of health is given by Andersen and Benham. Among their independent variables are a rating (good, fair, or poor) of the health of the family member with the poorest health, a count of family symptoms, and a measure of the absence of preventive care, all of which have

165

statistically significant and sizable regression coefficients. Grossman, in his comments on their paper, introduces an approach in which the demand for medical care is treated as a derived demand, derived from the demand for the commodity "good health." In his formulation, changes in health status operate by influencing the price of "good health" in the sense that if health deteriorates it becomes more costly to reach the desired level. The other authors follow the usual practice of either omitting health in the demand function (Silver) or of controlling for it (Rosenthal).

It would appear more reasonable that, if health is as important as it seems, its effects should be studied rather than avoided. This requires dealing with serious identification problems, since medical care can also influence health. Health is likely to be most important as a determinant of demand when we consider social rather than private demand because social demand contains elements of supply. Policymakers often seek to provide the greatest amount of medical care where health is poor. This fact may be an important source of difficulty in communications between economists and planners. Economists are quick to point out that little is known about the effectiveness of medical services in improving health, while usually offering no new contribution. Instead, they often put their effort into demand studies which omit health, a major consideration for public representatives in allocating resources. In studies of resource demand it is necessary to take into account the problems with which resources are intended to deal; for example, crime as a source of demand for police protection, births as a factor in family planning, and illiteracy as a determinant of the need for education.

When health is omitted from a demand analysis, its effects become subsumed under those of income, education, and other variables with which it is correlated. Some portion of health variation is random and becomes included in the error term. Part is endogenous — determined within the system of equations — and may be removed by simultaneous-equation methods. However, a substantial portion of health variation will still be predetermined. Individuals will differ in inherited qualities. The stock of health will vary as a consequence of environment and actions taken by a child's parents before he is old enough to plan for himself. Differences in the stock of immunities determined by exposure to disease and immunization as a child will influence health status. Health will vary as a consequence of conditions about which one has imperfect information and incomplete control. Furthermore, much of the variation in health can be treated as predetermined because we know too little about its determinants to include it in our models or because we lack data to represent the endogenous components adequately. It would be useful to begin with formulations which include health measures as independent variables and try to chip away at the proportion of health variation treated as predetermined as we learn more and acquire better data. In representing predetermined influences, lagged values of health can provide a useful measure. Separation of predetermined variation in health would make it possible to estimate the effects of changes in health on medical care demand and to obtain better estimates of the effects of other variables.

The effects of omission of health on other variables can easily be illustrated. Consider a range of income in which gains are associated with improvements in health. We would then tend to underestimate the income elasticities of demand.* In a comparison of income elasticities of different types of medical care, the problem of separating the effects of health and income is even more important than for total medical care. We know that hospitalization rates vary relatively little by income size class while physicians' office visits per capita vary considerably. This may well be because the latter reduce the demand for hospital services by virtue of their impact on health. If ambulatory care does improve health so as to reduce hospitalization, much of the observed effects of comprehensive financing may include large effects of health, rather than being price effects alone. If so, expansion of ambulatory care may be an independent alternative to comprehensive financing if a reduction in hospital inpatient loads is desired. If the effect of ambulatory care on hospitalization were estimated and the effect of health on the demand for hospital care were known, one could also estimate the implicit impact of ambulatory care on health. Many such hypotheses could be formed and tested. While controlling for health status may yield useful partial coefficients for some variables, it is necessary to go much further and not only estimate the partial effects of health but explore the resulting interactions among component variables and system relationships.

---

*If health and income are the only independent variables, the expected value of the regression coefficient in a simple regression of income on medical care is $E(b_{MY}) = b_{MY \cdot H} + b_{MH \cdot Y} b_{HY}$. Here $b_{MH \cdot Y} < 0$ and $b_{HY} > 0$.

PART IV

STRUCTURE OF INDUSTRY

Paul J. Feldstein and Sander Kelman
The University of Michigan

A FRAMEWORK FOR AN ECONOMETRIC MODEL OF THE MEDICAL CARE SECTOR

INTRODUCTION

In recent years the application of quantitative techniques to the study of various aspects of medical care has increased. These techniques have been used to supplement our subjective knowledge of the factors affecting the use and supply of medical care and the importance of each of these factors. However, studies which have been completed do not show the ultimate effects on medical care prices and output of changes in specific markets, such as the demand for hospital care or the supply of nurses, because a general formulation of the medical care market does not yet exist. In order to increase our understanding of how this market operates and the effects of various changes in it, it is necessary to construct a general market model and to estimate empirically the functional relations describing the entire market for medical care services.

There are good reasons why such a general market model has not been formulated and estimated; among them are the difficulties in defining and measuring prices and outputs in the market and specifying their interrelationships and the unavailability of data necessary to measure many important relationships. However, a first step must be made by defining theoretically the many relationships within the medical care market, if only to generate criticisms and thereby improve our knowledge. The purpose of this paper, therefore, is to make this start. We shall present a model of the medical care

A more detailed discussion of the model is available from the authors upon request. A larger version of the paper, which contains the data and sources used for giving empirical form to the model, is also available.

171

market together with parameters for the functional relationships. These parameters were developed both empirically and subjectively.

Such an econometric model will have several uses. First, the ability to forecast the effects of changes in variables, which stem from changes in government policy or from changes in the factors affecting supply or demand conditions, will enable planners to allocate resources more purposefully both toward the health field and within it. The availability of such a model will facilitate the evaluation of alternative government policies and, by providing more complete information, will help to improve decision-making. Second, the formulation of such a model in terms of specific functional relationships will serve also to indicate what types of data are needed to monitor the medical care sector for the purposes stated above. Finally, once such a model exists, it should be possible through the use of sensitivity analysis to assess future returns from additional research on the various parameters; i.e., more accurate forecasts can be obtained by reducing the variance of the parameters.

The purposes of this paper, then, are to formulate a model of the medical care sector, to specify this model in equation form, to describe how the parameters for the equations were developed, and to demonstrate the usefulness of such a model through a series of applications.

All of these objectives have not been fulfilled. Because we have not yet been able to achieve a convergence in our simulations of the model, we do not present the applications in this paper. They will, however, be presented in future publications. We hope that the model alone will stimulate discussion, so that an improved econometric model of the medical care sector may be developed.

A MODEL OF THE MEDICAL CARE SECTOR

Theoretical Formulation

In developing a model of any economic structure, there is always a conflict between allegiance to theoretical purity and the comfort of empirical compromise. The medical care sector is no exception. In principle we are talking about the total number of treatments for all the various diagnostic categories, each treatment weighted by the percentage probability of cure within a given period of time. The output concept is the sum of each of the above terms multiplied by their respective prices.

An analytic study of this sector, then, becomes an analysis of the determinants of supply of and demand for treatments for each of these diagnostic categories, the resulting demand for the services of various medical care institutions, and finally, the resulting demand for medical care resources:

manpower, drugs, and equipment. The determinants of the supplies of institutional and manpower services would also be investigated.

Consider, now, the supply of treatments for a particular diagnostic category of care. Although there are exceptions, each institution potentially has facilities to treat a given illness. Then, for each institution and each illness, there is a neoclassical production function relating various inputs to the resulting output level. This production function, together with the input prices, determines a least-cost expansion path, which implies a cost curve, and, together with the assumption of increasing marginal cost of expanding one treatment category relative to another in a given institution of fixed size, an upward-sloping supply curve. Hence for each illness category there is a supply curve of treatments for each type of institution in which such care can be dispensed.

On the demand side, the physician is the central agent in the delivery of care. In evaluating the patient's illness and sociodemographic and economic characteristics, the physician attempts to minimize the cost of treatment, within the constraints of his own income and leisure time objectives. He will select that institution or combination of institutional settings which will be consistent with both the needs and resources of the patient and these constraints. The prescribed medical package takes into account not only these factors and the different treatments by institutional setting but also their respective prices, the type and extent of the patient's insurance coverage, and his income level.[1] Hence, we have, for each diagnostic category, a separate demand equation. These, together with the supply curves, yield output solutions for the illness treatments in each institution. Such an analysis for each diagnostic category yields the solution for total expenditure on medical care, the demand for the services of specific institutions and medical care categories.

All of this can be criticized as too naïve an approach, but as a first approximation to the behavior of the medical care sector it is sufficient. It implies that the total demand for each of the institutions depends on the distribution of illnesses throughout the population, the productivity of each of the institutions in providing care, the relative prices of such care, level of income, and extent of insurance coverage.

We know, however, that illness-specific data on institution-specific utilization is not and probably will not be available. Hence, from the start we assume that the distribution of illness remains constant, and the relative institution-specific productivities in treating these illnesses remains constant. As a result, the utilization of institutions depends (in terms of economic variables) on prices, incomes, and insurance coverage, and we then turn to these as our basic level of aggregation in the study of the market for medical care.

Empirical Specification

Aggregate Level of Medical Care Activity

The model has three levels. The first level consists of (1) expressing the value of medical care as the sum of the values of medical care provided in each of the five institutional settings – hospitals, nursing homes, outpatient clinics, doctors' offices, and the patient's home – and (2) a Laspeyres price index based on this identity (equations 1 and 2). The second level is an analysis of the supply of and demand for the services of these institutions, and the third level shows the resulting derived health manpower demand and supply.

In what follows we shall elaborate upon the determination of output in the five institutional settings. The first two, acute hospitals and nursing homes, will have the same form, namely a stock-adjustment model; the last three will be explained by more conventional supply and demand equations.

Health Care Institutional Settings

Short-term general hospitals and nursing homes. With respect to hospitals and nursing homes, the measure of output which we shall use is patient days per thousand population, *PD*. There are two different ways of approaching *PD*. One is to recognize that *PD* is the product of average daily admissions per thousand population (*ADA*) × days in one year (365) × mean stay (average length of stay per patient in days), and to explain *PD* by seeking the determinants of *ADA* and mean stay. This approach, however, ignores the dynamics of a situation in which the provision of a service is greatly dependent on the accumulation of a stock of facilities. Thus, the second approach is to recognize that *PD* is also the product of the existing stock of beds per thousand population (*S*) × the average annual occupancy rate of those beds (*OCC*) × 365 (equations 3 and 13). This approach is much more appealing in economic terms because an explanation of *S* is tantamount to an explanation of the long-term determinants of the provision of hospital care, and an explanation of *OCC* is tantamount to an explanation of the short-term determinants of that provision, holding constant the long-term factors.

The equations for the determination of output in the nursing home sector are similar to those for hospitals. The dependent variable, however, is nursing home patient days and beds per thousand population *over age sixty-five*. Also a number of the independent variables are in terms of the population over age sixty-five. This is because approximately 90 per cent of the residents of nursing homes are over sixty-five and, hence, form the relevant population.[2]

For either hospitals or nursing homes, and under assumptions of constant morbidity and illness-specific incidence distributions, there is, we postulate, consistent with any constellation of a set of socio-economic variables, some desired provision of service, PD^*. Assuming proportionality between stocks and services, there is implied in the desired service a desired stock, S^*, where the factor of proportionality is the inverse of the optimum occupancy rate $\times$ 365 (equations 5 and 15). The desired stock, however, is unobservable, and hence we must look at the investment process to give empirical content to S^*. As a result, we posit that investment over the relevant period is proportional to the discrepancy between the desired stock at the end of the period and the actual stock at the beginning (equations 4 and 14).

The occupancy rate equation is basically a reduced form equation for the determination of the short-term fluctuation in facility services but is formulated in such a way as to account for the current state of long-term accumulation of facilities (equations 6, 7, 16, 17). The occupancy rate equation, together with the determinants of the stock of beds, then determines the output of short-term general hospitals and nursing homes.

Ordinarily, prices are determined by the intersection of supply and demand. In the analysis of hospital prices, however, we will assume that administrators set prices so as to cover expected average costs. To explain differences and changes in hospital costs, therefore, we consider the standard cost curve of conventional economics for the production of a standard unique product, a hospital patient day of care standardized for quality and service mix.

We recognize that the hospital product is not identical in all hospitals or over time, in spite of the impression given by the unit of output, patient day. Instead, hospitals vary greatly in both the quality and variety of services which they offer. We have tried to allow for these differences by including service mix as a variable. This variable is meant to serve two purposes: to measure complexity (the variety of services offered by the average hospital) and to measure the quality of care in the average hospital by assuming that the more complex the mix of services offered in the hospital, the higher the quality of services offered. Having adjusted for quality, we then analyze the cost for a standardized patient day. The determinants of cost for this standardized patient day depend upon absolute and relative wage rates, cost of capital, scale of output, and size of plant. The constellation of wage rates determines the employment of various manpower categories. The effect of a change in a particular wage rate on the average cost of the hospital patient day is not constant. The impact of a 10 per cent increase in the wage of one of the categories depends on the level of the wage, the level of employment of that factor, and the elasticity of substitution between that factor and the other factors. The greater the employment of that factor and the less elastic its substitutability, the larger the effect on average cost. Wages consist of nursing, paramedical, and staff physician salaries. Empirically, they take on the values which they receive in the manpower sector of the model.

Cost of capital is taken to mean the annual depreciation charge against the existing stock of physical capital. Included in the cost of each hospital patient day is an allocation of this charge. This cost depends on the expected life of assets (and hence the depreciation rate), the capital intensity of hospital operations (the stock of capital relative to output), and the hospital administrator's treatment of the Hill-Burton subsidy program (equations 10, 11, and 12).

Finally, we come to the level of output (PD_H) as a determinant of hospital cost. Theoretically, there are three effects which changes in output can impose on hospital costs. First, if occupancy rates tend to fall, average costs will rise, raising price, but this is a temporary phenomenon and can be ignored. Second, if output tends to rise over time, capital and labor costs also tend to rise. Since we have specifically treated these phenomena, that is not a behavioral consideration motivating the appearance of output in the cost equation. Finally, over time, part of the increase in output results from an increase in the availability of larger facilities. As has been pointed out, larger facilities enable hospitals to operate at higher *long-run* occupancy rates and to achieve economies of scale which reduce the average cost of a patient day of hospital care. Hence average size, not output, is the relevant variable (equations 8 and 9). Equation 8 presents the estimated cost of a hospital patient day of care, including the associated cost of physician services.

Doctors' office visits. For the demand side it is necessary to consider both economic and sociodemographic factors. Economic factors are income, insurance coverage, welfare payments, and prices; sociodemographic factors are age, sex, and degree of urbanization. Variables are included for one of two reasons: they generate demand for either general or specific types of health care, that is, scale effects, substitution effects, or both. Scale effects arise from those factors associated with either morbidity (age, sex, and urbanization) or the relaxation of income constraints (income relative to the general medical care price level, and the over-all level of health insurance coverage). Substitution effects arise from factors associated with the feasibility of certain types of delivery under differing population arrangements (urbanization), institution-specific insurance coverage, and relative prices (equation 18).

For the supply of doctors' office visits we assume a neoclassical production function in which drugs, capital, nurses, paramedical personnel, and doctors are combined. We do not treat capital and drugs specifically in this model, and hence we begin with a production function involving the remaining three inputs and their respective wages. The economic conjugation of these two sets of information results in an expansion path and, consequently, a least-cost function. In the case of the Cobb-Douglas production function, the cost function depends on the relative and absolute output elasticities, the level of technology, and the relative and absolute wage rates. (In this cost-minimizing model of producer behavior, the relative wage rates are set equal to, and hence account for, the relative marginal productivities.) Assuming further that price and cost are monotonically related by the elasticity of demand, the supply relation then depends on the price of a doctor's office visit and the same set of factors affecting cost.

Because they contribute not only organizational talent but also productive efforts, doctors can be considered as both entrepreneurs and direct factors of production. Hence, to the extent that rate of return to the clinical practice of medicine gives rise to a certain stock of physicians and to the extent that the annual income differential between private practice and hospital staff practice gives rise to a certain distribution of that stock, the number of physicians in offices and, hence, the number of doctors' office entrepreneurs is largely determined by the market for manpower. Instead of a wage figure, however, the number of physicians in private practice is used to formulate the supply relationship (equations 19, 20, 21).

Outpatient visits. The demand for outpatient visits is specified as having the same form as that for doctors' office visits (equation 22). Similarly, the reasoning behind the supply relation of outpatient visits per thousand population follows the same logic as that of the supply of doctors' office visits, with a few minor exceptions (equation 23). In doctors' office visits, services of the doctor are, in fact, those of the entrepreneur, and are accounted for by the stock of doctors, whereas in outpatient clinics the doctor's service is strictly that of a hired factor and is accounted for by the wages of hospital staff physicians.

Theoretically, then, the model consists of the supply and demand equations of both staff and non-staff clinical physicians, based mainly on staff and non-staff wages. This formulation, however, leads to a complication which we wish to avoid. To avoid explicit treatment of the two segments of the profession, we use, as a surrogate for wages paid to the staff physician, the annual income earned by the average clinical physician. Staff physicians are a very small proportion of total clinical physicians, and there is a substantial degree of competition between private and non-private practice for doctors; consequently, the differential in income from the two types of practice must reflect the psychic advantages of pursuing one type of practice over another, and little else. As a result, we would expect the wage paid to staff physicians to follow closely, albeit at a lower level, the changes in the income earned by physicians in private practice.

Despite specific neglect of the problem of capital accumulation apart from the accumulation of beds, we cannot allow the supply of outpatient visits to depend merely on certain current costs. Capital costs are a large part of any hospital's or quasi-hospital's total costs and should be taken into account in an analysis of a supply function. We look at the problem of capital accumulation as a constraint on the supply of outpatient visits. This can be viewed as analogous to the inclusion in the supply of doctors' office visits the stock of physicians in private practice, for this stock represents a flow of capital into offices in response to the expected rate of return to private practice. Although the market for doctors' office visits does not operate in the same way as that for outpatient visits, indirectly there is a great deal of similarity. If we think of those socioeconomic variables discussed in the section on short-term hospitals as giving rise to a demand for facilities and, hence, to a flow of capital to finance those facilities, inclusion in the supply function of the stock of short-term general hospital beds per thousand population acts as a surrogate for the capital constraint on outpatient facilities.

Home care. Defining home care as any medical care received in the home presents some difficulties because it would appear that anything from taking an aspirin to performance of open heart surgery might be included. However, in terms of medical care we view the home as a substitute facility for other institutions, so that we shall consider as home care only those activities which in the other settings would also be termed medical care. No one goes to the hospital or to a doctor's office merely to take an aspirin. He may, after examination and diagnosis, take an aspirin, but it is the former, not the latter, activity which constitutes the *raison d'être* of the other settings: if he were to have a house call by his physician after which he was given an aspirin, this would be considered home care because of the house call, not the aspirin. Let us then consider home care to be medical treatment in the home where medical manpower or machinery are hired.

The demand for home care, in days per thousand population, depends largely upon the same variables as the demand for services in the other settings. We assume that it is an inferior good and hence that the demand is negatively related to both price and income. Furthermore, it is negatively related to all forms of health insurance other than that which covers home care. The prices for care in alternative settings are, of course, assumed to be positively related to the demand for home care. Finally, marital status and family size are assumed to be factors complementary to the purchase of home care and, hence, assumed to exert a positive effect on the demand for home care (equation 24).

We shall argue that the supply side of home care ought to be neglected. First, it is not an institution. No administration is responsible for organizing the inputs, scheduling the admissions, etc. It is merely a "scene" where medical care is dispensed; it could be an institutional setting in the same sense as the others only if the supply side included a model of the housing sector. Furthermore, the home care supply concept lacks meaning because the price of home care is essentially taken to be the price of the inputs hired to dispense medical care in the home (equation 25).

Health Manpower

We now come to the third level of the model, the derived demand for the various categories of health manpower and their supply. We start with the demand(s) for manpower. The derived demand for a factor of production is, theoretically, the demand relationship between that factor and its wage. The specific form of this demand function depends upon the assumptions made about the markets for the final product and the factors of production and upon the production function for the product. For example, in the Cobb-Douglas production function the demand for a specific factor depends directly on the total expenditure for the other factors (itself related to the wage paid to other factors) and on the output elasticities of the other factors and the wage of the factor in question. Furthermore, for each factor there is a derived demand curve for each institutional setting. Hence, the total derived demand is the horizontal summation of these five curves.

One set of variables appearing in our derived demand function for a particular health manpower category is comprised of the outputs of the five institutional settings. If, as before, we assume that all output elasticities are equal, and hence their ratios unitary, we can neglect them in this treatment. We specify that the wages of the respective labor inputs enter into each derived demand relation and take the expected signs. Finally, although physicians and paramedical personnel are within the institutional medical care sector, nurses are not: a number are employed by local school systems. As a result, in the derived demand for nurses we include a measure of the output of the school systems.

In the empirical form of the derived demand equations there is yet another adjustment to be made. We shall assume that nurses and paramedical personnel are largely incapable of adjusting their daily or weekly hours to suit their own preferences; that is, they are considered to be institutional employees and their weekly hours to be fixed and uniform. The implication of this is that the determination of the number of full-time (equivalent) nurses and paramedical personnel is tantamount to the determination of the hours of service which they render. With doctors, however, this is not the case. There is, in fact, evidence that in the short run doctors operate on a backward-bending supply curve.[3] Hence, the dependent variables in the nurse and paramedical equations will be in terms of numbers employed per thousand population, whereas the equation for doctors will be in terms of annual hours of patient care rendered by doctors per thousand population (equations 26, 34, 46).

Nurses. We turn now to the determination of the supply of these manpower categories, beginning with nurses. The stock of nurses consists of all trained nurses, even if they are working elsewhere, for if nursing wages rise sufficiently, they will return to nursing. The total stock of nurses is equal to the lagged stock plus the recent increment per thousand population (equation 28). The increment is equal to the current number of nursing school graduates plus the net in-migration of trained nurses, minus the number of deaths and retirements among the stock of nurses (equation 29). It is stated that the number of employed nurses per thousand population is some proportion of the existing stock (equation 27).

The nursing force participation rate is expected to vary inversely with the proportion of the stock of nurses who are married and under forty years of age and with the relative wages paid in other occupations for which nurses could be qualified, and directly with the real wage paid to nurses (equation 33). The number of nursing school graduates is considered to depend upon the weekly incomes of nurses relative to that of a possible alternative occupation such as teaching (a proxy variable for the relative rate of return), the amount of scholarship dollars per nursing student (which would affect the rate of return to girls entering nursing schools), and the number of females per thousand population graduated from high school three years previously. This variable is the pool from which some percentage will enter nursing school. The larger this number, the larger will be the number of nursing graduates (per thousand population) several years hence (equation 30).

Inasmuch as most of the net inflow of nurses appears to be from Canada, we specify that this variable depends on the relative nursing wage in the U.S. and Canada less 1 (equation 31). Since it is believed that nurses retire from the stock either because of age or inadequate wages, we include as explanatory variables in the retiree equation the proportion of employed nurses over the age of sixty and the nursing wage relative to the Social Security retirement benefits that a nurse receives if she retires (equation 32).

Physicians. As has been stated previously, we measure the supply of physician services not in numbers of physicians but in hours of service devoted to patient care per year per thousand population. This we undertake by separately explaining the hours per physician per year and the stock of physicians; this is similar to the determination of hospital *PD*, which was the product of a long-term and a short-term supply phenomenon (equation 35).

First, we consider the determination of the supply of hours per physician per year. Traditionally, such a variable depends on the wage rate, but in a non-monotonic fashion; that is, we have come to expect backward-bending supply curves, at least in the long run, for most forms of labor. Hence, it would seem that the supply of hours depends on physicians' hourly compensation and annual level of income where the effects are expected to be positive and negative, respectively. Note that the three variables are linked by a multiplicative identity (income equals hours times the wage rate). As a result, it can be shown that the supply of hours depends simply on the hourly wage rate or on annual income, where the coefficient on the explanatory variable is a combination of the coefficients on the two hypothesized explanatory variables. Since equations appear in terms of the real weekly income of physicians, we will formulate the supply of physician hours of service in those terms. The sign on income in the hours equation depends on the relative magnitude of the effects of income and the hourly wage in the behavioral relation (equation 36).

We turn next to the determination of the stock of physicians. Behaviorally, the supply of factors has traditionally depended on wages or, in the case of factors involving large investments, on the rate of return. However, the present model is basically one of short-run forecasting of an investment process with a rather long period of gestation. In such a situation the rate of return is relevant over only a substantially long period of time, so that it is not suitable for use in this study.

Furthermore, the institutional aspects of the market for physicians are such that the rate of return is of only minor empirical importance. The usual behavioral assumption in a factor supply model is of free entry in response to the rate of return, or of differential rates of return for different prospective occupations, so that in the long run, assuming no psychic income differentials, rate of return differentials are eliminated. However, entry into the profession is not free, and the number of entrants is substantially less than the number who desire to attend medical school. Moreover, the inducement to become a physician is to a considerable extent based on non-economic factors such as social status. The decision usually is made at least eleven years before the return begins. Such an early decision, if based upon a rate of return consideration, implies either a rather long-term expectations model or knowledge that the rate of return will be held constant, in which case it becomes statistically superfluous. It might be postulated that the desired rate of return is the important determinant of medical school capacity, which again implies a rather constant rate of return in the long run, and hence is of little value for statistical investigation.

Consequently, for the period of analysis in this model, capacity of domestic production, and not the rate of return, must be judged the important determinant of physician supply. In fact, as long as the capacity of medical schools remains substantially beneath the number of qualified students which would be generated by rate of return considerations, it becomes a behaviorally superfluous variable. The implication of this fact is that attempts to augment the supply of physicians by directly increasing the rate of return will merely increase the rate of return to the existing number, which has been determined by capacity.

Since we assume that the capacity constraint will be effective in the above sense for at least the next decade, we specify the number of entrants to be identical to capacity (equations 37, 38, 39, 40).* Some specification of the dynamics of medical school capacity is required. We offer two alternative forms, one positive and the other normative. First, the American Medical Association has stated that medical schools will continue to increase the number of graduates enough to keep the physician-population ratio constant. Although population has been increasing at a rate of 1.6 per cent, recent data show that medical school entrants are increasing at a rate of only 1.4 per cent per annum. However, graduates of foreign medical schools have been contributing an increasing number and presumably a larger proportion of physicians to our supply, and it appears that the AMA assumes that this source will continue to account for a 0.2 per cent annual increase. We then can translate the AMA statement to mean an increase of 1.4 per cent per annum in medical school capacity (equations 41, 42).

The second approach to this problem is to ignore the politics of medical school expansion and to consider it as merely a problem of money. The costs of alternative public programs to expand the provision of health care then can be compared. Such an approach is considered normative in the sense that it assumes that what is desirable and economically possible is also politically possible. We assume, then, that the average cost of expanding the capacity of medical schools is $30,000 per entering student (equations 42a, 43, 44, 45).

Paramedical personnel. We turn, finally, to the supply of paramedical personnel. This category is made up of many different occupations, and little training is required. Therefore, we specify the supply of paramedical personnel to depend upon only the real wage and the wage relative to that of retail trade employees (equation 47).

Operational Implementation

What follows is a brief discussion of the empirical work currently being pursued on the model. We first assume a linear form for each of the nonproportional behavioral equations. Then, taking assumed values for the beta coefficients[4] of each independent variable in each equation and ranges of the data for the period 1955-1965, we are able to generate a set of a priori regression coefficients for the structural equations.

Our purpose, however, is to find the total direct and indirect effects of the exogenous variables, including the policy instruments, on the endogenous variables of the system. In a linear model this effect is obtained from the reduced form, but since ours is not a linear model, such an approach is not possible. What we seek, then, is a set of elasticities defined as the percentage

---

*Some of the variables and equations affecting the supply of doctors, such as foreign medical school graduates, death and retirement, etc., although not discussed in the text, should be self-explanatory; see the larger version of this paper for further analysis.

increase in an endogenous variable associated with a 1 per cent permanent increase in an exogenous variable. These elasticities are obtained by iterative processes, letting one exogenous variable change at a time.

Such a set of elasticities is useful for assessing the merits of various policy instruments because these elasticities show the final effects of the policy instruments on such things as total medical care output (MC) and the price level (P_{MC}). For instance, by starting with the 1965 values of the system, increasing the value of hospitalization coverage by 10 per cent, iterating the model until it converges, and noting what percentage increase results in P_{MC}, one obtains some idea of the cost of extending hospitalization insurance to a larger proportion of the population. A similar treatment is possible for all of the other exogenous and endogenous variables.

EQUATIONS FOR AN ECONOMETRIC MODEL OF THE MEDICAL CARE SECTOR

Aggregate Equations

(1) $MC = [P'_H PD_H + P_{DO}DOV + P_{OP}OPV + P_{HC}HC]POP$
$\qquad + P_{NH}PD_{NH}POP_{65}$

(2) $P_{MC} = \big([P'_H PD_{H-1} + P_{DO}DOV_{-1} + P_{OP}OPV_{-1} + P_{HC}HC_{-1}]POP_{-1}$
$\qquad + P_{NH}PD_{NH-1}POP_{65-1}\big)/MC_{-1}$

Market for Care by Institution

Short-Term General Hospitals

(3) $PD_H = 365 \cdot S_H \cdot OCC_H$

(4) $S_H = \gamma S_H^* + (1-\gamma)S_{H-10}$

(5) $S_H^* = f(AGE,\ MAR,\ SEX,\ URB,\ \dfrac{Y}{CPI},\ INS_H,$
$\qquad INS_H \cdot INS_{DO},\ INS_H \cdot INS_{OP},\ \dfrac{WEL}{CPI}, AVG_{H-10},$
$\qquad S_{NH}AGE)$

(6) $OCC_H = f(S_H^{*\#},\ AVG_H,\ P'_H, \dfrac{P_{OP}}{P'_H}, \dfrac{P_{DO}}{P'_H}, \dfrac{P_{NH}}{P_H}, \dfrac{P_{HC}}{P'_H})$

(7) $S_H^{*\#} = S_H^* - S_H$

(8) $P'_H = 1.3P_H$

(9) $P_H = f(\dfrac{DEP}{PD_H \cdot POP}, \; W_N, \dfrac{W_{par}}{W_N}, \; \dfrac{W_{MDp}}{W_N}, \; AVG_H, \; MIX)$

(10) $DEP = \dfrac{1}{L} V$

(11) $V = C \cdot S_H \cdot POP$

(12) $C = f(MIX, \; P_{con})$

Nursing Homes

(13) $PD_{NH} = 365 \cdot S_{NH} \cdot OCC_{NH}$

(14) $S_{NH} = \eta S^*_{NH} + (1 - \eta) \; S_{NH-5}$

(15) $S^*_{NH} = f(URB, \dfrac{Y}{CPI}, \dfrac{WEL}{CPI}, \; INS'_{NH}, \; AVG_{NH-5})$

(16) $OCC_{NH} = f(S^{*\,\#}_{NH}, \; AVG_{NH}, \; P_{NH}, \dfrac{P_{NH}}{P_H}, \dfrac{P_{NH}}{P_{HC}})$

(17) $S^{*\,\#}_{NH} = S^*_{NH} - S_{NH}$

Doctors' Office Visits

(18) $DOV^D = f(\dfrac{Y}{CPI}, \; INS_{DO}, \; INS_H \cdot INS_{DO}, \; INS_{OP} \cdot INS_{DO}, \; P_{DO},$

$\qquad\qquad \dfrac{P_{DO}}{P'_H}, \dfrac{P_{DO}}{P_{OP}}, \dfrac{P_{DO}}{P_{HC}}, \dfrac{WEL}{CPI}, \; AGE, \; SEX, \; URB)$

(19) $DOV^S = f(P_{DO}, \; W_N, \dfrac{W_{par}}{W_N}, \; MD_{PP})$

(20) $MD_{PP} = MD_P - MD_{HP}$

(21) $MD_{HP} = 0.022 \; S_H \cdot MIX$

Outpatient Visits

(22) $OPV^D = f(\dfrac{Y}{CPI}, \; INS_{OP}, \; INS_{OP} \cdot INS_H, \; INS_{OP} \cdot INS_{DO}, \; P_{OP},$

$$\frac{P_{DO}}{P_{OP}}, \frac{P_{OP}}{P'_H}, \frac{P_{OP}}{P_{HC}}, AGE, \frac{WEL}{CPI}, URB, SEX)$$

$$(23) \quad OPV^S = f(P_{OP}, W_N, \frac{W_{par}}{W_N}, \frac{W_{MDp}}{W_N}, S_H)$$

Home Care

$$(24) \quad HC^D = f(\frac{Y}{CPI}, \frac{WEL}{CPI}, INS_{HC}, INS_{HC} \cdot INS_{DO},$$

$$INS_{HC} \cdot INS_{OP}, INS_{HC} \cdot INS_H, P_{HC}, \frac{P_{DO}}{P_{HC}}, \frac{P_{OP}}{P_{HC}},$$

$$\frac{P_{HC}}{P'_H}, \frac{P_{NH}}{P_{HC}}, MAR, FAM)$$

$$(25) \quad P_{HC} = 0.01 P_{DO} + 0.032 W_N$$

Market for Manpower Services

Services by Professional Nurses

$$(26) \quad N^D = f(PD_H, PD_{NH}, OPV, DOV, HC, SC, W_N, \frac{W_{par}}{W_N},$$

$$\frac{W_{MDp}}{W_N})$$

$$(27) \quad N^S = KS_N$$

$$(28) \quad S_N = S_{N-1} + \Delta S_N$$

$$(29) \quad \Delta S_N = G + M_N - R$$

$$(30) \quad G = f(\frac{W_N}{W_T}, HSG_{-3}, SCH)$$

$$(31) \quad M_N = f(\frac{W_N}{W_c} - 1)$$

$$(32) \quad R = f(N_{60}, \frac{W_N}{RET}, \frac{W_N}{CPI})$$

$$(33) \quad K = f(SMY, \frac{W_N}{CPI}, \frac{W_N}{W_T})$$

Services by Practicing Clinical Physicians

$$(34) \quad HRS_{MD}^D = f(PD_H, PD_{NH}, OPV, DOV, HC, W_{MD_p}, \frac{W_{MD_p}}{W_{par}},$$

$$\frac{W_{MD_p}}{W_N})$$

$$(35) \quad HRS_{MD}^S = HRS/MD_p \cdot MD_p$$

$$(36) \quad HRS/MD_p = f(\frac{W_{MD_p}}{CPI})$$

$$(37) \quad MD_p = MD_{p-1} + \Delta MD_p$$

$$(38) \quad \Delta MD_p = MSG + RMG_N - \Delta MD_{NP} - DR$$

$$(39) \quad MSG = MSE_{-4} - D_{-\Sigma 4}$$

$$(40) \quad MSE = MSC$$

$$(41) \quad MSC = MSC_{-1} + \Delta MSC$$

$$(42) \quad \Delta MSC = 0.014 MSC_{-1}$$

$$(42a) \quad \Delta MSC = \frac{SUB}{\$30,000}$$

$$(43) \quad D_{-\Sigma 4} = 0.11 \; MSE_{-4}$$

$$(44) \quad FMG_N = f(\frac{W_{MD_p}}{W_{FOR}} - 1)$$

$$(45) \quad DR = 0.02 MD_p$$

Services by Paramedical Personnel

$$(46) \quad PAR^D = f(PD_H, PD_{NH}, OPV, DOV, HC, W_{par}, \frac{W_{par}}{W_N}, \frac{W_{MD_p}}{W_{par}})$$

$$(47) \quad PAR^S = f(\frac{W_{par}}{W_R}, \frac{W_{par}}{CPI})$$

List of Variables

Endogenous

C	construction and equipment cost per bed of U.S., non-federal, short-term, general and other special hospitals
$D_{-\Sigma_4}$	number of dropouts per thousand population from medical school class entering four years previously
DEP	total depreciation charges per year in U.S., non-federal, short-term, general and other special hospitals
DOV	number of doctors' office visits per thousand population per year
DR	number of practicing physicians per thousand population died or retired
ΔMD_p	increase in number of practicing physicians per thousand population
ΔMSC	increase in number of first-year medical school spaces per thousand population
ΔS_N	increase in stock of nurses per thousand population
FMG_N	net inflow of foreign medical school graduates per thousand population
G	number of nursing school graduates per thousand population
HC	days of home care received per thousand population
HRS_{MD}	annual hours of patient care by practicing physicians per thousand population
HRS/MD_p	annual hours of patient care by practicing physicians per physician
K	proportion of stock of nurses actively employed as nurses
M_N	net immigration of foreign-trained nurses per thousand population
MC	contribution of medical care sector to GNP
MD_{HP}	number of physicians with hospital practice per thousand population (interns, residents, and hospital staff physicians)
MD_p	number of practicing physicians per thousand population

MD_{pp}	number of physicians in private practice per thousand population
MSC	total first-year medical school spaces per thousand population
MSE	number of first-year medical school entrants per thousand population
MSG	number of medical school graduates per thousand population
N	number of employed nurses per thousand population
OCC_H	occupancy rate in U.S., non-federal, short-term, general and other special hospitals
OCC_{NH}	occupancy rate in nursing homes
OPV	number of outpatient visits per thousand population
P_{DO}	price per doctor's office visit
P_H	hospital charge per patient day
P'_H	hospital charge per patient day plus separate billings by physicians and surgeons
P_{HC}	cost of a day of home care
P_{MC}	Laspeyres medical care price index (1960 = 1.00)
P_{OP}	price of an outpatient visit
PAR	number of employed paramedical personnel per thousand population
PD_H	hospital patient days per thousand population
PD_{NH}	nursing home patient days per thousand population over age sixty-five
R	number of nurses retiring and dying during current year per thousand population
S_H	stock of hospital beds per thousand population
S_H^*	desired stock of hospital beds per thousand population
$S_H^{*\#}$	shortage of hospital beds per thousand population
S_N	stock of trained professional nurses per thousand population
S_{NH}	stock of nursing home beds per thousand population over age sixty-five

S^*_{NH}	desired stock of nursing home beds per thousand population over age sixty-five
$S^{*\,\#}_{NH}$	shortage of nursing home beds per thousand population over age sixty-five
V	current undepreciated value of fixed hospital assets
W_{MD_p}	weekly income of practicing physicians
W_N	weekly income of nurses
W_{par}	weekly income of paramedical personnel

Exogenous

AGE	proportion of population over age sixty-five
AVG_H	average size of short-term hospitals (in beds)
AVG_{NH}	average size of nursing homes
CPI	consumer price index
ΔMD_{NP}	increase in the number of non-practicing physicians per thousand population
FAM	average family size
HSG	female high school graduates per thousand population
INS_{DO}	proportion of the population covered by insurance for doctors' office visit fees
INS_H	proportion of the population covered by hospitalization insurance
INS_{HC}	proportion of the population covered by insurance for the costs of home care
INS_{OP}	proportion of the population covered by insurance for outpatient visits
L	average lifetime of hospital physical assets, in years
MAR	proportion of females over age fourteen who are married
MIX	short-term hospital service mix
N_{60}	proportion of employed nurses over age sixty
P_{con}	construction cost index

P_{NH}	price of a nursing home patient day
POP_{65}	thousand population over age sixty-five
POP	thousand population
RET	weekly retirement benefits (Social Security)
SC	number of public school children per thousand population
SCH	nursing school scholarships as proportion of tuition covered
SEX	proportion of the population over age fourteen which is male
SMY	proportion of S_N married and under age forty
SUB	federal subsidies to aid medical school construction
URB	proportion of the population urban
W_c	weekly wage paid to professional nurses in Canada
W_{FOR}	weekly income of physicians practicing in foreign countries
W_R	weekly income of retail trade personnel
W_T	weekly income of schoolteachers
WEL	public assistance for medical purposes per thousand population
Y	median family income

NOTES

1. Paul J. Feldstein, "Research on the Demand for Health Services," *Milbank Memorial Fund Quarterly* 44, no. 3 (July 1966):128–62, provides a more complete discussion of the factors influencing physicians' choice of treatment methods, as well as a review of research on patient characteristics.

2. National Center for Health Statistics, *Characteristics of Residents in Institutions for the Aged and Chronically Ill*, ser. 12, no. 2 (Washington, D.C.: U.S. Department of Health, Education, and Welfare, 1963), Table 1, p. 22.

3. *Medical Economics*, December 11, 1967, p. 75.

4. A. S. Goldberger, *Econometric Theory* (New York: John Wiley and Sons, 1964), pp. 197–98.

Peter E. de Janosi
The Ford Foundation

COMMENT

In contrast to macroeconomic Keynesian models which tend to fall into a broadly standardized pattern, specific sector or industry models are being constructed in a great variety of forms. Industry models, it appears, depend very much on the objectives of the model builder, on the underlying accounting scheme, and on the nature and organization of the industry. Macromodels or industry models alike, however, do share one characteristic: they offer a description of economic activity in terms of a system of mathematical equations. And with the help of statistics – theory and data – empirical content is given to the system, which in turn has its basis in economic theory.

I

The formulation of various types of equations making up the system – specification – involves the translation of propositions derived from economic theory into explicit mathematical relationships. But the equations (or the model) are not meant to include all conceivable variables, and even the best and most complete system must always remain an abstraction of the workings of the real world.

The choice of variables is rarely settled by theoretical considerations alone, as economic theory unfortunately does not offer us enough guidance, especially in health economics. Thus the model-builder should and does test a number of alternative formulations, and he is wise to remain flexible and open-minded during the specification process. Specification will also require a statement about the exact form of the mathematical equation (e.g., linear, logarithmic, parabolic). While at one time computational convenience was perhaps the model-builder's prime consideration, the existence of high-speed computers now permits him more latitude.

191

The model Feldstein and Kelman have specified is first of all a large one, embodying a wide variety of theoretical considerations and formulations. The over-all medical care sector is divided into several markets for care and manpower services, and in each there are demand and supply equations for short-term general hospitals, nursing homes, doctors' offices, outpatient clinics, home care, professional nurses, practicing clinical physicians, and paramedical personnel.

For each of these separate though related markets Feldstein-Kelman have postulated certain relationships, and perhaps it is here that one can make some initial comments about the choice of variables. I hesitate to do so because I realize that it is easy to suggest variables in addition to those proposed by Feldstein-Kelman. Thus, for example, nowhere in the model can one find variables measuring the use of drugs or the use of medical capital equipment. But to suggest that some variables ought to be included is not helpful; the critical question is whether other variables would be useful and effective. And an answer to this question cannot be given in the abstract.

The Feldstein-Kelman declamatory approach to the specification process unfortunately invites the kind of discussion I am hesitant about. They have specified by decree, and are not sufficiently sensitive to the tentative nature of what economic theory has to offer in the health field. At the same time it is surprising that they give little indication that they have considered the respectable amount of empirical work that has been accumulating in the health care sector. A willingness to draw on existing knowledge and to experiment with alternative uses of variables is sorely missed.

Another general question concerns the rationale for the authors' choice of five institutional settings in which medical care is supplied and demanded. How independent are the markets and how meaningful is it to analyze them separately? It should be noted that Feldstein-Kelman are careful to allow for a degree of interdependence between the institutional settings – for example, through an insurance coverage variable – but it would be helpful to have an explicit consideration of the pros and cons for using these five institutional settings before a large general model is estimated.

Of the five markets the short-term general hospital subsector receives the most careful and ingenious attention. For example, the treatment of hospital beds in terms of a stock adjustment model may well show considerable advantages over a more conventional economic approach. Yet it also should be pointed out that the explanatory variables – income, age, insurance, etc. – appear to influence directly only the desired stock of the hospital beds; their impact on the occupancy rate is consequently exerted through the stock equation. We will have to await empirical tests before we know whether doing so will yield good results.

Let me skip to two other sectors. First a minor point on the supply and demand for doctors' office visits: equation 18 is formulated to explain the demand for doctors' office visits per thousand of population (DOV^D) per year with twelve explanatory variables. The complexity of this equation is staggering, and one naturally wonders about the explanatory strength of some of the variables. It was also surprising to note that the dependent variable was measured per thousand of population, yet one of the explanatory variables — income — was simply median family income. Either the labeling is incorrect, or some adjustment ought to be made for the fact that the scales of the two variables are different.

The other sector I want to comment on is the demand and the supply sector for professional nursing services. It appears that the supply equation 27 as shown in the paper gives a misleading impression of simplicity. It is simply a definitional, not a behavioral, equation. If one substitutes into K (percentage of nurses actively employed) and S (trained professional nurses per thousand of population), the behavioral equations explaining K and S, the result will be a rather complex equation. Indeed, it has a curious form and shape and certainly is not a linear equation at all.

II

Under "normal" circumstances a model-builder will confront the system of equations with data of time series and/or cross-sectional nature. This confrontation and the estimation of the parameters are of great interest, and indeed proper estimation techniques have been favorite subjects for econometricians. We need not go into these topics here; it is enough to say that Feldstein-Kelman will have to face the issues sooner or later, and there is little doubt they will do so well. Yet I cannot help but wish that in this paper they had been more explicit about the stochastic nature of the equations and about the statistical problems.

Be that as it may, Feldstein-Kelman face two immediate problems: one is that much of the data simply are not available; the second is that the statistical estimates were not ready for the conference even where data were available. Knowing the authors' ingenuity, I assume that they will overcome the former problem as easily as the latter.

In closing, let me raise and answer tentatively two broader questions that arise from reading the Feldstein-Kelman paper. The first of these deals with sensible (I purposely do not say optimal) research strategy in model-building. Should one start with small models, or is it better to take the plunge and build a large one? I am not aware of the existence of any rational guidelines that will help to answer the question, but the Feldstein-Kelman model in its present form seems to at least one reader too large, given the current state of knowledge and our data base. The second issue of concern is what we might ultimately learn about the health care industry with models. The Feldstein-Kelman model in its present incarnation has not yet offered new economic insights, but I continue to be hopeful that further model explorations (on a bit less grandiose scale and with greater empirical content) will produce small but positive bits of information about what we do know and what we do not know. In model-building the proof of the pudding is not only in the eating but also in the cooking.

W. John Carr
Harvard University

ECONOMIC EFFICIENCY IN THE ALLOCATION OF HOSPITAL RESOURCES: CENTRAL PLANNING VS. EVOLUTIONARY DEVELOPMENT

A great deal of effort has been expended in recent years to improve the allocation of hospital resources through the establishment and operation of area-wide planning agencies.[1] The use of centralized planning bodies of this sort to influence or direct the allocation of resources among otherwise independent organizational entities is certainly at variance with traditional American reliance upon market forces to assure efficient production and distribution by competing firms. The question thus arises: under what sets of conditions may central planning and control rather than market methods of allocation result in a more efficient distribution of hospital resources?

In order to shed some light on this question, two basic types of economic models will be constructed in this paper, one of a completely centralized planning system and the other of a pure market system. Simulation analysis will be utilized to determine the relative efficiency of these two methods of resource allocation under conditions likely to be encountered in the hospital field.

Under the central planning system, decisions regarding hospital size and location will be made on the basis of parameter estimates which contain errors. In contrast, under the market system, decisionmakers will be assumed

This research was sponsored by Grant HM 00302-02, U.S. Public Health Service. The advice and encouragement of Gerald D. Rosenthal, Project Director, are gratefully acknowledged. Funds were also provided by Grant CRD-457-8-303 from the Social Security Administration. Thanks are due to Paul J. Feldstein for valuable comments. D. A. Breault was primarily responsible for the computer programming required by this study, and additional programming aid was received from H. A. Droge and Gregory George. The project has also benefited from the research assistance of Marjory Markel, Carl Penndorf, and Richard Boleman.

to have no knowledge of the relevant economic parameters, size and location being determined by an evolutionary trial-and-error process.[2]

PLANNING MODEL

Assumptions

In order to construct the planning and market models, it will be necessary to identify the services produced by hospitals, draw from the conclusions of positive economics regarding their demand and supply, and specify the effect of alternative production arrangements on welfare. For simplicity, only three basic types of services produced by short-term general hospitals will be considered: (1) inpatient care, (2) outpatient care, and (3) visits to inpatients.* In addition, the assumption will be made that hospital care is differentiated in such a way that J distinct types of service may be distinguished on the basis of medical quality, degree of amenity provided, ethnic atmosphere, and the like.

With regard to demand, it will be assumed that potential consumers of inpatient care, outpatient care, and visits to inpatients are uniformly (or randomly) distributed over an unbounded flat plane with density D persons per square mile. The aggregate demand for each of these services will be considered constant with parameters U_I, U_O, and U_v representing utilization rates in patient days, outpatient visits, and visits to inpatients, respectively, per person per year.†[3] An equal number of persons in any given area will be considered to have an absolute preference for each of the J types of services mentioned above. Within each of the J categories, consumers of inpatient and outpatient care will select the alternative having the lowest effective price, while visitors will travel from the (residential) locations to which the patients they visit have been assigned.‡[4]

The cost of hospital services will be divided into hospital and travel components. It will be assumed that each of the J types of service must be produced in a different hospital and, for simplicity, that there are no hospital cost differences attributable to them. So far as the hospital cost function is concerned, although many problems of adjusting for qualitative differences in output remain, there is a fairly substantial amount of statistical evidence that

---

*Hospitals also produce services such as education, research, and opportunities for the expression of altruistic behavior.

†The actual demand for these services is undoubtedly affected by price and other variables.

‡The term "visitors" will include patients' physicians as well as their friends and relatives. A study of the Hospital of the University of Pennsylvania has indicated that the proportion of trips made by inpatients, physicians, and other visitors is approximately constant regardless of distance to the hospital, which suggests that the latter groups travel, on the average, about the same distance as the patients they visit.

the average cost curve for inpatient care is U-shaped, reaching a minimum at an average daily census level of about 200 to 350.[5] Assuming that the marginal cost of both outpatient visits and visits to inpatients is constant, this function may be represented by the equation:

$$(1) \qquad C_H = A_1 + B_o I + C_o O + D_o V + E_1 I^2,$$

where C_H is total cost incurred by the hospital, I is number of patient days of inpatient care, O is number of outpatient visits, V is number of visits to inpatients, and $A_1, B_o, C_o, D_o,$ and E_1 are parameters of the equation. Since it will be shown that these services are produced in fixed proportion, this equation may be reduced to:

$$(2) \qquad C_H = A_1 + B_1 S_{PD} + E_1 S_{PD}^2,$$

where $B_1 = B_o + C_o O/I + D_o V/I$ and S_{PD} is size in terms of inpatient days. Dividing by S_{PD} to obtain average cost per unit of composite output,*[6] we obtain:

$$(3) \qquad C_{H_A} = A_1 S_{PD}^{-1} + B_1 + E_1 S_{PD}.$$

The travel cost incurred by inpatients, outpatients, and visitors may be divided into distance-related, time-related, and terminal components.[†] It will be assumed that straight-line travel is possible in any direction and that cost per unit distance may be represented by:

$$(4) \qquad C_{x_1} = C_{x_o} + 2\frac{C_t}{RT}\left(\frac{1}{L} + \frac{U_o + U}{U_I}\right),$$

---

*Another factor which should be taken into account is cost arising from the residential location preferences of hospital employees. However, under certain plausible conditions this cost will tend to be constant per unit of composite output.

†Assuming an automobile is used, the distance-related component would consist primarily of the marginal cost of automobile operation and certain road costs; the time-related component would consist mainly of the value of time spent in traveling; and the terminal component, which will be considered constant per unit output and ignored herein, of parking charges and the like.

A theoretical analysis of the value of time has been formulated by Gary S. Becker.[7] Unfortunately, the psychological qualities ascribed to time by this theory are wholly inaccurate, and it has led to the erroneous belief that in the absence of certain rents, externalities, and discontinuities, the value of time in all uses must be equal to the wage rate.

Clearly, one may be willing to pay twenty dollars per hour to avoid sitting in a dentist's chair (with the dentist drilling) at the margin but may require payment of two dollars per hour at the margin to leave a beach (on a warm day). Now, substitute sitting

where C_{x_1} is total travel cost per mile, C_{x_0} is distance-related travel cost per mile, C_t is time-related travel cost per person per hour, L is length of inpatient stay in days, R is rate of speed in miles per hour, and T is number of one-way trips per inpatient day, given by:

$$(5) \qquad T = 2 \left(\frac{1}{L} + \frac{U_o}{U_I} + \frac{U}{P_v U_I} \right) ,$$

where P_v is number of persons per visitor trip.*

Under conditions of perfectly inelastic demand, the entire resource-allocation welfare effect of a difference in cost may be related to the resources drawn away from other areas of the economy. Cost per unit output will thus be used as an index of welfare (and price will be set equal to average cost), but it should be emphasized that the results of the analysis are subject to numerous qualifications of welfare economics.[8]

Construction of Model

Under the above assumptions, it may be shown that the optimal hospital service areas are hexagon-shaped and arranged in a honeycomb pattern, under certain conditions, and that there will be J such independent systems of hospitals.[9] Given the shape of the service area, it is possible to find the relationship between the average distance traveled and the hospital size, and thus to calculate aggregate (hospital plus travel) cost per unit output in terms of size (S_{PD}) and the environmental parameters $(A_1, B_1, T, C_{x_1}, U_I, D, J,$ and E_1).[10]

The size of a hospital will be equal to the size of the area it serves times the density of the population it serves (D/J) times the utilization rate (U_I). In the case of a hexagon:

$$(6) \qquad S_{PD} = 2\sqrt{3} \, \frac{U_I D Y_H^2}{J} ,$$

where Y_H is the distance from the center of the hexagon to the nearest point of any side.

---

in a dentist's chair (without novocain) for work and find a wage rate (W) and hours of work that will make an individual indifferent with equal income between this alternative and his present employment. If he accepts the alternative, will he act as if the value of time in all uses is W?

In seeking to maximize utility, an individual may be thought of as balancing off various monetary and nonmonetary costs and benefits. The benefits need not accrue in the same time periods in which the costs are incurred. For these reasons the value of time in different uses, as conventionally measured, will not generally be equal.

*For simplicity, the number of persons per inpatient trip and per outpatient trip is assumed equal to 1.

The average distance traveled by patients and their visitors is equal to:*

(7)
$$X_H = \frac{4 + 3 \ln 3}{6 \sqrt{3}} Y_H.$$

Substituting this value of X_H in the equation for average travel cost per patient day:

(8)
$$C_T = TC_{X_1} X_H,$$

we obtain:

(9)
$$C_T = \frac{4 + 3 \ln 3}{6 \sqrt{3}} TC_{X_1} Y_H.$$

In order to find the average travel cost in terms of hospital size, we may solve equation 6 for Y_H and substitute the resulting value in equation 9.

Setting $K_1 = \dfrac{4 + 3 \ln 3}{6 \sqrt{2} \sqrt[4]{27}}$:

(10)
$$C_T = K_1 TC_{X_1} \left(\frac{U_I D}{J}\right)^{-\frac{1}{2}} S_{PD}^{\frac{1}{2}}.$$

Adding the average hospital and travel components of cost (C_{H_A} and C_T) to obtain aggregate average cost (C_A):

(11) $C_A = A_1 S_{PD}^{-1} + B_1 + K_1 TC_{X_1} \left(\dfrac{U_I D}{J}\right)^{-\frac{1}{2}} S_{PD}^{\frac{1}{2}} + E_1 S_{PD}.$

The size at which the cost associated with hospitalization is minimized may be determined by setting the derivative of C_A with respect to S_{PD} equal to zero and solving the resulting equation transformed to a quartic, by radicals:

(12)
$$S_{PD} = \left[\frac{\sqrt{u} + \left(\dfrac{2w}{A_1 \sqrt{u}} - u\right)^{\frac{1}{2}}}{2}\right]^{-2}$$

*This equation is derived in the Appendix to this paper.

where

$$(13) \qquad u = v - \frac{4}{3} \frac{E_1}{A_1 v},$$

$$(14) \qquad v = \left[\frac{1}{2} \left(\frac{w}{A_1}\right)^2 + \sqrt{\frac{1}{4} \left(\frac{w}{A_1}\right)^4 + \frac{64}{27} \left(\frac{E_1}{A_1}\right)^3} \right]^{\frac{1}{3}},$$

and

$$(15) \qquad w = \frac{K_1}{2} TC_{x_1} \left(\frac{U_I D}{J}\right)^{-\frac{1}{2}}. *$$

---

*The second-order condition for a minimum is:

$$(16) \qquad S_{PD} < \left(\frac{8A_1}{K_1 TC_{x_1}}\right)^{\frac{2}{3}} \left(\frac{U_I D}{J}\right)^{\frac{1}{3}}.$$

The problem of minimizing aggregate average cost in the more general case of price-responsive demand (with an L-shaped firm cost curve and hexagonal market area) has been considered by Mills and Lav,[11] but the conclusions they reach are incorrect because transportation cost is not included in the analysis except as a determinant of quantity demanded.

There also appears to be some confusion regarding the criteria that should be used to determine an optimal level of output and allocation of resources in this case. This problem may be approached in the following manner. Assume that price discrimination is utilized to offset marginal travel cost so that each consumer pays the same effective price. Average cost per unit output (C) – consisting of firm and travel components – may then be regarded as a function of firm size (S) and quantity demanded per consumer (Q):

$$(17) \qquad C = f(S,Q)$$

Determine optimal firm size by setting the derivative of C with respect to S equal to zero:

$$(18) \qquad \frac{\partial C}{\partial S} = f_S(S,Q) = 0.$$

Introducing this size into equation 17 after multiplying by S, taking the derivative of CS with respect to Q to obtain expected long-run marginal cost, and setting it equal to price (P):

$$(19) \qquad \frac{\partial CS}{\partial Q} = f_Q(S_{f_S(S,Q)=0}, Q) = P.$$

Solving this equation and the demand equation $P = g(Q)$ simultaneously for P and Q, we obtain a Pareto-optimal solution, provided the other conditions for Pareto optimality are satisfied. Cases in which the population is mobile would, in principle, require a tax equal to marginal travel cost in order to ensure an efficient distribution of residential locations.

Estimates of Environmental Parameters

Estimates of average values of the environmental parameters to be utilized in the analysis may be found in Table 1. So far as possible, these refer to the conterminous United States and to non-federal, short-term, general and special hospitals other than psychiatric hospitals in 1963.

Monte Carlo Analysis

If the values of the parameters were known with certainty, the size obtained by solving equations 12–15 would minimize the cost of hospitalization. But planners are usually presented with estimates of parameters which are subject to random error and which may be biased. In this case, the value of size obtained by solving equations 12–15 will, in general, not be optimal, and higher costs will be incurred because the hospitals constructed will be too large or too small.

In order to investigate the effect of errors in the estimates of the parameters upon cost, it will be assumed that the estimated values of the parameters shown in Table 1 are true values known with certainty. Independent, normally distributed random errors, with zero mean and given variance, will be added to the assumed true values of the parameters, the degree of error being measured by the ratio of the standard error of the estimate to the parameter mean, herein termed the coefficient of variation of the estimate (CVE). By repeatedly introducing these erroneous estimates into equations 12–15, solving for size, introducing the solution into equation 11 along with the assumed true values of the parameters, and solving for cost, it is possible to determine the average effect of the errors on size and cost.*

---

*The rationale for using equations 12–15 to determine optimal size in the presence of errors in the estimates of the parameters is that the expected value of the derivative of cost with respect to size is equal to the derivative of the expected value.[12] However, the derivative of equation 11 will provide a biased estimate of the true derivative of cost in this case because it is a non-linear function of the individual parameters, and its expected value will thus not, in general, be equal to its true value. An additional bias will result if the estimates of the parameters entering this equation in a multiplicative manner are not statistically independent.

A correction for these biases may be made by using a Taylor series to obtain a polynomial approximation of the derivative of equation 11. The first n terms of the Taylor series will be a function of the means, variances, covariances, and higher order central moments and product central moments of the parameter estimates.[13] By introducing estimated values of the parameters into the Taylor series and subtracting the higher order terms from the first term, one may obtain a more nearly unbiased estimate of the derivative of cost.

Effects on welfare of incorrect estimates of aggregate demand resulting from errors in U_I and D will not be explicitly considered. It will be assumed that aggregate capacity can be appropriately increased or decreased at the indicated level of cost, which would be the average result under plausible assumptions. In the case of price-responsive demand, more meaningful measures of aggregate-capacity welfare effects could be obtained, but they would be small if errors in the demand-parameter and population-density estimates were small, as would be likely under conditions similar to those hypothesized here.

Table 1: Estimates of Environmental Parameters

Parameter	Symbol	Estimate	Source
(1)	(2)	(3)	(4)
Base Estimates			
Population density (persons per square mile)[a]			
City	D_1	16,014	b
Suburban	D_2	2,158	b
Rural	D_3	50	b
Inpatient utilization rate (patient days per person per year)	U_1	1.0386	c,d
Outpatient utilization rate (visits per person per year)	U_0	0.4602	c,d
Visitor utilization rate (visits per person per year)[e]	U_v	3.9643	c,d,f,g
Number of types of hospitals	J	4	g
Hospital constant cost (dollars per hospital per year)	A_1	155,979	h
Inpatient long-run marginal cost, constant component (dollars per patient day)	B_0	31.48	h
Outpatient long-run marginal cost (dollars per visit)	C_0	4.32	h
Visitor long-run marginal cost (dollars per visit)	D_0	0	g
Inpatient long-run marginal cost, variable component (dollars per patient day squared)	E_1	0.0000248	h
Total inpatient days	ΣI	192,905,000	c
Total outpatient visits	ΣO	85,471,000	c
Total visitors to inpatients	ΣV	736,291,000	c,f,g
Distance-related travel cost (dollars per mile)	C_{x_0}	0.0370	i
Time-related travel cost (dollars per hour per person)[j]	C_t	1.09	d,k
Length of inpatient stay (days)	L	7.6647	c
Rate of speed (miles per hour)	R	35	g
Persons per visitor trip	P_v	2	g
Constant	K_1	0.3772	—
Derived Estimates			
Aggregate long-run marginal cost, constant component (dollars per patient day)	B_1	33.39	—
One-way trips per patient day	T	4.9641	—
Aggregate travel cost (dollars per mile)	C_{x_1}	0.0921	—

[a]The city value is for Chicago, the suburban value is for Cook County excluding Chicago, and the rural value is for those parts of Illinois lying outside standard metropolitan statistical areas, all for 1960.

[b]U.S., Bureau of the Census, *County and City Data Book, 1967* (Washington, D.C.: U.S. Government Printing Office, 1967), pp. 2, 82, 92, 432, 448, 484.

[c]*Hospitals* 38, no. 15 (August 1, 1964):484, 504, 506, 520.

[d]U.S., Bureau of the Census, *Statistical Abstract of the United States, 1965* (Washington, D.C.: U.S. Government Printing Office, 1965), pp. 5, 11, 237.

[e]In calculating the visitor utilization rate, the figure of 1.79 (non-physician) visitor groups per inpatient day reported by Coughlin, Isard, and Schneider (see n. 4 to text) for the Hospital of the University of Pennsylvania was utilized along with an estimate of two adult-equivalent visitors per group.

[f]*Ibid.*, pp. 35, 48.

[g]Rough guess.

[h]Carr and Feldstein (see n. 5 to text) and American Hospital Association data. The figures shown are weighted averages of the five service-capability-group regression coefficients.

[i]Wilfred Owen, *The Metropolitan Transportation Problem*, 2d ed. (Washington, D.C.: The Brookings Institution, 1966), p. 125. The figure shown is an estimate of the marginal monetary cost per mile for automobile travel.

[j]An empirical estimate of the average relative value of time spent in commuting for upper-level English civil servants (46 per cent of the wage rate) by M. E. Beesley (see n. k below) was applied to the U.S. wage rate in manufacturing industries to calculate the value of time spent traveling to and from hospitals. Although the value of commuter time may tend to overstate the value of time spent making non-routine trips, it should be noted that trips to the hospital are often made under conditions of pain and anxiety. Also, the higher morbidity and rare fatalities that result as a direct consequence of the time required to get to hospitals should be taken into account. A review and discussion of estimates of the value of travel time may be found in James R. Nelson, "The Value of Travel Time," in *Problems in Public Expenditure Analysis*, ed. Samuel B. Chase, Jr. (Washington, D.C.: The Brookings Institution, 1968), pp. 78–126.

[k]M. E. Beesley, "The Value of Time Spent in Travelling: Some New Evidence," *Economica* 32, no. 126 (May 1965):174–85.

It was initially assumed that each of the derived parameters, A_1, T, C_{x_1}, U_I, D, and E_1, was subject to the same degree of error, the coefficients of variation of the estimate being set equal.* Independent, normally distributed random errors were added to the given parameter values, and the resulting estimates were utilized in equations 12–15 to obtain an estimate of optimal size. This estimate of size was then introduced into equation 11 along with the assumed true values of the parameters in order to determine the cost incurred. For each of the three hypothesized values of population density, the above process was iterated 10,000 times for each value of the coefficient of variation of the estimate from 0 to 0.5 in steps of 0.05.[†] The means and standard deviations of cost were then determined and are presented in graphic form in Figure 1. Lines *AA*, *BB*, and *CC* in each panel refer to the city, suburban, and rural population density levels, respectively.

*B_1 is not used in determining optimal size, and no error term was added to J because it may take only integral values.

[†]In the construction of the model, it was implicitly assumed that the parameters were positive, as negative values would be untenable or absurd. Positivity was assured in the Monte Carlo analysis by setting the value of each parameter equal to one one-hundredth of its assumed true value if it fell below that amount. As expected, this "Bayesian constraint" condition did not occur over the lower range of the CVE, but

Fig. 1. Relationship of cost of hospitalization (C_A) to coefficient of variation of estimate (*CVE*).

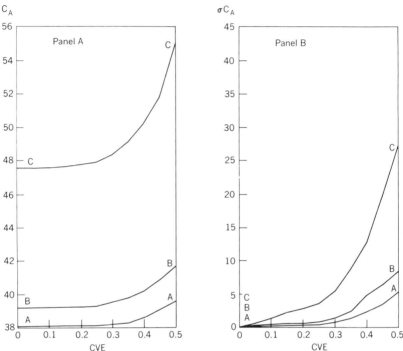

The relationships of average cost incurred under the planning model to the coefficient of variation of the estimate shown in Panel A of Figure 1 are interesting because they indicate that levels of error corresponding to CVEs of 0.25 or less have a rather small effect on cost. Above this level, cost climbs quite rapidly, however, particularly in the rural population density case.* One may also be interested in the standard deviation of aggregate cost, shown in Panel B of Figure 1, because presumably only one value of C_A would obtain in a given planning situation.

occurred in about 2.4 per cent of the cases at the 0.5 level of the CVE. Also, size was set equal to an average daily census of 1 if it fell below that amount. This condition, which could otherwise give rise to extremely high values of cost, occurred in only 0.003 per cent of all cases. Inequality equation 16 was also tested, but, as is intuitively evident, it was never violated.

*At first glance, the cost resulting from errors in the parameter estimates may appear rather low in the city and suburban cases. But it should be noted that each $2 per patient day amounts to about $400 million per year on a nationwide basis, an amount approximately equal to Harberger's 1954 per capita estimate of the allocative welfare loss due to monopoly in all manufacturing applied to the current population.[14]

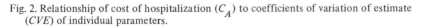

Fig. 2. Relationship of cost of hospitalization (C_A) to coefficients of variation of estimate (*CVE*) of individual parameters.

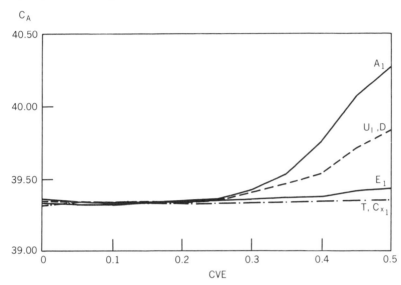

In order to determine the effect of errors in the individual parameters upon size and cost, the CVE relating to each individual parameter was stepped from 0 to 0.5, while the CVE's of all other parameters assumed subject to random error were held constant at 0.2 in each case. The average-cost results, which refer to the suburban population density level, are shown in Figure 2. Over the upper range of the CVE, errors in A_1 have the greatest effect upon C_A. Errors in U_I and D have an intermediate-level effect, and errors in E_1 and, particularly, in T and C_{x_1} have very little effect.

Errors in the parameter estimates may be broken down into systematic and random components. The systematic component or bias (of unknown direction or extent) may be reduced through better design of the statistical procedures utilized or improvements in the (economic) assumptions underlying their use. In the case of random variation, there is the possibility of trading increases in sampling cost for decreases in the cost of project operation. Monte Carlo analyses of the type conducted above should be of value in this regard because they make it possible to determine the relationship betewen the cost of project operation and the sample size, and thus the cost of sampling, relating to each parameter.

MARKET MODEL

In order to construct a simulation model of the market process from which estimates of cost and efficiency may be obtained, it will be necessary to make some assumptions about the market behavior of hospitals in addition to the assumptions already made about environmental conditions. Theoretical ideas relating to the market behavior of firms will thus be explored and, when feasible, examined, using hospital data.

Theoretical Considerations

We may approach the theoretical and empirical study of market allocation by asking two basic questions. First, is there any evidence that hospital facilities, in the fairly recent past, were efficiently (and systematically) distributed with respect to size and location? Second, assuming that there is some evidence for an efficient distribution, what factors account for the efficiency?

Since the model developed above describes a relationship between optimal size and the environmental parameters, the first question may be approached by determining whether the relationship defined by the model holds empirically. In order to do this, it will be necessary to take account of only those parameters which have a substantial effect upon optimal size and which vary greatly among hospitals or localities. Both population density (D) and the A_1 parameter of the hospital cost equation appear to meet these requirements.*

We will thus attempt to predict the size of hospitals from A_1 and D and will compare the relationship obtained with that indicated by equations 12–15. In order to accomplish this, E_1 in equations 12–15 will initially be assumed equal to zero. We then obtain:

$$(20) \qquad S_{PD} = \left(\frac{2A_1}{K_1 TC_{x_1}} \right)^{\frac{2}{3}} \left(\frac{U_I D}{J} \right)^{\frac{1}{3}}$$

Taking the logarithm of both sides and rearranging:

$$(21) \qquad \ln S_{PD} = \frac{2}{3} \ln \frac{2}{K_1 TC_{x_1}} + \frac{1}{3} \ln \frac{U_I}{J} + \frac{2}{3} \ln A_1 + \frac{1}{3} \ln D .$$

Thus, given values of S_{ADC} (size measured by average daily census), A_1, and D, we may fit a regression equation of the form:

$$(22) \qquad \ln S_{ADC} = a + b \ln A_1 + c \ln D.$$

If hospitals are efficiently distributed, we would expect the value of b to be 2/3 and the value of c to be 1/3 if E_1 is, in fact, zero (and there is little or

---

*One of the major conclusions of the cost study by Carr and Feldstein (see n. 5 to text) was that the value of A_1 increases with increased capability to provide a wide range of complex medical services. In other words, hospitals which are capable of providing a great variety of diagnoses and treatments exhibit a greater degree of initial economies of scale than those capable of producing only a relatively simple set of services. (Differences in A_1 were not considered in the Monte Carlo analysis primarily because it appears that variations in cost due to errors in the parameters attributable to differences in A_1 will largely cancel out in a given planning area.)

no substitution effect, associated in the model with variations in J correlated with D). However, a sensitivity analysis based upon equations 12-15 indicated that if E_1 has its estimated value, the value of b in equation 22 would be reduced to about 0.59, the relationship between A_1 and S_{ADC} remaining almost linear in the logarithms, and the value of c would be expected to lie somewhere between 0 and 1/3, depending on the size range covered. The value of a should then be greater than the value of the first two terms of equation 21 minus ln 365, or −4.7149, because size varies less with A_1 and D than indicated by that equation.

A regression in the form of equation 22 was fitted to 1965 data from 1,946 hospitals in 215 standard metropolitan statistical areas:*

(23) $\ln S_{ADC} = -3.4669 + 0.6669 \ln A_1 + 0.0560 \ln D$ $(R^2 = 0.709)$.
                    (0.0099)   (0.0103)

These results are broadly consonant with the hypothesis that hospital sizes are distributed efficiently, with 71 per cent of the variance of hospital size being related to differences in economies of scale and in population density.

Taking the above results as evidence for efficiency, let us proceed to ascertain its source. Following Alchian,[15] we may consider a process by which firms with differing characteristics are submitted to an economic environment for selection by survival. Adaptive behavior will be brought into the analysis by considering the results of imitation and rational thought.

There are both altruistic and egoistic motives leading to the creation of new hospitals and expansion of the capacity of old ones. These are reflected in the interests of the major groups of hospital decisionmakers: physicians, administrators, and trustee-philanthropists.[†] Whatever are the desires of these diverse individuals, their satisfaction is almost certainly dependent upon the utilization of constructed facilities. Furthermore, if constructed facilities are not utilized, there is the disutility associated with advocating or being involved in a project which fails.

Utilization is dependent upon either growth in demand (or current inadequacy of supply) or the achievement of greater efficiency than competing

---

*The hospital data were obtained from the American Hospital Association. The value of A_1 for each hospital was obtained by applying the reported number of facilities and services to constant-cost values derived (by linear interpolation) from the five service-capability-group regression equations in Carr and Feldstein (see n. 5 to text). Population density data for 1960 were obtained from U.S., Bureau of the Census, *County and City Data Book, 1967* (Washington, D.C.: U.S. Government Printing Office, 1967), pp. 432-63. The number in parentheses below each regression coefficient is the standard error of that coefficient. R^2 is the coefficient of determination.

†Joseph P. Newhouse has hypothesized that the consensual maximand (for nonproprietary hospitals) is a function of the quantity and quality of service produced. The values of quantity and quality are then determined by production tradeoff and indifference curves relating the two and a revenue constraint.[16]

institutions. As neither of these factors is predictable with certainty, those contemplating projects which would increase aggregate capacity must make decisions under conditions of risk. Such decisions, in principle at least, ought to be analyzable in terms of the von Neumann-Morgenstern utility index, in which different individuals have differing subjective probability distributions of potential outcomes, place different subjective values upon them, and have different attitudes toward risk as defined by their utility functions.[17] The amount of capacity constructed thus depends upon the supply of capital and entrepreneurial time. Entrepreneurship is likely to be supplied by those already engaged in the hospital field, while capital is available from a variety of sources.*

In order to determine the effects of some of the above factors upon the quantity of facilities constructed and to obtain an estimate of capacity expansion under conditions of constant utilization for the simulation analysis, hospital construction over the 1951-1960 decade was analyzed. The coefficients of a regression equation relating a bed construction variable to three independent variables were estimated, using state data.[†]

The dependent variable (BC) consisted of bed capacity in late 1950 plus beds constructed from late 1950 to late 1960 per thousand population in 1960 minus bed capacity per thousand population in late 1950. It thus represents the gross change in bed capacity per thousand population from late 1950 to late 1960.[‡]

The first independent variable (BR) was constructed to reflect the perceived need for additional bed capacity over the decade. It consisted of bed capacity per thousand population required to service the level of utilization in

---

*A recent survey has indicated that 28.4 per cent of all funds for hospital construction were obtained from private contributions, 22.6 per cent from long-term borrowing by the hospital, 19.3 per cent from federal grants under the Hospital Survey and Construction (Hill-Burton) Act, 13.7 per cent from bonded indebtedness of a taxing agency, 9.3 per cent from hospital reserves, and 6.7 per cent from other sources.[18]

[†] Data from each of the forty-eight conterminous states and the District of Columbia were utilized. Data relating to the District of Columbia, Maryland, and Virginia were combined because of the extent to which hospital service areas cross their borders.

[‡] The number of beds added was determined from changes in the number of beds reported to the American Hospital Association in each individual, non-federal, short-term, general and other special hospital over the 1951 to 1960 decade. Data for 1948, 1949, 1951, or 1952 were utilized for hospitals which did not report in 1950, and 1958, 1959, 1961, or 1962 data were utilized for hospitals which did not report in 1960. The bed capacity of new hospitals was determined at the time of entry or at the earliest possible year thereafter, and again in 1960 (or 1958, 1959, 1961, or 1962 if non-reported in 1960), so that subsequent increases in capacity could be accounted for separately. The hospital data were obtained from the Guide Issues of *Hospitals*, vols. 23-37 (1949-1963); the population data were obtained from U.S., Bureau of the Census, *Statistical Abstract of the United States, 1955* (Washington, D.C.: U.S. Government Printing Office, 1955), p. 14, and *Statistical Abstract of the United States, 1965*, p. 11.

late 1958 minus actual bed capacity per thousand population in late 1948.* (Each independent variable was lagged approximately two years to allow time for decision-making and construction.) If perception of the need for additional beds was correct on the average, the coefficient of this variable in the linear regression equation utilized should be close to +1.

The *BR* variable is, in part, a function of utilization, and its use in the regression equation which follows is thus subject to the criticism that utilization may be dependent upon bed capacity. The resolution of this issue, known as the Rosenthal-Roemer controversy, involves a number of difficult econometric problems and will not be considered in detail here.[19] However, given the widespread dislike of the hospital-patient role and the fact that cash is still a fairly important source of hospital payment, it appears that no capacity constraint on utilization need be invoked to explain current patterns of hospital use.[†]

The second independent variable (ΔU) consisted of the percentage change in total (*not* per thousand population) utilization from late 1948 to late 1958.[‡] It was hypothesized that the availability of entrepreneurial talent, hospital reserve funds, and borrowing capacity would be an increasing function of the size of the industry, while the amounts necessary to maintain a given rate of growth would be an increasing function of the growth rate itself. The expected sign of this variable was therefore negative.

*Under conditions of stochastic demand, the total number of beds required to provide comparable service for a given amount of utilization is a function of the sizes of hospitals because small hospitals must generally operate at relatively low levels of occupancy to maintain a given probability of running out of space. The average actual relationship between empty beds (*EB*) and bed capacity (*B*) was determined by Carr and Feldstein using 1963 data from 3,147 voluntary, short-term general hospitals:

$$(24) \qquad \ln EB = -0.1411 + 0.7191 \ln B \qquad (R^2 = 0.595).$$
$$(0.0106)$$

An assumed desired average number of empty beds in the hospitals of each state was determined from the 1958 average hospital daily census in the state and from equation 24. The average number of empty beds was then added to the 1958 average hospital daily census in the state, and this sum was multiplied by the number of hospitals to obtain an estimate of required bed capacity. Required bed capacity per thousand population in 1958 was then determined, and actual bed capacity in 1948 was subtracted from it to obtain the value of the *BR* variable.

The hospital data were obtained from the Guide Issues of *Hospitals*, vols. 23, no. 6 (June 1949):38, and 33, no. 15 (August 1, 1959):388; the population data were obtained from *Statistical Abstract of the United States, 1955*, p. 14, and from *Statistical Abstract of the United States, 1960*, p. 10.

[†]In a study of hospital care in New England in 1962 being conducted by Alex M. Burgess, Jr., W. John Carr, Osler L. Peterson, and Gerald D. Rosenthal, it was found that cash constituted 26.33 per cent of total payments for patient care.

[‡]Data were obtained from the Guide Issues of *Hospitals*, vols. 23, no. 6 (June 1949): 38, and 33, no. 15 (August 1, 1959):338.

The availability of capital from charitable, non-federal tax revenue and Hill-Burton sources was indicated by total per capita income over the 1949–1958 decade (Y).* On the assumption that the direct effect of income outweighs the negative relationship between income and Hill-Burton appropriations, the expected sign of this variable is positive.

The following regression results were obtained:

(25) $BC = 1.1303 + 1.0146\ BR - 0.01151\ \Delta U - 0.02961\ Y\ (\bar{R}^2 = 0.492).$[†]
$\qquad\qquad$ (0.2046)   (0.00260)   (0.01990)

As was anticipated, the coefficient of the BR variable was almost $+1$ and the coefficient of the ΔU variable was negative. Unexpectedly, the coefficient of the per capita income variable (Y) was negative, although not significantly different from zero. The negative sign may have occurred because the effect of Hill-Burton expenditures on hospital construction was greater than the direct effect of income or because construction cost is positively correlated with income.

In order to determine the rate of change in bed capacity when utilization remains constant, the values of BR and ΔU in equation 25 were assumed equal to zero, and Y was given its national average value. Dividing the resulting value of BC by 1950 bed capacity, we obtain an autonomous increase in capacity of about 19 per cent over the decade, or an annual rate of autonomous capacity growth of about 1.75 per cent.[‡]

According to Stigler's survivorship principle, changes of this sort should result in selection of the more efficient institutions for survival.[§][20] Effective operation of the survivorship mechanism, however, requires that patients (or someone involved in the hospital selection process, e.g., physicians) choose hospitals according to a set of consistent and transitive preferences.[‡] If com-

---

*Data were obtained from *Statistical Abstract of the United States, 1951*, p. 264; *Statistical Abstract of the United States, 1955*, p. 291; *Statistical Abstract of the United States, 1958*, p. 311; and *Statistical Abstract of the United States, 1960*, p. 312.

[†] $\bar{R}^2$ is the corrected coefficient of determination.

[‡] If utilization increases over time, the rate of growth in bed capacity in excess of that required by the growth of utilization will be reduced because the coefficient of ΔU has a negative sign. Substituting the national average values of all three independent variables in equation 25 and subtracting the national average value of BR from the resulting value of BC, we obtain a rate of excess growth of about 10 per cent over the decade, or a little less than 1 per cent on an annual basis. This suggests either that occupancy rates fell considerably over the decade or that bed capacity was taken out of hospital service. Direct comparison of the late 1950 to late 1960 hospital data used previously indicates that about 11 per cent of the bed capacity in existence in late 1950 or constructed from late 1950 to late 1960 was lost over the decade.

[§] It is important to distinguish, as Stigler does, between efficiency related to the viability of firms and social efficiency.

[‡] In view of the fact that a large proportion of hospital charges are incurred for "hotel service," routine nursing care, and the amount of time spent living in the hospital

petition is effective in this sense, one would expect high-cost hospitals to encounter financial difficulties and eventually change their characteristics or leave the industry. In order to investigate the effect of deviations from optimal size upon financial condition, it was initially assumed that the hospital industry was perfectly competitive within each product market and that all product-dependent cost variations were measured by the A_1 and B_1 terms of the hospital cost equation.

Under perfectly competitive conditions, net revenue per patient day (NR_{PD}) should be equal to cost per patient day at the optimal size level ($\hat{S}_{PD}$) minus cost per patient day at any given value of size (S_{PD}). Substituting values of $\hat{S}_{PD}$ and S_{PD} in equation 11 in turn (ignoring the E_1 term), subtracting cost at the given size level from cost at optimal size, and rearranging terms:

$$(26) \quad NR_{PD} = A_1(\hat{S}_{PD}^{-1} - S_{PD}^{-1}) + K_1 TC_{x_1} \left(\frac{U_I D}{J}\right)^{\frac{1}{2}} (\hat{S}_{PD}^{\frac{1}{2}} - S_{PD}^{\frac{1}{2}}).$$

Assuming that there is some approximation to perfect competition in the real world, a regression equation may thus be estimated in the form:

$$(27) \quad NR_{PD} = a + bA_1 (\hat{S}_{ADC^{-1}} - S_{ADC^{-1}}) + cD^{-\frac{1}{2}} (\hat{S}_{ADC^{\frac{1}{2}}} - S_{ADC^{\frac{1}{2}}}).$$

If net revenue generally decreases as hospitals deviate from optimal size, the values of b and c should be positive.

Utilizing data for the 1,946 hospitals used in deriving equation 23 and values of $\hat{S}_{ADC}$ predicted from that equation, we obtain:

$$(28) \quad NR_{PD} = -1.4028 + 0.001127 A_1 (\hat{S}_{ADC^{-1}} - S_{ADC^{-1}}) + 17.42D^{-\frac{1}{2}}$$
$$\qquad\qquad\quad (0.000468) \qquad\qquad\qquad\qquad\qquad\qquad (2.93)$$

$$(\hat{S}_{ADC^{\frac{1}{2}}} - S_{ADC^{\frac{1}{2}}}) \ (R^2 = 0.019).*$$

This equation indicates that to the extent that hospitals deviate from optimal size they generally encounter increasing financial difficulty.

---

environment, it seems reasonable to expect patients to develop preferences among hospitals. Furthermore, there is some evidence that patients take an active role in the hospital-choice process. In a recent study of a large eastern medical center, "patient contrivance" was found to be the most important factor in hospital choice for about one-half of the private and semi-private admissions.[21] In addition, physicians, as individual entrepreneurs, have an incentive to affiliate with hospitals which their patients or prospective patients prefer, in addition to taking account of their own personal preferences.

*The net revenue data utilized consist of gross (patient plus other) revenue minus total expense per patient day.

The above results lend support to the hypothesis that the survivorship principle is operative. More direct evidence may be found in Table 2, which portrays the transition probabilities of hospital bed capacity over the 1951 to 1960 decade. The rate at which the institutions in various ranges of bed capacity left the hospital field (i.e., were dropped from American Hospital Association registration as short-term institutions) ranged from about 35 per cent of all hospitals in the 6- to 24-bed class down to about 2 per cent in the 200- to 299-bed class and back up to about 7 per cent in the 500-bed and over group.* Although no adjustment was made for variations in effective (hospital plus travel) cost arising from the complexity of service provided or population density, it is quite evident that those hospitals in the general range of relatively low effective costs were best able to survive.

Table 2 also indicates the size distribution of increases in bed capacity for both new hospitals and additions to existing ones. About 32.5 per cent of the

Table 2: Transition Probabilities of Hospital Bed Capacity, 1951–1960[a]

Bed Capacity, 1951	Bed Capacity, 1960								
	0	6–24	25–49	50–99	100–199	200–299	300–399	400–499	500 and over
(1)	(2)	(3)	(4)	(5)	(6)	(7)	(8)	(9)	(10)
0	0	.16	.39	.25	.12	.05	.02	b	.01
6–24	.35	.39	.22	.04	b	0	0	0	0
25–49	.20	.05	.48	.25	.02	0	0	0	0
50–99	.09	b	.06	.56	.27	.01	b	0	0
100–199	.06	0	0	.05	.58	.26	.05	b	0
200–299	.02	0	0	.01	.09	.51	.25	.09	.03
300–399	.03	0	0	0	0	.12	.51	.28	.06
400–499	.05	0	0	0	.02	0	.07	.52	.34
500 and over	.07	0	0	0	.01	0	.01	.07	.85

[a]This table is based upon the late 1950 to late 1960 American Hospital Association data mentioned previously.

[b]Less than 0.005 but greater than 0.

*In 1965 about 50 per cent of all hospitals dropped from American Hospital Association registration simply went out of business, while 22 per cent were unable to meet even the minimal standards required for registration and had become hospitals only in a very marginal sense; see *Hospitals* 40, no. 15 (August 1, 1966): 436. (Merged hospitals were not assumed to have left the field for purposes of this paper.) For a statement of American Hospital Association registration requirements, see any recent Guide Issue of *Hospitals*. As might be expected, relatively new hospitals were particularly prone to the hazards of competition. About 24 per cent of all hospitals which left the field in the 1951–1960 decade were less than ten years old in late 1950 or were constructed between late 1950 and late 1960. In contrast, about 17 per cent of all hospitals extant in late 1960 were less than twenty years old at that time.

total growth in bed capacity over the 1951-1960 decade was provided by new hospitals (at time of entry) and about 66.5 per cent by additions to existing institutions.

In addition to the blind forces of the survivorship mechanism, imitation and rational thought may play a role in bringing about efficiency in the hospital care market. Existing firms which have survived the rigors of competition for long periods of time are likely to be more efficient on the average than entering firms with more widely varying characteristics. Thus imitation is likely to improve the chances for survival of new firms. Because of the substantial difficulties involved in distinguishing the effects of imitative behavior from other factors, no empirical study of imitation in the hospital field will be undertaken here, but a simple form of imitation will be built into one version of the simulation model.

Rational thought also undoubtedly plays a role in determining hospital size and location. As a simple example, it is most unlikely that a hospital operating at a much lower than optimal occupancy rate would expand bed capacity. It does not appear, however, that rational thought has extended to the explicit use of economic analysis in the selection of size and location, although some reasoning of this sort does occur.

Simulation Analysis

The complexity of the market process made the development of an algorithmic market resource allocation model infeasible. Therefore, a market simulation model was developed which, by its nature, could only be applied to a finite number of patients in a finite area. Thus the assumptions of the market model provide only an approximation to the assumptions of the infinte area, uniform population density planning model, but the differences (outlined below) should not affect the efficiency comparison very substantially.

So far as demand is concerned, patients were assumed to be distributed randomly (with given expected density) over a given square area.* As each patient (with randomly determined locational coordinates) entered the market over time, he selected a hospital among those not yet full (of the one of the four types preferred) for which the sum of hospital price and travel cost was minimum.

---

*Two assumptions of the planning model are violated here, but probably not too seriously. First, optimal hospital service areas within the hypothesized square area will not be hexagonal. Square service areas would be possible, however, and calculations indicate that travel costs incurred with square areas are only about 1.5 per cent higher than those incurred with hexagonal areas for a given firm size. Second, the random locational distribution of patients may affect the nature of the service areas somewhat and may result in a shift of optimal conditions between time periods.

On the supply side, the basic hospital and travel cost assumptions used in the planning model were assumed to obtain. In order to avoid the problem of simultaneous determination of price and output, hospital price was initially set equal to cost at bed capacity output levels, and total bed capacity was set equal to total quantity demanded. The simulation analysis was then run through a number of time periods, with additions to capacity, and in each successive time period hospital price was set equal to cost at the output level attained in the previous period.* Although this assumption was made primarily to avoid the simultaneous determination problem, it is also realistic in that there are time lags both in price changes and in responses to them.† In the initial model, hospital decisionmakers were assumed to act randomly or, with a minor exception, in a deterministic manner based only upon the present state of a firm parameter. This general type of behavior will be characterized by the term "perfect stupidity" to distinguish it from adaptive behavior.[22]

The hospitals were initially assigned locations with coordinates (latitude and longitude) drawn independently from a uniform probability distribution. Their sizes were determined from a negative exponential probability distribution, which was used because it is the uncertainty-maximizing distribution for a given total quantity of something (beds) distributed among a given number of individuals (hospitals).[23] The parameter of the negative exponential distribution, which determines the average value of hospital size, was selected arbitrarily, as noted below.‡ The size of a randomly selected hospital was adjusted so that total bed capacity equaled total quantity demanded.

In subsequent time periods, aggregate bed capacity was increased by the establishment of new hospitals and the expansion of the capacity of existing ones. In each case, the new hospitals were generated by the method outlined above. The average number of new hospital beds added in each time period was set equal to 32.5 per cent of the total number to be added, in accordance with the empirical relationship noted above. The remainder was distributed among previously existing hospitals in proportion to their bed capacities. The assets represented by bed capacity were assumed to require replacement after twenty years. Capacity in each hospital was replaced only to the extent that it would otherwise have fallen short of the patient census.

---

*For simplicity, it was assumed that the costs attributable to unutilized capacity in each time period and any profits or losses attributable to differences between prices and costs were reflected in hospital reserve accounts or in transactions with non-patient entities.

†Such delays may also occur in the planning system when parameter values change, but they are inherent in the operation of the market even when parameter values remain constant.

‡The upper end of the negative exponential distribution was truncated, so that no hospital with a bed capacity larger than 10 per cent of the total patient census was created.

Patients with newly selected random locational coordinates were assigned to the hospitals in each time period. Those hospitals which received no patients in a time period were assumed to have permanently left the field. In practice, the least efficient hospitals were found to leave the field very quickly.*

In each of the simulation analyses reported below, one day of experience was simulated every five years over two hundred years of time.† The travel plus hospital costs (*not* prices) incurred in providing patient care and the cost of additional facilities were calculated in each time period.

The first simulation analysis was based upon the experience of 4,314 patients per time period (enough to fill twenty-five hospitals of optimal hexagonal service area size) in the suburban population density case. The average size of newly entering hospitals was arbitrarily set equal to the optimal size (172.57 beds), and an increase in capacity of 0.1168 beds per unit patient census every five years was assumed in accordance with the above findings on autonomous growth. The patient-cost results of this simulation for the first hundred years of evolutionary experience are shown by Line *AA* in Figure 3.

Fig. 3. Relationship of patient cost to time and initial hospital size.

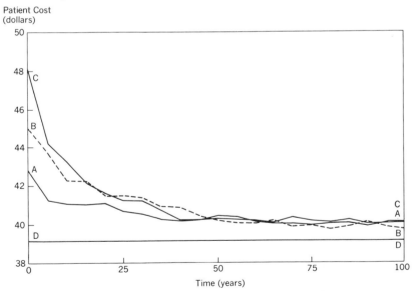

*A more realistic, and complicated, alternative would have involved basing survival on financial flows and a bankruptcy criterion. For the development of optimal firm strategy in this case, see Borch.[24]

†Note that the five-year time periods utilized imply a five-year lag in response to price determinants.

In addition to patient costs, average gross costs of $1.28 per patient day were incurred for facilities provided by autonomous growth and not required for the direct care of patients.* Part of these costs should be recoverable, particularly when hospitals go out of business before their assets are fully depreciated. Note, however, that an additional social disorganization cost is incurred when a hospital closes completely.

In order to assess the effect of differences in average initial hospital size upon cost, the initial size was set equal to one-half (86.28) and one-fourth (43.14) its optimal value. The results, shown by Lines *BB* and *CC*, respectively, in Figure 3, indicate that although costs in these cases were higher in the initial time periods, they declined to about the same average level.

On the assumption that the parameter values have remained constant and that the hospital market has had time to adjust to them, it is the long-run average equilibrium values which should be compared with the costs incurred under the planning method. In the final hundred years of market operation, average patient costs of $39.87 (standard error equals $0.01) were incurred in the above three simulations.† This compares with a cost of $39.26 under a perfect resource allocation system, shown by Line *DD* in Figure 3.

A second set of simulation analyses was undertaken to determine the effect of population density upon market efficiency. Patient costs for the rural, suburban, and city population density levels were $51.01 (standard error equals $0.05), $39.94 (standard error equals $0.02), and $38.49 (standard error equals $0.01), respectively, in the final hundred years of operation. Costs incurred under the corresponding perfect resource allocation systems would be $47.62, $39.26, and $38.06, respectively.

In order to determine the effects on patient costs of variations in the intensity of competition, additions to capacity were set equal to one-half, one, and two times the previously utilized empirically determined value. The resulting patient costs in the final hundred years were $40.27 (standard error equals $0.05), $39.94 (standard error equals $0.02), and $39.92 (standard error equals $0.02) in the suburban population density case. Thus, the increase in competitive pressure appeared to have an effect on patient cost over the lower range of intensity values, but not over the upper range. Increases in the intensity of competition are, of course, accompanied by proportional increases in the cost of additional facilities constructed (less whatever facility costs are recovered). There would, presumably, be some time distribution of competitive pressure for which the discounted sum of additional facility and

---

*A construction and equipment cost of $20,000 per bed was assumed.[25]

†The standard errors of cost presented in this section must be considered with caution because they are affected by autocorrelation. In the two-hundredth year the average hospital patient census was 205 (standard deviation equals 66) and the average hospital bed capacity was 246 (standard deviation equals 55).

patient cost is minimized.* The Hill-Burton program, assuming that it has some effect on the quantity of facilities constructed, provides a policy instrument for affecting the degree of competition.

The above simulation analyses were based upon the model characterized by perfect stupidity. In order to allow for adaptive behavior, simple forms of imitation and rational thought were added. Imitative behavior was provided by setting the size of each new hospital (after the initial time period) equal to the size of a randomly selected, previously existing institution. Rational thought was brought into play by increasing the capacity of only those hospitals which were full. Patient costs of $40.03 (standard error equals $0.01) were incurred in the suburban population density case with the empirically determined level of autonomous capacity growth. This compares with an average patient cost of $39.94 under the perfect stupidity assumption. This is a surprising result, with some rather bizarre implications for public policy.

Under current conditions, patients often pay only small proportions of their hospital bills personally and thus are less likely to choose efficient institutions. In order to determine the effect of "cost pass through" to insurance companies and other third-party payers, hospital price was set equal to 26.33 per cent of its previous value (the proportion found to be paid by cash). Patient cost in this situation was $40.01 (standard error equals $0.03), as compared with the $40.03 cost level attained in the comparable case above. Thus, third-party payment of this magnitude does not appear to have much effect on the efficiency attained.

CONCLUSIONS

The primary purpose of this paper was to compare the efficiency attainable under market and under planning resource allocation methods. It appears that at relatively low (but probably attainable) levels of parameter error, the planning method has the potential of being more efficient in a technical sense. But the alternative to the market is not some theoretically perfect planning scheme. It is, rather, a system of basing decisions on an abstraction of a complex reality operating within a political-bureaucratic context.

There are formidable technical difficulties involved in the construction of realistic planning systems. Reliable evidence on costs and consumer preferences must be obtained and combined to produce resource allocation decisions by some algorithmic or heuristic means. Furthermore, there is always the possibility that some important variable will be overlooked completely. The market, whatever its inefficiencies, has the advantage of automatic opera-

---

*In the biological case, the cost of achieving a given genetic change, in terms of the number of selective deaths required, is largely independent of the intensity of the process over a wide range.[26]

tion. The efficiency of bureaucratic planning organizations may also be questioned.[27] For example, it is well known that governmental regulatory agencies often, if not generally, favor the interests of producers in regulated industries over those of consumers.[28]

It is possible, of course, for these potential objections to be overcome, and a number of currently operating hospital planning groups appear to be doing so effectively. Furthermore, the absolute amount of potential savings which could result from an efficient planning system appears to be very large. But it is to be hoped that public policy measures will be judged on the basis of results rather than intentions.

APPENDIX

The hexagonal service area shown in Panel A of Figure 4 can be divided into sections such as ABC, shown in greater detail in Panel B. The average distance traveled by patients (X_H) may be found by taking the limit of the sum of the distances to the hospital, at A, times the elements of area in ABC and dividing by the total area (A_{ABC}). This may be readily accomplished by using polar coordinates.

Fig. 4.

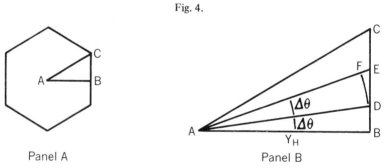

Panel A   Panel B

In the limit, as $\Delta\theta$ approaches zero, the area of sector ADF approaches $\frac{1}{2}Y_H{}^2 \sec^2 \theta \Delta\theta$. Likewise, the average distance traveled by patients within ADF approaches the distance from A to its centroid, $\frac{2}{3}Y_H \sec \theta \cos \frac{1}{2}\Delta\theta \dfrac{\sin \frac{1}{2}\Delta\theta}{\frac{1}{2}\Delta\theta}$. Multiplying the average distance traveled by the area of the infinitesimal element ADF and integrating from B to C:

$$(29) \quad X_H A_{ABC} = \frac{1}{3}Y_H{}^3 \int_0^{\frac{\pi}{6}} \sec^3 \theta \, d\theta$$

$$(30) \qquad = \frac{1}{6} Y_H{}^3 \left[\frac{\sin \theta}{\cos^2 \theta} + \ln \tan \left(\frac{\pi}{4} + \frac{\theta}{2} \right) \right]_{0}^{\frac{\pi}{6}}$$

$$(31) \qquad = \frac{4 + 3 \ln 3}{36} Y_H{}^3.$$

Dividing by the area of ABC, $(\sqrt{3}/6) Y_H{}^2$:

$$(32) \qquad X_H = \frac{4 + 3 \ln 3}{6 \sqrt{3}} Y_H.$$

NOTES

1. See James H. Cavanaugh, "The Rise of the Areawide Planning Agency: A Survey Report," *Hospitals* 39, no. 15 (August 1, 1965):52–56, for statistics on the growth and present extent of areawide planning activity.

2. Armen A. Alchian, "Uncertainty, Evolution, and Economic Theory," *Journal of Political Economy* 58, no. 3 (June 1950):211–21, provides a pioneering discussion of the role of the evolutionary process in economics.

3. See Gerald D. Rosenthal, *The Demand for General Hospital Facilities* (Chicago: American Hospital Association, 1964), for empirical evidence on the case of inpatient care.

4. See Robert E. Coughlin, Walter Isard, and Jerry B. Schneider, *The Activity Structure and Transportation Requirements of a Major University Hospital* (Philadelphia: Regional Science Research Institute, 1964), particularly pp. 42–44.

5. W. John Carr and Paul J. Feldstein, "The Relationship of Cost to Hospital Size," *Inquiry* 4, no. 2 (June 1967):45–65; Harold A. Cohen, "Variations in Cost among Hospitals of Different Sizes," *Southern Economic Journal* 33, no. 3 (January 1967):355–66; and Martin S. Feldstein, *Economic Analysis for Health Service Efficiency* (Amsterdam: North-Holland Publishing Co., 1967), particularly pp. 56–89. For references to studies reaching somewhat different conclusions, see Carr and Feldstein, "The Relationship of Cost to Hospital Size," p. 50, n. 11.

6. See Millard F. Long and Paul J. Feldstein, "Economics of Hospital Systems: Peak Loads and Regional Coordination," *American Economic Review* 57, no. 2 (May 1967):119–29, for an analysis in which costs arising from the stochastic nature of demand, ignored herein, are considered.

7. Gary S. Becker, "A Theory of the Allocation of Time," *Economic Journal* 75, no. 299 (September 1965):493–517.

8. E. J. Mishan, "A Survey of Welfare Economics, 1939–59," *Economic Journal* 70, no. 278 (June 1960):197–265. Of particular relevance here is the fact that the market prices of the factors of production may not reflect the value of their marginal products in all alternative uses; moreover, other conditions required for Pareto optimality may not be satisfied.

9. See Walter Christaller, *Die zentralen Orte in Süddeutschland* (Jena: G. Fischer, 1933), in which the advantages of a hexagonal market area were apparently first recognized (translated by Carlisle W. Baskin as *Central Places in Southern Germany* [Englewood Cliffs, N.J.: Prentice-Hall, 1966]; see, particularly, pp. 63–64 of the translation). A much more complete development of this idea was later presented by August Lösch, who concluded that under conditions of price-responsive demand and profit maximization, free entry would result in hexagon-shaped market areas and that these

areas would be optimal in the sense that demand per unit area would be maximized. See his *Die räumliche Ordnung der Wirtschaft* (Jena: G. Fischer, 1940), the second edition of which was translated by William H. Woglom as *The Economics of Location* (New Haven, Conn.: Yale University Press, 1954); see, particularly, pp. 105–14 of the translation. It has subsequently been proven that under Lösch's assumptions free entry need not result in hexagonal, or space-filling, market areas; see Edwin S. Mills and Michael R. Lav, "A Model of Market Areas with Free Entry," *Journal of Political Economy* 72, no. 3 (June 1964):278–88. In addition, Walter Isard has noted that under certain cost and demand conditions the hexagonal shape may not be optimal; see his *Location and Space-Economy* (Cambridge, Mass.: M.I.T. Press, 1956), pp. 242–43. But it appears likely that the conditions required for non-hexagonal market areas to be optimal will seldom be met in real-world situations, and the hexagonal shape will be assumed optimal in this paper.

10. See R. G. Bressler, Jr., *City Milk Distribution* (Cambridge, Mass.: Harvard University Press, 1952), pp. 244–51, and Jerzy Mycielski and Witold Trzeciakowski, "Optimization of the Size and Location of Service Stations," *Journal of Regional Science* 5, no. 1 (Summer 1963):59–68, for less complicated cost-minimization models somewhat similar to that constructed in this section.

11. Mills and Lav, "A Model of Market Areas."

12. See Harold Cramér, *Mathematical Methods of Statistics* (Princeton, N.J.: Princeton University Press, 1946), pp. 67–68, for a proof.

13. See A. A. Sveshnikov, ed., Scripta Technica, trans., *Problems in Probability Theory, Mathematical Statistics and Theory of Random Functions* (Philadelphia: W. B. Saunders Co., 1968), pp. 136–37, for an equation based upon the first three terms of the series.

14. See Arnold C. Harberger, "Monopoly and Resource Allocation," *American Economic Review* 44, no. 2 (May 1954):77–87.

15. "Uncertainty, Evolution, and Economic Theory."

16. See "Toward a Rational Allocation of Resources in Medical Care" (Ph.D. diss., Harvard University, 1968), pp. 39–70.

17. See C. Jackson Grayson, Jr., *Decisions under Uncertainty: Drilling Decisions by Oil and Gas Operators* (Boston: Division of Research, Harvard Business School, 1960), pp. 279–319, for an interrogative determination of the utility functions of business decisionmakers. The hospital case is more complicated in that potential outcomes are not readily measurable in common units of value (e.g., dollars), but this does not appear to be an insuperable problem.

18. See Jeffrey Lynn Stambaugh, "A Study of the Sources of Capital Funds for Hospital Construction in the United States," *Inquiry* 4, no. 2 (June 1967):3–22.

19. See M. W. Reder, "Some Problems in the Economics of Hospitals," *American Economic Review* 55, no. 2 (May 1965):472–80.

20. George J. Stigler, "The Economies of Scale," *Journal of Law and Economics* 1 (October 1958):54–71.

21. Raymond S. Duff and August B. Hollingshead, *Sickness and Society* (New York: Harper & Row, 1968), p. 112.

22. See Roy E. Murphy, Jr., *Adaptive Processes in Economic Systems* (New York: Academic Press, 1965), for an abstract treatment of evolutionary and adaptive mechanisms in economics. The properties of some general evolutionary models are explored in Lawrence J. Fogel, Alvin J. Owens, and Michael J. Walsh, *Artificial Intelligence through Simulated Evolution* (New York: John Wiley & Sons, 1966), and in Frederick E. Warburton, "A Model of Natural Selection Based on a Theory of Guessing Games," *Journal of Theoretical Biology* 16, no. 1 (July 1967):78–96.

23. See Nicolas Rashevsky, *Mathematical Biology of Social Behavior*, rev. ed. (Chicago: University of Chicago Press, 1959), pp. 72–75, for a derivation, which is formally identical with the derivation of the Boltzmann energy distribution.

24. Karl Henrich Borch, *The Economics of Uncertainty* (Princeton, N.J.: Princeton University Press, 1968), particularly pp. 181–201.

25. Millard F. Long, "Efficient Use of Hospitals," in *The Economics of Health and Medical Care*, ed. S. J. Axelrod (Ann Arbor: The University of Michigan, 1964), pp. 211-26.

26. J. B. S. Haldane, "The Cost of Natural Selection," *Journal of Genetics* 55, no. 3 (December 1957):511-24.

27. John Jewkes, *Public and Private Enterprise* (Chicago: University of Chicago Press, 1965), and John S. McGee, "Pricing in Publicly-Controlled Industries: U.S.A.," in *Price Formation in Various Economies*, ed. D. C. Hague (New York: St. Martin's Press, 1967), pp. 68-81.

28. See Ray H. Elling, "The Hospital-Support Game in Urban Center," *The Hospital in Modern Society*, ed. Eliot Freidson (New York: The Free Press of Glencoe, 1963), pp. 73-111, for an interesting account of how a series of citizens' committees were influenced by hospitals intent on achieving their own ends.

Jerome Rothenberg
Massachusetts Institute of Technology

COMMENT

First and foremost, despite some difficulties which I shall discuss, the Carr paper is a good one. It displays much highly imaginative work. It is ambitious and raises knotty but significant issues that will have to be faced if progress is to be made in research in this important area.

A. The central theme is the efficiency in the provision of hospital services of central planning compared with a form of competitive, decentralized decision-making like a free market. One is led to ask why the theme is relevant within the context of a market economy: what is there about the hospital sector that makes central planning a live issue?

Let us consider some reasons for preferring central planning to decentralized market planning in any sector within a market economy.

1. A sector contains a few units which are large in relation to the total size of the market area, and the basic investment has high durability. Thus entry is not free, mistakes by the existing large units can have a substantial effect on over-all sector performance, and such mistakes can take a long time to correct.

2. Important externalities are involved: some of the decision-making units in the sector can fail to take into account the full effects of their behavior upon other units in the sector.

3. Individual units do not possess enough information to enable them to achieve their own ends.

4. Individual units reveal systematic non-optimal behavior in terms of their own goals.

The relevance of these factors for the hospital service sector is as follows.

222

1. Significant fewness applies for small and moderate-sized communities, where the total number of hospitals is small, but this factor is less applicable for very large metropolitan areas with many hospitals.

2. Important externalities are involved in this sector: because of their locations, some hospitals affect the services of other hospitals.

3. The problem of securing information adequate for single-hospital-unit management seems to be unimportant.

4. Because of the internal structure of incentives, systematic and persistent departures from optimal behavior by individual hospitals may well be an important characteristic of the sector.

Thus, there are real grounds for asking whether central planning may not increase the efficiency of over-all resource use in the hospital sector. In his model Carr blurs this issue by assuming away the first and second characteristics and arguing that, in the presence of the evolutionary adaptation of his survivorship mechanism, the last characteristic is not important. His comparison may thereby pass by some of the key facets which make the basic theme relevant.

B. Carr's comparison is between the asymptotic performance of central planning and market analogue models, which may be seriously misleading. When adjustment processes take a long time, the appropriate criterion is present-discounted value, not asymptotic behavior. In Carr's comparison the evolutionary process shows substantial deviations for at least fifty years. We must not take the exact number of calendar years too seriously, but, given reasonable response lags and the high durability of plant capital, we should expect the adjustment process to be a very long one.

Asymptotic performance may be a good proxy for present-discounted value even where adjustment processes are long if the alternatives being compared have essentially the same time shape of adjustment toward their asymptotes, and if the parameters of the system change infrequently relative to the rate of adjustment to any change. In the systems being compared, the relative rates of adjustment differ extravagantly — indeed, excessively. Moreover, the parameters of the health care systems can be expected to vary considerably within periods of adjustment like those required in Carr's simulation process. Thus his basis of comparison is inappropriate.

If the basis is changed to that of present-discounted value, the outcome may be radically different from what Carr suggests. The evolutionary process looks considerably less efficient than the central planning model, even under Carr's characterization of the two. Moreover, we should in fact wish to see this characterization modified to permit a fairer comparison. The decentralized system shows an efficiency adaptation over time, and one would expect the central planning system to do so too. Central planners can be expected to learn from experience to correct notably poor information. Information adaptation will take place as a result of performance feedback. So, instead of being stationary, the planning process should show improvement over time. The addition of this improvement makes the evolutionary process look even more inferior.

C. The decentralized simulation model rests on the survivorship mechanism as the operational analogue of an actual market system. Carr asserts that all that is required for effective operation of the survivorship mechanism is that patients "choose hospitals according to a set of consistent and transitive preferences." This is not so. Over and above this, such choices must carry a bias that consistently favors the more efficient over the less efficient resource use – in particular, the more efficient over the less efficient hospital. There are reasons for believing that some of the biases are efficiency-irrelevant and some are even efficiency-decreasing. Mere survival and growth need not denote unambiguous improvements in efficiency. The survivorship mechanism cannot successfully carry an evolutionary hospital system toward improved efficiency because of inherent defects, four of which I shall discuss.

Effect of fewness. The two major policy variables for allocative efficiency treated in the model are hospital size and location. For both variables inefficiencies are transmitted through high costs, mediated by either underutilization or inefficient operation. The basic presumption of Carr's treatment is that hospitals displaying inefficiency will be squeezed out by the lower prices of better located and/or better sized hospitals. This is most likely to occur if there are many small hospitals in the community and strong competition is possible with the trial-and-error entry of a variety of many different locations and sizes. Such conditions are far from common, however.

Substantial economies of scale are possible for some service types, especially in the upper quality grades, and, as a result, in small and middle-sized communities a few large units will come to dominate the market. Their particular size-location mixes will impose severe constraints on potential competition. New units are restrained from entering the market to compete because of the radical decrease in patient census per hospital that would result from entry of any unit large enough to capture economies of scale. Thus, hospitals which are inefficient because of size or location often continue unchallenged by new entrants. Moreover, lack of a profit maximization motive obviates internal pressure to improve efficiency.

A situation in which there are high entry barriers because of the existence of substantial economies of scale is perhaps extreme. With even moderate entry impacts, however, a number of questions bearing on survivorship can be discerned. If economies of scale are sufficient to give each new entrant a noticeable impact on units already in operation and there is a lumpiness in entry, then under some combinations of demand and cost circumstances, lowest-cost operation of existing units may require suboptimality in size, location or type, or over or underutilization. Entry cannot be infinitely graded in all dimensions to supplant existing units which are suboptimal in a given dimension. Entry by a unit closer to optimality in the relevant dimension would result in discrepancies for the entrant in the other dimensions because of the non-trivial entry interaction, which would lead to higher operating costs. In these circumstances, suboptimality for an existing unit in some dimension, or even underutilization, does *not* imply a relatively high-cost operation with poor survivorship prospects.

Suppose there are a finite number of size-location-type configurations. The survivorship process may not lead to the lowest over-all cost for the system as a whole because, in the instance just noted, the survivorship sequence depends on just which units are initially present: it is not invariant but history-bound. With a given set of units, if the most efficient size for some type is very large, then an entrant of that size may supplant a number of smaller units, and the new assortment may not leave enough business for a further entrant of that or of the next largest and succeedingly efficient size. The resulting pattern might then show one very large and efficient hospital and a number of smaller and much less efficient ones, with a total operating cost higher than that of a pattern of several hospitals of the second rank. The wrong *sequence* of survival confrontations can lead to local but not general optima when economies of size and lumpiness are important. Survivorship is not always a dependable process for progress toward efficiency.

Effect of non-profit status and availability of charitable contributions. Both of these work against internal incentives that promote efficiency. Carr's argument (in the original paper) deprecates this. There he asserted that "at some point the marginal cost of obtaining contributions will equal the amount obtained. This may occur even at rather low levels of average cost of solicitations." The argument is in the context that such contributions do not really ease the market discipline on hospitals to be efficient.

The assertion is misleading and does not afford aid to the larger argument. At the equilibrium solicitation level it is marginal contributions that equal marginal cost. Average contributions will generally exceed marginal cost at this point, and total contributions may substantially exceed total solicitation cost. Thus, net contributions *can* help to insulate an inefficient hospital from the rigors of the market. One of the two efficiency levers of the survivorship mechanism, the internal budget constraint, is directly weakened, and the other, patient patronage, is indirectly weakened by the rupture of any necessary linkage between patient charges and rate of utilization. Thus inefficiencies may induce neither internal reform nor loss of patient patronage. Gradually the market may be supplanted.

The mechanism is further divorced from over-all system efficiency if especially efficient hospitals fail to reduce patient charges but use the earnings differentials mainly to try to raise the size of the contributions they seek.

Effect of demand bunching. A systematic tendency for patient choices to bunch in favor of high-quality hospitals confounds the market tendency to favor efficient low-cost hospitals. Bunching comes about as follows. Carr distinguishes between hospital service type (quality) and efficiency. He assumes that the same number of individuals prefer each service type. This is not a reasonable assumption, however, if the service types are in fact qualities. Instead, it is likely that, except for the effects of patient charges, waiting lines, etc., there will be among patients an approximation to a unique, consensual preference ordering for these types, with higher quality types being preferred to lower quality types.

Assume initially that, as a result of competition, patients have distributed themselves among hospitals so that the differential patient charges between hospital types equals the patients' equilibrium marginal rate of substitution between these types. They will be indifferent among different types at the margin. A substantial third-party payment of hospital bills, largely by insurance groups and public welfare agencies, is then introduced. The portion of charges that patients must pay becomes less than the total bill, and typically the differential in this resulting patient's share between different hospital types is less than the prior equilibrium marginal rate of substitution. Since high-quality types are generally preferred to low-quality types, the decreased price differential makes the former a bargain. Because of the presence of third-party payments, many more patients are systematically induced to choose the high-quality types.

Thus there will be a bunching of demand across hospital types for reasons of quality rather than efficiency. In some instances more efficient but lower quality hospitals will lose business to higher quality but less efficient hospitals. These service types are to some extent correlated with size because certain high-quality types require minimum absolute scales to warrant the relevant specialization, variety, and profundity of care. Therefore, the bunching tendency will be associated with size distribution. Larger, high-quality hospitals will be favored over smaller, low-quality ones without respect to differences in efficiency.

The bunching of demand on high-quality types means that some hospitals with excess capacity will be passed over in favor of units already filled. Patients whose illnesses permit waiting for admission will lengthen the queue for care in the high-quality hospitals. Thus, overutilization may persist side by side with underutilized capacity.

It is quite likely that the process of selection in this competitive but non-profit-maximizing market will not uniformly favor efficiency. Substantial third-party payments will result in selection tendencies sometimes significantly at odds with efficiency.

Evidence on growth and decline. Carr adduces from the growth characteristics shown in his Table 2 that small, inefficient hospitals exhibit market selection vulnerability. This conclusion seems unwarranted. The data indicate that, except for the extreme size classes, hospitals in the smaller size classes are neither more likely to become smaller nor less capable of growing larger. Indeed, the probability of increasing by one size step is about the same for all non-extreme classes, and the probability of decreasing one size step is actually greater for the larger size classes than for the smaller. Moreover, the findings with regard to the smallest hospitals may have more to do with quality than with efficiency. Quality level preferences of patients, in conjunction with third-party payments, could account for the evidence. In summary, the connection between market selectivity and efficiency is by no means paramount, reliable, or sometimes even observable.

D. Planning errors among city, suburban, and rural densities show up as quite large, due mainly to an assumption that was used in arriving at the estimate of travel costs (the same average speed for all trips regardless of the population density associated with a particular trip). Surely one would expect speed to vary inversely with density and the differences to be substantial. If so, total travel time per trip (including parking) will vary far less among different density areas than is shown here because the greater distances necessary in low-density areas will be offset by the faster speeds relative to high-density areas. As a result, planning errors will differ less among the three types of area.

E. The assumption of fixed proportions among inpatient care, outpatient care, and visits is suspect. One would expect the proportions to differ in hospitals of different size and in hospitals of different service types. Since differentials in treatment vs. travel costs are involved, this could significantly affect the optimality of size and location.

F. The measurement of the bed requirement variable is unsatisfactory. Here it is measured as (Bed Capacity/1,000) in 1958 for each state. It should actually be measured on a community, or at most regional, basis. Beds in widely separated parts of a state, other than in really small states, are not substitutes for the same hospital need.

G. In the regression analysis of bed capacity expansion the variable, change in total utilization, is used and shows a highly significant negative coefficient. Despite its significance, its conceptualization is weak. It is not at all clear that this is a usefully interpretable variable to employ. In the explanation of bed capacity retirements, with less than 50 per cent of the variance explained, the residuals are large. It might be instructive to examine them explicitly to test whether the trend toward excess growth is real, or whether perhaps the predicted excess is offset by high residuals in the opposite direction.

In conclusion, I wish to repeat that, although I have noted a variety of difficulties in Carr's paper, they are for the most part honorable ones, stemming from the very ambitiousness of the approach. The work shows subtlety, imagination, and technical prowess. Its reach is fascinating and instructive. I find it a welcome addition to our literature.

Carl M. Stevens
Reed College

HOSPITAL MARKET EFFICIENCY:
THE ANATOMY OF THE SUPPLY RESPONSE

INTRODUCTION

As with other industries, the economic efficiency of the hospital industry may be evaluated in terms of market structure, conduct, and performance. Market performance may be described and measured in terms of various properties. In this paper, I am mainly concerned with one central property: an efficient or optimum rate of output, defined as an efficient supply response to demand events. Because of the special nature of the demand for hospital services, this may be put in terms of an efficient or optimum industry capacity.*

Ceteris paribus, attention to an efficient rate of output is, of course, attention to only one of a number of interdependent dimensions of efficient market performance. Thus, for example, whatever the rate of output of hospital services, sector performance will not be efficient unless that output is secured at least cost. This dimension of hospital market performance has

Research for this paper was supported by Grant CH-00372-01, U.S. Public Health Service. The author wishes to express his thanks to his research assistants, Joanne Osterud and Barbara Rockefeller, for valuable assistance in locating data and in making computations, and to his colleague, Mildred Howe, for helpful comments upon the analysis.

*Medical services are "different" from the ordinary run of goods and services. These differences have not, by and large, been adequately reflected in economic analysis of the sector. The remedy is to build the analysis from the ground up, as it were. What is required is an analysis which proceeds sequentially from an initial step which would analytically characterize the nature of demand. I have included a brief Appendix addressed to this topic.

received much more attention than the dimension of optimum rate of output, upon which I have chosen to focus this inquiry.*

In what follows, I shall present some direct measures of output (capacity) in terms of beds and patient days for the hospitals in the metropolitan Portland area. Of more analytical significance, however, are the measures presented in terms of a .01 probability of shortage criterion. This criterion is one commonly employed in evaluation of the performance of the hospital sector. I have been led to conclude that a rate-of-output efficiency criterion of this genre is not only operationally tractable but is also conceptually appropriate, given the nature of demand for hospital services.[†]

Generally, in economic analysis of market efficiency (including the hospital industry) it has been difficult to evaluate market performance directly, and economists have turned to an examination of market structure and market conduct. Accordingly, I shall examine the nature and the structure of the decision-making process which determines the hospital's rate of output or capacity – the supply response to demand events. The basic data for the analysis were obtained by extensive interviews with hospital administrators and members of their staffs.[‡]

In my opinion, an examination of the hospital management decision-making process is central to understanding and evaluating the performance of this sector. In dealing with the hospital sector and the larger medical services industry of which it is an integral part, we are dealing with, from the economist's point of view, an unfamiliar mixture of ordinary market, atypical market, quasi-market, and non-market institutions. An analytical context of this kind requires particular attention to market structure and conduct before conclusions may be reached about market performance and remedies for inefficiencies.

Identifying the Output of the General Hospital Sector

This analysis is concerned with voluntary (i.e., non-governmental), non-profit, short-term general hospitals. Such hospitals are usually multiproduct enterprises, with some commitment to patient care, medical education, medi-

---

*Efficiency in the sense of least-cost combinations of inputs involves much more than how any one hospital at any one point in time produces whatever mix of services it has defined as its output. It involves management of the health care production function "in the large."

[†] See the Appendix, which affords a brief rationale for this conclusion.

[‡] The administrative staffs of six of the largest of the twenty hospitals in the Portland metropolitan area were interviewed. Together, these six hospitals had about 1,700 beds – slightly over half of total bed capacity in the area. A complete study of hospital management decision-making structure should, of course, include interviews with the other components of the hospital management "triangle," i.e., the governing board and staff physicians. I hope to carry these out at a future date.

cal research, and public health. For purposes of this analysis, direct patient care — sometimes referred to here as "hospital services" — will be regarded as the output of the general hospital sector.*

THE THEORY OF THE HOSPITAL AS A FIRM: MANAGEMENT STRUCTURE AND DECISION-MAKING

The Role of Motivation Postulates in the Analysis

Since the hospitals with which we are concerned are non-profit enterprises, there would appear to be a prima facie case that some alternative to profit maximization† will be required as a model. We might begin to construct such a model by defining an alternative postulate of the hospital's goals or objectives, which could be regarded as its "success criteria."

Without attempting to spell out the reasons for it or offering examples, I would judge that we cannot reasonably expect to synthesize from generally prevailing characterizations of hospitals' objectives formulations that will yield much by way of deductions about their economic behavior; that is, we cannot expect to get as much analytical "mileage" out of motivation postulates as in, say, the conventional theory of the business firm. Analysis will have to depend more upon empirical generalization about economic choice behavior and less upon deducing propositions about such behavior from underlying postulates about objectives. Nevertheless, considerations relating to the objectives of the components of the hospital management triangle may be relevant in a general sense to the analysis of the hospital sector.

The Management Triangle

Hospital management is well described as a triangle: the governing board of trustees or directors, the hospital administrator, and the staff physicians.[1] Because of the management triangle, it is misleading to regard "the hospital" as *a* decision unit. It is true that it is, in a general sense, an organizational unit. There is a governing board and an administrator employed by and responsible to it. However, from another point of view, the hospital is basically a facility used by its staff physicians (who share in its management) in

---

*This analysis is concerned with the character (e.g., rationality) of the output decision-making process in the general hospital sector. In spite of the fact that to some extent the several outputs of the hospital might be regarded as joint products, a basic reason for separating them for analysis is that different criteria for efficient resource allocation apply to each of them.

†While not profit maximizers, hospitals are subject to budget constraints and pursuant to this may be regarded as cost minimizers (for any given quantity and quality of output). To the extent that this is true, the conventional theory of cost and production will be useful in an analysis of the hospital's economic behavior.

their own practice of medicine. It is a facility used jointly by a group of independent businessmen who themselves have a direct financial relationship to the patients admitted to and billed by the hospital. Ray E. Brown has offered this characterization of the triangle: "There are other important tension areas that are unique to the hospital. No other form of organization can equal the obstacles to tranquillity that are present in the medical staff-administrative-trustee triangle. The picture of third-party independent contractors responsible for specifying the services rendered to the clientele of an enterprise, at once dependent upon the enterprise for carrying out their orders, but independent of the enterprise with their relationships with the enterprise's clientele, is not found in any other type of enterprise. While they are not stockholders in the hospital, they have a deep, abiding proprietary interest because their livelihood, to an ever-increasing extent, is dependent upon the hospital."[2]

According to Gordon, the really unique features of the hospital, as compared with other organizations, stem from the relationship of the licensed, practicing, self-governing medical staff to the board, the administrator, and other components of the organization.[3] This relationship is predicated upon the legal position of the physician. Medicine legally can be practiced only by those licensed to do so. The hospital itself cannot lawfully practice medicine, nor can it lawfully control the professional practices of its physicians.[4] It is these circumstances which result in the relatively independent status of physicians in the hospital. Administrators may have little real authority over the physicians, and the only coercive sort of power available to the boards studied by Gordon was that of appointment and reappointment to the staff, an ultimate weapon which is seldom used.

The view of the physician as an independent professional entrepreneur who uses hospital facilities is central to conceptualization of hospital management structure. Such a view is not, of course, intended to imply that the individual physician is in every sense "independent" of the other organizational components that make up the hospital. In addition to his link to hospital administration as such, all physicians collectively comprise the medical staff, which is increasingly adopting a committee and administrative organization of its own, thus tending to bring professional group discipline closer to the decisions of the individual private physician.[5] The hospital board has final responsibility for the operation of all phases of the institution, a categorical statement which, while true, is not very informative about the effective role of the board in hospital management.[6]

The position of the administrator in the hospital has been, and still is, somewhat ambiguous. In the past it has been common to characterize him as low man on the management totem pole. However, there have been important historical changes. Hospital administration is emerging as a full-scale profession and, as the hospital becomes more complicated, the increasingly professional administrator becomes more central to the decision-making process.[7]

The foregoing broad generalizations afford a useful initial orientation. They make it clear, for example, that the hospital as a decision-making "unit" is atypical of enterprises with which economists are most familiar and at least suggest the nature and sources of the difference. The central point here is the role of the relatively independent professional physician in the hospital organization.

Not much would be gained by trying to refine these generalizations as generalizations. What is required to understand the implications of hospital-management structure for resource allocation is an examination of the way in which, in practice, the various components of the decision-making structure relate to specific resource allocation decisions, in particular, for present purposes, the decisions which determine the rate of output (capacity) of the hospital sector.

THE ANATOMY OF THE SUPPLY RESPONSE TO DEMAND EVENTS

The capacity of the hospital sector in a given service area will be determined by those decisions which determine the capacity of the individual enterprises and the number of enterprises in the sector. We may ask what decisions determine such a basic enterprise parameter as the capacity of a hospital. The concept of an equilibrium rate of output may readily be defined in the case of the profit-making enterprises characteristic of other sectors, and market behavior such as an increase in supply in response to an increase in demand may quite readily be rationalized. But why should the hospital, as a non-profit enterprise, have a preference for any particular rate of output (capacity) over another? Similarly, why should the non-profit hospital respond to an increase in demand by an increase in rate of output – indeed, why should such an enterprise be expected to respond in any particular way to any particular change in the market data confronting it?

The foregoing questions arise naturally from a conceptual format of hospital market structure which places the patients and potential patients on the demand side of the market and "the hospitals" on the supply side. Although, of course, the demand for hospital services is derived from demand by patients and potential patients, a more useful analytical format can be provided by recognizing that it is the staff physicians who are, in a proximate sense, on the demand side of the market for hospital services. In light of this consideration, one might say that the optimum capacity for any given hospital (in any short run) is determined by the requirements of the staff physicians who are using it as an adjunct to their own businesses. This leads to the conclusion that some balance must be maintained between the capacity of the hospital and the size of its medical staff. But it does not explain why any given capacity, with its commensurate staff, should be regarded as a preferred or equilibrium position, rather than some smaller or larger capacity, each accompanied by an appropriately smaller or larger commensurate staff. The mere requirement for a short-run balance between staff demands and capacity is not enough to preclude the possibility that the size of each hospital, and hence the capacity of the hospital sector, is related arbitrarily to total market demand.

My findings suggest that the supply of hospital services is rather systematically related to market demand, the non-profit character of the hospital notwithstanding. The crucial link between the hospitals as suppliers and the market is to be found in the staffing policies of the hospitals. The institutions which were the subject of this research (and I was informed that the same is true for the West Coast generally) followed open-staff policies; i.e., they were willing to admit to staff membership all "qualified" physicians who requested staff privileges.*

Given the open-staff policy, the supply-response mechanism may now be sketched as follows. In a given hospital service area the demand for medical services generally, including hospital services, increases over time, and along with it, the supply of physicians increases. These physicians seek staff privileges with the hospitals in the service area and, pursuant to the open-staff policy, are accommodated. This means, however, that the pre-existing capacity of the hospitals will prove too small to accommodate their demands. They will then bring pressure to bear upon the hospitals to expand capacity, and the hospitals will respond to this pressure and attempt to restore the balance between capacity on the one hand and the demands of the hospital staff on the other.

Broadly speaking, this is the picture of the supply-response mechanism which emerged from my investigation of the sample of hospitals in the metropolitan Portland area, and there was general agreement among the administrators I talked with that this was indeed the way to account for and to describe the supply response. I do not mean to imply, however, that the

---

*These hospitals recognize three categories of staff members: active, the regular staff with full admitting privileges; courtesy, physicians who may occasionally admit a patient under special circumstances and if he can be accommodated; associate, younger men just joining the staff and in a kind of probationary state prior to acquisition of active staff status. Sometimes the term "unrestricted" is used to refer to the arrangements which I have called "open" staff policy. Open-staff policy does not, of course, mean that any physician who applies for staff privileges will be accepted. The medical staff in each hospital has certain standards which must be met. It may be noted that this quality screening may serve as a kind of surrogate for control of quantity of staff; that is, given an open-staff policy, different degrees of rigor could be used in applying quality standards, depending upon how current capacity fits with current staff requirements.

supply response on the part of the hospitals is no more than a "passive" accommodation to the demands of staff physicians and would-be staff physicians. Staff demands that are not "blue chips," so to speak, e.g., a demand for expansion not backed by hard evidence of an already high occupancy rate, would not be accommodated. Each of the hospitals I interviewed, in contemplating expansion, undertook studies and surveys designed to predict future demand for its facilities. The individual hospitals attempted to take account directly of many of the kinds of demand pressure which were being revealed to it via the mechanism of new staff acquisitions and the demands of existing staff. My net impression, however, was that it is the latter which is decisive, with the planning by hospital administration itself serving as a supplementary check upon other market cues.

This broad picture leaves a good bit to be explained. For example, why do the hospitals pursue open-staff policies which expose them to pressures for expansion? We will turn to this and related questions later. The important thing to note at this point is that this mechanism, as broadly described, does provide a direct link between market-demand events and decisions by individual hospitals about what capacity is to be deemed optimal. By recognizing this link, the mechanism introduces an element of economic logic into the supply side of the market for hospital services, in spite of the non-profit character of these enterprises; that is, the supply response of the hospital sector is predicated not upon some non-profit motive of the hospitals as enterprises per se, but rather upon the for-gain motives of the individual practitioners who want to use these facilities as a necessary adjunct to their own business operations.

The Open-Staff Policy and Hospital Accommodation of Staff Demands

There was general agreement among the hospital administrators interviewed that pressure from the medical staff was a decisive influence on expansion of capacity. As one man, whose hospital is in the midst of an expansion program, remarked, "The medical staff looks at it from the point of view of the economics of their practice – they put pressure on you." I gained the impression that hospital boards and administrators did not view expansion with equanimity. Capital funds are hard to come by and, if borrowed, expensive. Moreover, today's expansion, however financed, brings with it tomorrow's increase in current-account expense. Why, then, do the hospitals follow policies which result in pressures for expansion and accommodate these pressures when they manifest themselves? Is it out of the goodness of their eleemosynary hearts? Alternatively, do there exist a number of more particular pressures and imperatives in the situation which have this consequence?

My own investigations indicated that, to some extent, both of these factors are operating. I asked the hospital administrators this direct question:

"Assuming that the hospital has at some point achieved a satisfactory and workable balance between hospital capacity and the demands upon it made by the medical staff, why not simply close the staff and resist pressure for further expansion?" A part of the answer lies with the general orientation of the governing board. It does view the hospital as a service institution with responsibilities to the community. This does not, in the usual case, mean that it defines as its objective serving some given percentage of need in the service area. It does appear, however, that it would regard as inconsistent with this general service orientation a deliberate policy of refusal of staff privileges to qualifed applicants.

Thus, the board's conception of the hospital as a service organization and of its own responsibilities pursuant to this goal creates a disposition to accommodate physicians' pressures. Beyond this, however, a number of more particular pressures are operating, which serve to translate this disposition into actual expansion, and to determine the pace of such expansion. One of these is expansion via modernization. In principle, one might distinguish between straightforward expansion of capacity, for example, by adding additional general medical and surgical beds, and expansion via modernization. In practice, this distinction is somewhat blurred. Medical technology has been making rapid advances, and, in part because of quality competition in this industry, there is very strong pressure to modernize facilities, particularly ancillary facilities such as laboratories of various kinds, special diagnostic and treatment centers, and the like. Indeed, as one administrator put it, to stand pat in terms of modernization would be equivalent to closing the institution. It appears to be a fact of hospital life that modernization almost always entails expansion – initially, in heavier capital investment in ancillary facilities. From this expansion, in turn, is derived an increasing demand for beds. For example, installation of an intensive care unit for cardiac patients will lead to the processing of more patients and create a demand for more floor beds. Another example cited was the installation of a very modern facility for urological patients. In addition to better care per se, the facility permitted a surgeon to treat five patients in the time formerly required for two or three, thereby leading to an increased demand for surgical beds.*

---

*The relationship between the general medical and the surgical bed capacity and special diagnostic and treatment facilities has some interesting implications for utilization. One administrator pointed out that after the first four or five days of a patient's stay, at least for the kinds of patients in his hospital, the institution begins to lose money. In the first days the heavy volume of services is delivered and billed. As the patient remains, excess capacity, including unused (very expensive) personnel time in the ancillary facilities, may begin to be costly. Thus, both the medical staff utilization committee and the hospital administration itself may have a strong motivation for controlling length of stay.

In addition to requests from physicians to be admitted to staff membership, pressures for staff expansion may come from physicians who are already members of the staff. For example, staff physicians who add men to their own offices may now want staff privileges for them. More generally, as one administrator commented, "The life blood of the physician is referrals." For this reason there may be pressure from members of the existing staff in given specialties to admit more physicians in general, or even additional staff members in their own specialties, because the resulting prestigious and more visible service will attract more referrals.

Sometimes an effort to ensure that capacity already in place will be fully utilized may lead to some expansion. One administrator pointed out that of the several hundred staff physicians of various categories at his hospital, relatively few accounted for about one-half of the admissions. These men are very important to maintenance of a reasonable census which permits operation at or above the break-even point. Consequently, it is hard for the hospital not to accede to their demands for expansion.

Concern about future utilization also leads hospitals to think about replacements for the older members of the existing staff who may soon retire. If these men are now responsible for the major portion of admissions to a given service, and if no younger replacements have been provided for them, the service may tend to collapse upon their retirement. Thus, in order to ensure that today's capacity, fully utilized today, will be so utilized tomorrow, the hospital may add younger men, thereby causing a staff bulge and pressure on facilities.

A Few Qualifications

Growth of hospital capacity in a given service area depends not only upon the growth of existing organizations, the factor analyzed in this paper, but also upon the birth of new hospitals. For the metropolitan Portland area 84 per cent of the 1954-1966 total growth was accounted for by the expansion of existing institutions;* this can be explained by a theory of the growth of existing voluntary hospitals. For a more general theory of sector performance, however, an explanation for the founding of new hospitals is required.

*That is, if each hospital remained at the size it was in 1954 or in the year after that in which it was founded, only 16 per cent of the actual growth that took place by 1966 would be accounted for. Of the nine hospitals founded during this period, five were small proprietary hospitals which had, in 1966, an aggregate of only 300 beds (total beds in the area were 3,298). (Presumably, the general theory of investment in business enterprise explains the founding of these hospitals.) Of the remaining four, one was a small district hospital, one was the University of Oregon Medical School hospital, and one was the Bess Kaiser Hospital, an integral part of the Kaiser group practice health care system. Each of these is in a relevant sense a "special case" from the point of view of developing

It has been suggested that, despite its non-profit character, the hospital sector may exhibit some economic logic or rationality because its supply response operates through profit-making marketers, the physicians. The implication is that, so far as the supply response to demand is concerned, the efficiency of the hospital sector will depend upon the efficiency of the physician sector. Without undertaking an evaluation of the latter assertion, I would point out that establishing the market locus of the hospital sector supply response has some potentially interesting implications. It emphasizes the general interdependence of the sectors which comprise the medical care industry and suggests, among other things, that it may not be realistic to think in terms of planning for one sector, e.g., the hospital sector, without simultaneously taking into account relationships with other sectors. Indeed, given the hospital supply response mechanism developed herein, it is striking to note that at the same time that health manpower planners are pushing for a sizable increase in the number of physicians, hospital planners are contriving programs designed, in one way or another, to slow down and limit the growth of hospital sector capacity.

It might be argued that within the present institutional framework the way to plan the hospital sector would be to plan the physician sector, and to let the former take care of itself. For example, efficient creation and use of hospital capacity might be accomplished by eliminating the inefficient relative scarcity of physicians and removing financial and organizational barriers to free participation by physicians in whatever forms of health-care delivery systems they wish to try.

Given the picture in this section of the supply-response mechanism, it will be of interest to turn to the actual performance of the hospital sector market in the metropolitan Portland area.

DISCUSSION

Expected vs. Actual Market Performance

There is a general disposition in the literature to regard the performance of the hospital sector as haphazard. Ray E. Brown has noted that "there are those who argue that the hospitals of the nation have developed at random and that we have no rational system, but only a collection of uncoordinated

---

a general theory of growth of hospital sector capacity. One small voluntary hospital was also founded during the period.

Insofar as current market performance in the metropolitan Portland area is concerned, there was general agreement among administrators that the area's hospital capacity was determined by the individual decisions of each hospital and that the influence of areawide planning had, from this point of view, been minimal. The only "teeth" available to the area planning agency, namely, the rationing of Hill-Harris funds, are apparently not a controlling factor in decisions of individual hospitals.

principalities."[8] The supply-response model developed in Section III certainly would not lead us to expect random performance. Indeed, the central supply-response mechanism featured by the model would lead us to expect an orderly growth of industry capacity systematically related to the growth in general demand for medical services. In the model, increases in supply are seen as a function of the degree of demand pressure on capacity. A measure of such pressure, the theoretical pressure index, is here defined as the ratio of required occupancy rate to maximum occupancy rate, concepts to be defined in what follows.

Existing hospital facilities are, to a significant extent, non-price-rationed.* Staff physicians employ criteria such as the kind and severity of illness in deciding whether and when patients need hospital services. These criteria, established in accord with professional judgment, may be more or less restrictive of consumption of hospital services. The most restrictive of such criteria consistent with acceptable medical practice, as defined by staff physicians, may be called the "standard" criteria. The numerator of the theoretical pressure index, the required occupancy rate, is then defined as that rate which would result from application of the standard criteria.

The denominator of the theoretical pressure index, the maximum occupancy rate, is defined as that rate which, given the frequency distribution of the daily census by size, would be consistent with a given probability-of-space-shortage criterion, say, the hospital at full capacity on the average one day in one hundred (or five days in one hundred, etc.). An index value of 1.0 would indicate a required occupancy rate equal to the maximum rate, a position which may be regarded as an equilibrium one. An index value greater or less than 1.0 would indicate a required occupancy rate greater or less than the maximum rate, both disequilibrium positions.

Suppose, then, that in the service area for the time period in question the staff physicians in each of the hospitals have, on the average, maintained about the same standard criteria for ordering hospital services for their patients. If, with the passage of time, the demand for medical, including hospital, services increases, one may expect an upward drift in the pressure index. At some threshold level of the index, pressure generated by the medical staff upon the hospital for additional capacity will be accommodated (as put forth in the arguments developed in Section III), and there will be an increase in supply. This can be expected to bring about a decline in the pressure index — at the least, a halt or substantial slowdown of the increase. As this mechanism operates in the service area over time, if the staff physi-

---

*Although various features of this market (e.g., prepaid plans with no or nominal marginal user cost) tend to attenuate the effect, these services are also to some extent price-rationed. Thus in discussing non-price-rationing I am dealing with only a part of total rationing, albeit that part most central to the supply-creates-demand question.

cians tend to adhere to about the same admissions and retention criteria, and if the hospitals respond fairly quickly to medical staff pressures for additional capacity, then one may expect the pressure index in the service area to exhibit considerable long-run constancy, rising and falling somewhat in the short run with supply-demand adjustment lags but without significant departure from a central value.

Table 1 presents, among other data, the number of general acute and surgical beds in the metropolitan area and the weighted average observed pressure index for the years 1954-1966.* Figure 1 gives a graphic representation of these data. The theoretical pressure index, it will be recalled, has as its numerator the required occupancy rate, a rate which cannot be observed directly in the data. The observed pressure index has as its numerator the actual observed occupancy rate. Thus the observed pressure index presented in Table 1 and in Figure 1 is a surrogate for the theoretical pressure index. The two will be the same in the special case where the observed occupancy rate is the same as the required occupancy rate.

The observed pressure index exhibits approximately the behavior which would be expected of the theoretical index, based upon the supply-response model. The range of values over the thirteen years is not great, with a mean of approximately .90, a low value of approximately .83, and a high value of

Fig. 1. Pressure index and number of beds, Portland metropolitan area, 1954-1966.

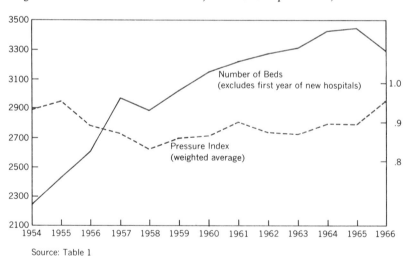

Source: Table 1

*For purposes of this table, the maximum occupancy rate was defined as that rate which would have been consistent with a capacity-or-above census one day in one hundred, i.e., a .01 probability of shortage criterion. For further information on calculation of the maximum rate, see Table 1, n. c.

approximately .96. Moreover, over these years the pressure index varied systematically, and in the way which might be expected, in relation to the growth in capacity of the hospital sector. During the first part of the period, from 1954 to 1958, during which the rate of increase in number of beds was most rapid, the pressure index showed a substantial decline from a 1954 value of .94 to a 1958 value of .83. Thereafter, as the rate of increase in capacity was slower, the pressure index showed a gradual increase, staying rather close, however, to its mean value. In the final year, 1966, when the number of beds declined, the pressure index responded by rising to its highest value for the period, .96.

On the face of it, this record of performance of the hospital sector in the Portland metropolitan area generally is in accord with what might be expected from the supply-response model. Thus, one analytical function of these data is to contribute to an affirmative judgment on the validity of the model. As a mild normative evaluation, I have suggested above that the structure of the decision-making process exhibited by the model is characterized by a certain economic logic and rationality.

There remains the question of how the record of market performance, per se, might be construed in terms of efficiency. Given the nature of demand for hospital services (see the Appendix), it might be contended that if the market performance record before us did indeed depict the behavior of the theoretical pressure index, then the supply response to demand in the market could be said to be efficient. It is, however, the observed pressure index that we have before us and must construe. We now turn to some considerations bearing on this question.

Does Supply Create Demand?

If the frequently cited "law" of hospital markets that "supply creates demand" is true, evaluation of observed market performance is difficult because, regardless of the efficiency of the supply response, relative constancy over time can be expected in the observed pressure index. One cannot "prove" simply by reference to the observed pressure index time series that this "law" was or was not at work. My own interpretation of this time series, considered in relation to the hospital sector capacity series, is that in this case the data suggest that the law was not operating, at least not very decisively, in the short run. For example, if for the early period of substantial fall in the pressure index one argues that supply was creating demand, one must allow for a considerable time lag in the demand response. In the final year, as has been pointed out, the number of beds declined and the pressure index moved up sharply, suggesting that whatever else is to be said for the hospital supply-demand law, it should make provision for asymmetry, namely, that although

Table 1: Selected Data on Hospital Facilities and Use, Metropolitan Portland Area,[a] 1954–1966

	1954	1955	1956	1957	1958	1959	1960
(1) Hospitals[b]	11	12	14	15	15	17	18
(2) Beds	2,249	2,430	2,611	2,962	2,891	3,062	3,151
(3) Average size	205	203	187	198	193	180	175
(4) Patient days	654,392	715,188	701,698	756,561	745,869	807,181	840,503
(5) Average patient days	59,490	59,599	50,121	50,437	49,725	47,481	46,695
(6) Average census	163	166	141	123	137	130	128
(7) Average occupancy rate	74.67	76.53	69.01	68.93	69.36	68.50	67.75
(8) Average pressure index (weighted)[c]	0.936	0.956	0.893	0.872	0.832	0.860	0.865
(9) Physicians and osteopaths	–	–	1,035	1,078	1,108	1,136	1,160
(10) Population	–	703,000	–	–	–	–	750,467

Table 1 –*continued*

	1961	1962	1963	1964	1965	1966
(1) Hospitals[b]	18	19	20	20	20	20
(2) Beds	3,226	3,284	3,316	3,433	3,452	3,298
(3) Average size	179	164	166	172	169	165
(4) Patient days	797,629	868,558	875,883	877,218	935,551	960,863
(5) Average patient days	41,981	45,556	43,794	43,861	46,778	48,043
(6) Average census	137	124	121	127	131	133
(7) Average occupancy rate	70.88	67.58	67.80	70.70	69.40	65.40
(8) Average pressure index (weighted)[c]	0.902	0.873	0.869	0.897	0.895	0.955
(9) Physicians and osteopaths	1,173	1,211	1,293	1,304	1,333	1,360
(10) Population	763,000	766,000	782,000	804,000	835,000	—

[a] Area includes Oregon counties Multnomah, Clackamas, Washington, and Columbia. The Hospital Planning Council for the Metropolitan Portland area defines the area to include Clark County, Washington, which, in 1965, had 15 per cent of the beds in the five-county total.

[b] Hospitals founded during period, year of establishment, and initial capacity were as follows: Hospital S, 1955, 31 beds; Hospital C, 1956, 43 beds; Hospital Q, 1956, 74 beds; Hospital R, 1957, 241 beds; Hospital A, 1959, 102 beds; Hospital G, 1959, 68 beds; Hospital I, 1960, 26 beds; Hospital T, 1962, 46 beds; Hospital E, 1963, 48 beds.

[c] Ratio of actual average occupancy rate to "maximum" occupancy rate, the latter defined as that rate which would have been consistent with a capacity census on the average day in one hundred. (The pressure index is a measure devised by Gerald D. Rosenthal; cf. *The Demand for General Hospital Facilities* [Chicago: American Hospital Association, 1964], pp. 44–52.) Calculation of the maximum rate is based on the common assumption that the daily census figures for the hospitals are Poisson-distributed. For purposes of this table, the maximum rates were estimated by use of a table provided by E. C. Molina, "Computation Formula for the Probability of an Event Happening at Least C Times in N Trials," *American Mathematical Monthly* 20 (May 1913):190–93.

Sources: (1)–(7), *Oregon State Plan for the Construction and Modernization of Hospitals, Public Health Centers and Medical Facilities* (Salem: Oregon State Board of Health, 1956–68), published annually; (9), *Report of the Board of Medical Examiners of the State of Oregon* (Portland: Board of Medical Examiners of the State of Oregon, Portland, Oregon, 1956–66), published annually; (10), *Population Trends and Projections 1955–1975 for the Metropolitan Portland Area*, Research Report No. 1 (Portland: Hospital Planning Council for the Metropolitan Portland Area, 1966), p. 2.

increases in supply may increase demand, decreases in supply do not eliminate demand.*

In the usual statement of the supply-creates-demand law, it is not clear whether the meaning intended is that increases in supply increase demand, in the sense of an outward shift of the demand schedule. If so, the law describes an unusual market phenomenon, which raises severe problems for evaluation of market performance. Alternatively, the law might be intended to say that increases in supply result in increases in amounts demanded, with the demand schedule remaining fixed. If so, the law is simply saying that the market for hospital services, like many others, tends to clear itself following an increase in supply. This behavior, of course, may be consistent with market efficiency, in that once capacity is in place, real marginal user cost may be low relative to alternatives.

In interpreting any given record of market performance, it obviously is important to know which, if either, version of the law is operating. To make this discrimination in the case of a conventional market for a conventional good, one might look at the price immediately before and after an increase in supply and at the accompanying increase in the amounts demanded or taken. If the post-expansion price were substantially the same as the pre-expansion price, one would argue that an outward shift in the demand schedule had occurred. (Whether the increase in demand was due to the increase in supply would remain an open question pending further investigation.) If, on the other hand, the post-expansion price were substantially lower than the pre-expansion price, one would argue that there had been a movement along the pre-expansion demand curve.

Conceptually, a similar approach can be used to make this discrimination for the hospital industry. However, in this market, "price" should be interpreted not in dollar terms but more generally, as the terms upon which individuals may consume hospital services. These terms are the previously mentioned criteria used by physicians in deciding the quantity of hospital services to order in behalf of their patients. They are non-price-rationing criteria, and use of a less stringent set of rationing criteria would represent a decrease in price.

My own impression is that the rationing criteria used by physicians and hospitals do vary. They tend to be less restrictive when occupancy is relatively low. Hence, one might expect that an increase in capacity would result

---

*The observed pressure index was devised by Rosenthal to test the supply-creates-demand "law." He used cross-sectional data for each of two years from hospitals in various states, working with the average size of hospitals in each state. He argued that if the law were really working he would observe approximately the same pressure index in each of the states. The substantial differences revealed in state-by-state values for the pressure index, he argued, suggested that the law was not in fact operative. The present time series approach brings additional evidence to bear on this point.

in an immediate post-expansion set of criteria less restrictive than those prevailing immediately prior to expansion, which may be construed as a short-
run fall in the "price," which clears the market. It would be accompanied by
an observed occupancy rate higher than the required occupancy rate and an
observed pressure index higher than the theoretical pressure index.

As has been suggested, whether or not this short-run behavior is efficient
depends in part upon the relative marginal real cost of delivering services in
this way rather than in some other way (to be distinguished from money cost
to the patient). In any case, this short-run adjustment via a decrease in
"price" (i.e., less stringent rationing criteria) and accompanied by an increase
in amounts of hospital service demanded is a very different market phenomenon than would be an adjustment via an increase in demand (i.e., in the
sense of an outward shift of the demand schedule). A high observed occupancy rate and high observed pressure index are not necessarily evidence of
real pressure on capacity, i.e., pressure which would lead to expansion of
capacity. It is the required occupancy rate and the theoretical pressure index
which are crucial from this point of view.

Whether, and in what sense, supply creates demand is a question fundamental to the economics of the hospital sector – to interpretation of data
depicting market performance, and to policy prescription. While the foregoing comments suggest that one cannot expect to infer the answer to this
question from simple, straightforward inspection of market performance
data, and also suggest the kind of information (i.e., evidence of "price"
change) that might be relevant to answering this question, they do not, of
course, resolve the basic empirical question.

APPENDIX: ANALYTICAL CHARACTERIZATION OF DEMAND FOR HOSPITAL SERVICES

Option Demand

Episodically, any individual may be said to have a current demand for
hospital services when, on the advice of his physician, he is admitted to a
hospital. (This is the demand concept which underlies measurement of hospital output in terms of patient days.) Of perhaps more importance for analysis
of hospital market organization, however, is the individual's continuing (non-
episodic) demand for the prompt availability of hospital services if and when
needed, that is, his "option" demand.[9] This is the demand concept which
underlies measurement of hospital output in terms of capacity – i.e., provision of standby as well as current account services.

Option demand in this sense may create special problems of market organization for goods which, like hospital services, have the following characteristics: they are of urgent importance; their purchase is infrequent and its

timing uncertain; their consumption may not easily be deferred; and expansion of their production requires considerable time and resources.

Demand for Reduced Risk of Death or Morbidity

Recognizing option demand as an important component of the total demand for hospital services is central to the analysis because it leads directly to the further recognition of the peculiar kind of probabilistic choice about resource allocation which is involved. It may seem fairly clear what the consumer with a current demand for hospital services is buying, but what do the option demanders "buy" when they make a trade-off between an increment to the stock of hospital facilities and the alternatives thereby foregone?

One way to get at this question is by introspection. What is an increment in the stock of hospital facilities worth to me? Reflection probably would yield the conclusion that it is worth whatever a reduction in the risk of my own death or morbidity is worth.* T. C. Schelling has pointed out that valuation of such risk reduction is very difficult.[10] In general, the reduction in risk which is to be valued in principle will be describable as a very small change in very small probabilities of the subsequent occurrence of anxiety-provoking events of extraordinary importance. For example, what is it worth to the individual to reduce the risk that he will die of preventable heart disease from .001 to .0001? As Schelling points out, in addition to the problem of actually measuring the risk reduction, the individual probably would find, even after considerable thought about the problem, that he had no readily identifiable preferences relevant to this kind of choice.

The Need-Demand Mix

I have pointed out that the peculiar choice problem which confronts the option demander of hospital services is such that he may find it impossible to state or to "reveal" in a reliable way his demand for such facilities. Where this is true, consumer demand in the ordinary sense cannot by itself be decisive for resource allocation. In a state of conflict, or otherwise unable to make a reliable choice, consumers may delegate to professionals the selection of what is "needed," reasoning that this may be the most feasible and reliable way to make the necessary choices.

This brings us to one of the crucial properties of the demand for hospital services, namely, the mix of "need" (professional preferences) and "demand"

---

*In cost-benefit analysis of medical activities the most popular current approach to measuring benefits is in terms of present value of increments to GNP yielded by preventing deaths or reducing morbidity. Without attempting to discuss the issue, I do not feel that this approach to valuation is really very relevant to medical resource allocation problems.

(consumer preferences) influences on the consumption side of the market.* The hospital industry, and indeed the medical services industry more generally, is one in which to an uncommon degree professional judgment about "need" supplements demand as a decisive influence in resource allocation. This circumstance is no mere artifact of the current mode of organization of the industry, but rather is inherent in the basic characteristics of demand for hospital services. Additional characteristics of demand, such as product uncertainty[12] and various public good externalities, reinforce the tendency to delegate consumption choices to professionals and attenuate reliance on conventional market equilibrium as a definition of optimum performance.

Output (Stock of Facilities) Norm

This Appendix thus far has set forth an analytical characterization of the nature of demand for hospital services. The problem now is whether we can infer from these characteristics anything about the kind of proposition, at least, which would be an appropriate statement of the economically efficient output norm.

Hospital output is frequently measured in terms of patient days. However, because of option demand, an adequate measure of output must include not only current consumption of hospital services but also units of stand-by capacity. Thus, hospital output can be conceptualized in terms of the capacity of the stock of facilities. The most frequently encountered rule for measuring adequacy of supply is based on a probable shortage criterion: the optimum stock of hospital facilities in a given service area is one such that the hospitals will be utilized to capacity, on the average, one day in every hundred (the .01 probable shortage criterion), or five days, or ten days, etc.

The probable shortage rule has much to recommend it. What the option demanders (the overwhelming majority of marketers at any given time) are interested in is the possibility of exercising tomorrow's consumption option "on demand." The probable shortage criterion is operationally meaningful from the point of view of such preferences because it poses the resource allocation question in a form appropriate to the potential consumers' concern. In fact, in order for the consumer to "judge" whether the market for hospital services is economically efficient, in the sense of effectively translating his preferences into market performance, he must have reason to believe, *ex ante* or on the basis of his episodic current consumption experi-

---

*Professional preferences are established pursuant to the professional concept of need, which, as Kenneth Boulding has pointed out, rests on some definition of homeostasis or maintenance of the client in a certain state.[11] The medical professional defines an ideal state of "health," which he has a professional interest in maintaining – and his client is then said to need whatever medical services professional judgment deems efficacious for maintenance of this state.

ence, if any, that it is meeting an "acceptable" probability of shortage criterion.

How is the representative consumer to "decide" whether a .01 or a .05 criterion is "worth it"? Or, put somewhat differently, on what basis is he to believe that the market is meeting an "acceptable" standard on this score? The foregoing discussion suggests that the consumer will make this decision by delegating it to a knowledgeable authority – the medical profession. The question here is not whether this delegation does, in point of fact, take place, but rather whether it is economically efficient – that is, does this mechanism translate relevant preferences into market performance? The basic characteristics of demand for hospital services are such as to suggest that the answer to this question is "Yes."

NOTES

1. Paul J. Gordon, "The Top Management Triangle in the Voluntary Hospital," *Hospital Administration* 9, no. 2 (Spring 1964):46–72, provides a good discussion of the hospital management triangle. He notes that, although there has been an abundance of literature on the management triangle relationship, reports of research on the topic have been limited.

2. Ray E. Brown, "Hospital Tensions Threaten Tenure," *The Modern Hospital* 72, no. 5 (November 1949):52.

3. Gordon, "The Top Management Triangle." My own research findings, based on interviews with hospital management, substantiate Gordon's research.

4. "Shaping the Doctor's New Role," *Medical World News*, May 31, 1968, p. 40A. It may be noted that court decisions in recent years have been attenuating the historical doctrine of "charitable immunity." These legal developments have some implications for hospital management structure.

5. Milton I. Roemer, "Growth of Salaried Physicians," *Hospital Progress* 45 (September 1964). An idea of the format for "representative" medical staff organization can be gained from sec. 4 of *Conditions of Participation for Hospitals* under the Medicare program, reproduced in "Hospital Medical Staffs' Requirements Listed," *The AMA News*, January 31, 1966. See also Donald R. Van Houten and Cecil G. Sheps, "The Role of the President of the Medical Staff: The Administrator's View," *Hospital Administration* 12, no. 3 (Summer 1967).

6. Frederick C. LeRocker and S. Kenneth Howard, "What Decisions Do Trustees Actually Make?" *The Modern Hospital* 94, no. 4 (April 1960):83, attempt to determine in more operational terms the role of the governing board in decision-making.

7. Douglas R. Brown, "A New Administrative Model for Hospitals," *Hospital Administration* 12, no. 1 (Winter 1967).

8. Ray E. Brown, "The Vital Framework of Area-Wide Planning," *Hospitals* 37 (March 1963):48.

9. See Burton A. Weisbrod, "Collective Consumption Services of Individual Consumption Goods," *Quarterly Journal of Economics* 78, no. 3 (August 1964):471–77, for a discussion of the "option demand" notion and some of its implications.

10. T. C. Schelling, "The Life You Save May Be Your Own," in *Problems in Public Expenditure Analysis*, ed. Samuel B. Chase (Washington, D.C.: The Brookings Institution, 1966).

11. Kenneth E. Boulding, "The Concept of Need for Health Services," *Milbank Memorial Fund Quarterly* 44, no. 4 (October 1966):203-4.

12. K. J. Arrow, "Uncertainty and the Economics of Medical Care," *American Economic Review* 53, no. 5 (December 1963):951.

Edwin S. Mills
The Johns Hopkins University

COMMENT

I believe an appropriate summary of the first part of Stevens' paper is to say that hospitals will expand to whatever capacity they can finance. In his paper Stevens concentrated on finance through the sale of services, but presumably he would agree that hospitals are no less willing to expand if financing comes from fund-raising or public subsidy. I believe that Stevens' theory is perceptive and plausible. Incidentally, the theory may be applicable to non-profit institutions other than hospitals, including universities.

Stevens' idea is strongly reminiscent of the revenue maximization theory of oligopolistic firms that has been put forward by Baumol and others. One of the unsatisfactory aspects of that theory is that it leaves undetermined the minimum rate of return on capital that constrains the firm's revenue. What rate of return would constrain a hospital? One hopes that it would be greater than zero, but how would one determine it?

I believe that Stevens places too much emphasis on the role of the doctor in determining demand for hospital services. The fact that, to some extent, the doctor makes the decision to demand the services, whereas the patient or the insurance company foots the bill, is intriguing. Other situations in which one person makes the decision and another pays the bill are the demand for prescription drugs and for college textbooks. This complex demand mechanism needs to be studied more, but it seems clear that the customer does have substantial influence on the demand decision. From Stevens' point of view the important fact is the number of beds demanded, whatever the mix of patient and doctor decision-making that explains the demand decision. What matters for the revenue maximization hypothesis is the number of people who will pay fifty dollars per day, and not the extent to which the patient or the doctor makes the decision.

249

Thus, demand, met and unmet, is the key to capacity expansion in Stevens' model. The "standards" he discusses are at best proxies for demand. Other measures might be delays in admissions and numbers of patients who must go for service to hospitals that are less desirable because they provide inferior medical services or are further away. It is potential increases in patients that induce capacity expansion, not increased staff. After all, the doctors do not occupy the beds.

Stevens' data refer mainly to industry, not firm, expansion, but revenue maximization is a theory of firm behavior. We hope that a given hospital will stop expanding when decreasing returns occur, but hospitals will be restricted to efficient sizes only if the demand mechanism is sensitive to price. I was interested in Stevens' data concerning the extent to which capacity expansion took place in existing hospitals. What, then, causes decreasing returns? And are there economies of multi-plant operation?

As in any industrial organization study, the extent of the relevant market should be discussed. In measuring potential demand it is important to know whether the metropolitan area constitutes the market area. For some services, e.g., emergency services, an area smaller than the metropolitan area may be important. Some people, especially those who live near the edge of the metropolitan area, may go outside it for service, and some people may come into a metropolitan area from other places, especially for highly specialized services.

In passing, let me note that I do not understand the notion of option demand that has been put forward by Weisbrod and others. To me, the value of a hospital is the sum of the utilities I will receive from the services it renders, each multiplied by the probability that I will want that service. If all those probabilities are zero, the hospital is worth nothing to me. I do not see the need to go outside the framework of expected utility maximization to understand this phenomenon.

The second part of the paper deals with the notion of optimum capacity from the point of view of society. This is a difficult concept, and I found Stevens' comments interesting. The discussion proceeds entirely in terms of the probability of excess demand. In the literature on water resources, shortage used to be measured in a similar way, by the relative frequency of inadequate supply. However, it is now recognized that duration, as well as frequency, is important. Ten days of water shortage may be much less serious if they are scattered through the year than if they occur in successive days at the end of August. I wonder whether duration is not important in shortage of hospital beds as well. If all beds are full on ten scattered days, nobody has to wait more than a day for a bed, but if days of shortage occur consecutively, somebody will have to wait much longer. This factor is important if a ten-day delay is more than ten times as costly as a one-day delay. The major point to be made about optimum capacity is that the value of additional capacity is measured by the costs borne by those who are subject to delays in hospital admission if capacity is not expanded. In some cases, the cost is that of going somewhat further for the needed service and is not particularly difficult to estimate. In other cases, delay may adversely affect health, in which case the problem is tougher.

I would assume that advocates of the notion that hospital supply creates its own demand simply mean that doctors lower standards for admission when there is excess capacity. Now the problem this raises is that the costs of delays are not simply proportionate to the frequency and duration of delays. When standards are low, presumably those who are refused admission bear less cost than do those who are refused admission when standards are high. This raises no problem in principle but makes life difficult for the practical fellow who must measure the costs of inadequate capacity. My final comment is that the lowering of standards when there is excess capacity may be perfectly desirable. Presumably, the marginal cost of providing additional service is less than average when beds are empty. Therefore, it may pay to admit some people for whom the costs of not being admitted are fairly low, but one cannot infer from full utilization of capacity the need for expansion.

PART V

PRODUCTIVITY AND COST

Richard M. Bailey
University of California, Berkeley

ECONOMIES OF SCALE IN MEDICAL PRACTICE

One of the most frequently quoted statements of John Maynard Keynes is that "the ideas of economists and political philosophers, both when they are right and when they are wrong, are more powerful than is commonly understood."[1] Another equally famous quotation from Keynes is that "soon or late, it is ideas, not vested interests, which are dangerous for good or evil."[2] In this paper I submit that there are a number of erroneous and possibly disastrous ideas circulating in this country concerning the supposed economies of scale to be found in the group practice of medicine. These ideas need to be discussed carefully, for they have formed the intellectual base for public policy decisions in recent years, decisions which may, in fact, work against an optimal allocation of medical resources, and physician resources in particular.

For several years the concept of multi-specialty group practice has been strongly advocated as economically preferable to the traditional forms of medical outpatient practice such as solo and small, single-specialty partnerships. The proponents of multi-specialty group practice have articulated rather well the alleged advantages, both professional and economic, of this form of organizational grouping of physicians. However, careful empirical research and sound documentation have seldom accompanied the elaborate justifications for group practice. Indeed, such a supporter of multi-specialty

Support for this research has been provided by Grant CH-00232, U.S. Public Health Service. Max Brown, my graduate assistant, was particularly helpful at all stages of preparation of this paper. My friends Burton Weisbrod and Richard Sandor made several valuable contributions to the arguments presented. None, of course, share the blame for any inadequacies in the paper.

groups as Rashi Fein has suggested that he has no obligation to prove that economies of scale exist in group practice. Rather, he concludes, "the burden of proof should be on those who would deny their existence rather than on others to demonstrate that they are present."[3]

My intent is not to prove anybody or anything right or wrong, as tempting as such a challenge might be. My goal is to contribute toward a better understanding of the medical service production process as it exists today. To achieve this end, this paper will review some of the current thinking on medical practice and the production of medical services, attempt to clarify some of the implicit theories and assumptions that are basic to current thought on the subject, and offer a new interpretation of the production process based upon my recent research findings.

THE "CONVENTIONAL WISDOM" ON ECONOMIES OF SCALE IN THE MEDICAL FIRM

It is easy to imagine that economies of scale *must* exist in medical group practice. Economists, in particular, are inclined to find the concept attractive, as they conjure up visions of the typical harried doctor and his nurse working at a multiplicity of tasks and being terribly inefficient in the process. Following quickly upon this vision, the economist sees a chart with a nice saucer-shaped, long-run average cost curve. He picks a point on the steeply sloping left side of the saucer and says "That's where the solo practitioner belongs." Visualizing the great opportunities for declining long-run average costs as one enlarges firm size and moves to the right on the curve, he quickly concludes that there must be a more efficient way to produce medical services than in firms of small size. *Ergo*, large group practices are the answer.

Such reasoning seems justified when considered in a general context. In our economy firms in many industries have found that large-scale operations result in lower unit costs because of indivisibilities of capital equipment, pecuniary externalities, and so on. This has been most obviously true in the heavy manufacturing industries, but recently it has been found that even some service industries, such as banking, benefit from scale economies. Such reasoning omits consideration of several important questions which may differentiate the medical service production process from that of other industries. (1) Do we have a commonly accepted concept of the product? (2) Can we use dollar measures of output as a proxy for "real" production, as we often do in other industries? (3) Do we really know much about the substitutability of factor inputs in the medical service production process? (4) Even if the potential for substitutability of factor inputs exists, can we explain the failure of physicians to avail themselves of opportunities to use lower cost inputs on grounds of scale alone?

Apparently, those who profess that economies of scale exist in medical practice either do not consider these questions important or have never bothered to ask them. They have assumed that the generally accepted theories of production are as applicable in medicine as elsewhere. Klarman has suggested that one of the reasons why no one has seriously attempted to measure economies of scale in group practice is that only a small minority of physicians in private practice work in such organizations.[4] Although this observation is certainly accurate, serious proposals that hold significant long-run implications for the future structure of medical practice are being made with increasing frequency. For example, in a report dated February 28, 1967, Secretary of Health, Education, and Welfare Gardner specifically recommended to the President the encouragement of group practice.[5] One year later, the *Economic Report of the President* cited group practice as yielding significant gains in efficiency.[6] Such conclusions seem to be based on a naïve extrapolation of certain basic economic principles to an industry about which few economists are well informed. The facts to support such policies do not exist.

I am willing to acknowledge that economies of scale may exist in certain aspects of the medical services production process. The question raised here is not whether they exist but where they are to be found and how significant they are. We must have some idea of their size before we can decide what kind of an answer group practice offers in the way of increased physician productivity. I submit that the most important public policy issue is how we can increase physician productivity, not how we can achieve internal economies of scale in the practice of medicine. Although the literature often treats these topics as integrally related, they are not. It is the intent in the next section of this paper to shed some light on these topics.

CONCEPTUAL DIFFERENCES BETWEEN PHYSICIAN PRODUCTIVITY AND ECONOMIES OF SCALE

Although the terms "productivity" and "economies of scale" are generally thought to be well understood by economists, they have been abused with great regularity when applied to the health field. Productivity — a rate concept — is concerned with the question of how much output can be obtained from a unit of input. Since the physician is usually viewed as the scarce resource in the production of medical services, the analysis will focus specifically upon average physician productivity. The methods by which the physician can combine his input activities with other resources to produce a given type of medical service define his production function. Assuming a constant state of technology, we might expect to find physicians producing at different rates (even within organizations of similar size) for a number of reasons:

method or technique may vary, quality of education may differ, assistants may not be similarly trained, office layout may or may not be conducive to an orderly work flow, and so on. With an improvement in one or any of these factors average productivity may increase, either because a given physician is moving closer to his production frontier or because a general technological advance has been made.

Measures of physician productivity necessarily must include inputs and outputs. The inputs customarily considered important in the production of medical services in the physician's office are heterogeneous; they include such factors as man hours, both of medical and paramedical personnel, and capital equipment, including land and buildings. The output measures that have been used most frequently by economists include office visits, hospital visits, and house calls. The adequacy of these output measures has been questioned by many observers. Some argue that no output measure is satisfactory unless it includes an indication of the impact of the service on the patient's health. Others believe that some specific evaluation of the quality of the service (usually defined by health professionals as meeting certain input standards) is necessary. Others want to look at an incident of illness, measure all inputs received by the patient in the course of treatment, and count recovery from the illness as the final output. Without pausing to take issue with each and every position that has been advanced, I shall merely note that customary output measures focus upon what the physician produces, not the effects upon the patient.

For certain analytical purposes it may be quite legitimate to attempt to measure the success of medical services in restoring the patient's health. Such analyses inevitably evaluate the final product of the medical firm in terms of its ability to contribute to consumer utility. But for the purpose of applying positive economic analysis to the medical services production process, it is inappropriate to muddy the waters with so many variables and relationships that the meaningful factors cannot be identified and isolated. The concept of the production function of the medical firm has never been postulated in anything resembling a specific form. We assume that the patient purchases services from the physician with some expectation that these services will improve his health, but the physician does not produce health. His output in this paper is largely considered to be office visits. Thus measures of average physician productivity are defined as output of office visits ÷ input of physician man hours.

The concept of economies of scale also deals with inputs and outputs but broadens the picture to include a description of how *all* input factors are combined in firms of various size to produce the final output(s). The key point is this: it is to be expected that the proportions of factors used will differ in firms of different scale producing the same type of good or service, primarily because of the indivisibility of certain factors which cannot be acquired in all sizes with similar efficiency. Because of factor indivisibility, the theory posits that in most industries large firms will receive increasing returns to scale. At some point in growth, these internal factor indivisibilities become inconsequential, and constant returns to scale set in. Finally, at some later stage of growth, decreasing returns to scale occur, with additional inputs yielding less than a proportional quantity of output.

The economies of scale referred to above are present only in the internal operations of firms. There are, however, a growing number of externally produced services which are increasingly important to the medical firm. Most references to economies of scale in medical practice have emphasized the opportunity of large group practice to realize internal economies; very little attention has been given to the significance of economies that are available outside the firm. We will return to this issue later.

Whereas our discussion of physician productivity did not mention dollars, the ultimate criterion to be applied in any search for economies of scale is lowest per-unit costs. Confusion often arises when we apply this criterion to medical practice because the physical volume of output is rarely defined precisely. But how can we measure lowest per-unit costs if we do not know what the unit is? Some economists have proceeded to discuss economies of scale as if this were an unimportant point. They have somehow reasoned that large organizations can produce medical services more cheaply than small ones because there may be greater division of labor in medical groups. Since such specialization often leads to higher productivity and lower unit costs in other industries, medical groups must be able to have lower unit costs. The indivisibility of capital equipment which can produce a high volume of output at low unit cost is also advanced as an argument in this case.

Problems frequently arise in specifying the source of economies of scale in any industry because of the presence of multiple-product firms. Size generally brings with it the development of a broader product line and the internalization of manufacturing, marketing, or distributing functions previously handled by others. Therefore, when we analyze firms of a different size in a given industry with the intent of finding scale economies, it is not self-evident that direct comparisons are possible. For example, can we say that a large, multi-specialty group practice is comparable to a solo practice? Must we not carefully distinguish between common products made by each firm and then further analyze the production process to see where differences exist? With this overview of the concepts of physician productivity and economies of scale, let us turn to some specific issues.

THE "CLASSICAL VIEW" OF ECONOMIES OF SCALE IN MEDICAL PRACTICE

Rashi Fein observes the maxim that because of factor indivisibility a firm cannot buy half a machine, nor is it efficient for a small firm to buy a machine and use it at less than full capacity.[7] He further notes that some physicians, namely, solo practitioners, may do without some equipment. His conclusion is that such physicians are less productive.[8] This argument seems to imply that unless a doctor has the equipment needed in his office his patients will be denied its use. But what if it is available in a large hospital department across the street, even in another private office in the same building? If the doctor sends his patient across the street or down the hall for a chest film or a blood count, is he operating at a lower productivity level? In my opinion, the literature focuses on a minor issue, ownership of these tools of production. What impact on physician productivity does the ownership variable have?

From other sources we find statements that add to the confusion about the supposed advantages of group practice: "Business end of medicine in hands of business staff. Doctors can devote more time to medicine, and hence be more productive."[9] In the first place, this statement assumes that the solo practitioner cannot delegate administrative matters to a staff (of possibly only one or two persons). It also ignores the many business services which can relieve the physician in small-scale practice of many of his business duties — computerized billing services; bookkeeping, accounting, and tax services; dictation services; and employment agencies providing part-time assistants as needed. These external economies made possible by the growth of the medical services industry are not insignificant. Moreover, even if the physician could devote more time to medicine in a large group practice because others were carrying the administrative duties, do we know that he would use his time this way? Further, increased use of a factor (in this case, physician man hours) does not necessarily increase its productivity. It may act to increase total production, but the production rate may not change much.

In the *Report to the President on Medical Care Prices* which was cited earlier, we find the statement: "There is evidence that . . . physicians with more assistants are more productive."[10] Even if this statement were true, it says only that the marginal product of an assistant is greater than zero. Unhappily, the source of the evidence is not disclosed. No one can be sure whether the report is asserting a cause-and-effect relationship or a coincidence. To begin with, there are good reasons for questioning the evidence used to prove an increase in productivity. This argument is that since the gross income of physicians using more assistants increased faster than fees, average productivity must have increased. But what if income rose because more doctors offered and sold additional services to their patients, such as laboratory or X-ray tests? Certainly these services generate additional gross income, but they do not speak to the issue of physician productivity. Moreover, even if average productivity did increase, did it increase because the ratio of paramedical personnel to physician rose? This would have to mean that paramedical man hours were substituted for physician man hours. Has this really occurred, or are the additional paramedical people simply used to provide new and additional services which were formerly supplied elsewhere?

In the conventional thinking about group practice, there is apparently an implicit assumption that we are dealing with a one-product firm and a single production process; that is, most analysts have accepted the patient visit, or perhaps something more abstract such as the patient's health, as the sole final output of the physician's office. Laboratory, X-ray, and paramedical personnel services in various associated activities have been regarded as inputs, not outputs. These analyses of the medical firm seem to be based on the assumption that the final measurable product, the patient visit, can be produced in a variety of ways, depending upon the number of inputs at the physician's disposal. In general, there has been complete neglect of the fact that the large multi-specialty group practices are in reality multi-product firms. Comparable medical specialists functioning in large medical groups may produce many services similar to those of the solo practitioner, but the total number of services produced in the various medical practices tends to be correlated with size. The "classical view" has not recognized these differences in output mixes and instead has expressed the production process in such a way as to imply that the final products are similar and only the inputs vary. Thus one might say that the "classical view" of the product of any medical firm engaged in producing personal medical services could be denoted in the traditional form of a production function with multiple inputs and one output.

Broadly speaking, each firm's input factors could be divided into the classical categories of capital and labor, i.e.: $(K_1, K_2, K_3, \ldots, K_x; L_1, L_2, L_3, \ldots, L_y)$, where K_1 is floor space, K_2 is laboratory equipment, K_3 is X-ray equipment, etc., and L_1 is physician hours, L_2 is medical assistant hours, L_3 is technician hours, etc. Of course, we would expect the total number of components in the input vector to vary directly with the size of the firm.

We could now, at least conceptually, describe each firm's production function as: $f(K_1, \ldots, K_x, L_1, \ldots, L_y) = y$. Here a significant point needs to be understood. This traditional view of the production process implies considerable substitutability of inputs that can be used to produce outpatient personal medical services. Physician time is deemed the scarcest and most expensive input; thus, to the extent that either capital or man hour inputs of paramedical personnel can be substituted for physician man hours (as occurs, it is implied, in large, multi-specialty group practices), physician productivity is increased. To the extent that large medical firms are expected to have a greater division of labor and more specialized capital equipment, we could also reason that they would be able to capture increasing internal returns to scale. I believe this concept of the production function to be inadequate for measuring economies of scale in medical practice and will now attempt to state my understanding of that process.

A NEW INTERPRETATION OF ECONOMIES OF SCALE IN MEDICAL PRACTICE

The decision to treat certain service industry factors as inputs or outputs is always difficult to make. As I pointed out above, it appears that most economists concerned with production by the medical firm have settled upon the patient visit as the only acceptable output measure.[11] In so doing, they have implied that the final product of the medical firm may be achieved by varying methods and that by increasing firm size, opportunities for substitution of low-cost for high-cost inputs are increased.[12] I reject this view and advance the idea that a simpler but more useful analysis is to realize that the medical firm produces a range of products. These products may be denoted by the output vector $(Y_1, Y_2, Y_3, \ldots, Y_n)$, where Y_1 might be examination by a physician, Y_2 might be a laboratory test, Y_3 might be an X-ray examination, and the like. As one would expect, the total number of components in the output vector will vary with the size of the firm. A firm with a single physician will have fewer components than will a large, multi-specialty group practice.

For a number of reasons, based upon both historical observation of the organization of the medical service industry and recently acquired knowledge (to be discussed later), I treat each of these products of the medical firm as having a separate and unique process function; that is to say, there is one process function for routine medical examinations, another for complete medical histories and physical examinations, and still other sets for laboratory tests and X-ray examinations. We might label these "physician products" (where the dominant input is physician time) and "ancillary products" (where the dominant input is paramedical personnel time).

In solo practice few products are offered, the most significant of which is examination by the physician. (Hospital visits are also significant products offered by all physicians, but we exclude these from present consideration because we are concentrating primarily on the economic entity of the physician's office.) Conceptually speaking, even different kinds of examinations conducted by the physician, such as a routine or annual physical examination, are different products and are generated by separate production relationships. However, the differences are slight, perhaps varying only by the physician's man hour input. In creating these physician's products, opportunities for substituting other factor inputs for the physician's man hour input may be minimal. The few other products offered by a firm with only one physician are usually relatively simple laboratory tests.

In the small firm the function which describes the production of these products is highly labor-intensive. Because high-volume laboratory equipment is indivisible, few solo physicians possess it. The same argument applies to X-ray apparatus. Because the laboratory must necessarily be labor-intensive in the small firm, we can hardly expect much more than constant returns to scale and constant unit costs, notwithstanding certain externalities. This means that total production for the firm, and hence revenue, is bounded by the amount of the intensive factor, labor. Thus we would expect a profit-maximizing small medical practice to have a high level of labor factor input.

As we move along the spectrum toward larger firms with more physicians, it is natural to find a more diversified product line. The relationships among these various products deserve careful consideration. For the moment, let us consider these products in terms of sets. All those generated by the physician, such as examinations, might be one set, all those from the laboratory another set, and all those from X-ray yet another set. The point here is that no product in any one set is necessarily a joint product with another in any other set; that is to say, most laboratory tests involve no inputs common to examinations by the physician, nor are the two products generated simultaneously by the same person. No technical connection exists between the production of physicians (M.D. examinations) and laboratory tests. Phrased in yet another way, we could say that the addition of a certain laboratory test to the product line of the firm alters in no way the function of the physician with regard to patient examinations. Whether a doctor sends a patient across the hall, across the street, or across the town for a laboratory test, the technique he uses for examining that patient is not affected. It has been developed and internalized by years of medical school and postgraduate training and is not easily changed.

Production within a given set, however, may be characterized as assorted; that is, given the inputs, there may be any number of different products. In an office with the standard line of medical equipment and supplies believed to be indispensable to his specialty, the physician can create a wide range of diagnostic and therapeutic products. Moving to another set of products, we can easily see that a technician, given the basic equipment and supplies of a laboratory, can produce a number of different laboratory tests. There is also a degree of joint production in each of these sets.

To summarize what has been established so far, we can say that a firm's production should be described by constructing the process functions for each of the firm's outputs. Thus, production might be characterized as follows:

$$Y_1 = f^1(K_1, \ldots, K_n, L_1, \ldots, L_m)$$
$$Y_2 = f^2(K_1, \ldots, K_n, L_1, \ldots, L_m)$$

$$\cdot$$
$$\cdot$$
$$\cdot$$

$$Y_x = f^x(K_1, \ldots, K_n, L_1, \ldots, L_m)$$
$$Y_{x+1} = g^1(K_{n+1}, \ldots, K_r, L_{m+1}, \ldots, L_t)$$
$$Y_{x+2} = g^2(K_{n+1}, \ldots, K_r, L_{m+1}, \ldots, L_t)$$

$$\cdot$$
$$\cdot$$
$$\cdot$$

$$Y_{x+z} = g^z(K_{n+1}, \ldots, K_r, L_{m+1}, \ldots, L_t)$$

$$\cdot$$
$$\cdot$$
$$\cdot$$

etc., where Y_1 through Y_x are the assorted products generated by the physician, such as patient examinations, consultations, and so forth. Each f denotes a different technical relationship, in the sense that the production function for specific physician products requires varying amounts of physician and paramedical man hour inputs and various inputs of capital. Products Y_{x+1} through Y_{x+z} are generated by the laboratory. Again, each g denotes a different technical relationship among factors. This description is repeated for each set of products offered by the firm. The technical relationships existing in the production of the $Y_1 - Y_x$ physician products are assumed fairly constant for all physicians in a given specialty for the reasons mentioned before. These technical relationships might not hold so much in the production of ancillary products for obvious reasons of indivisibility of capital.

Having at least identified the various production processes of the medical firm, we may discuss how the specific form might change as a result of firm size. How the functions might appear for a solo physician firm has been noted: a small product line with labor-intensive production functions and constant returns to scale. As the firm grows in number of physicians and total output, certain products may be added to the line that can bring increasing returns to scale and decreasing unit costs. Many of the laboratory products can be generated on this basis with the very sophisticated, high-volume equipment available today.

What is happening in the larger medical groups becomes very clear when terms are defined in the same way as the firm's production has been described. First of all, new products are added to the line as the firm grows. The motive behind this diversification is not always clear. It may be based on the belief that vertical integration increases efficiency, but efficiency of what? We have already seen that production in the laboratory has no direct connection with physician production. Some small gains in average physician productivity in the larger firms may arise from better timing and sequence of patient flow, but this possibility raises a whole new question of demand structuring which is too complex to be considered at this point. Perhaps the motive for vertical integration is financial: with a high volume of patients, the large firm may be able to utilize the same type of high-volume equipment found in the nearest hospital or commercial laboratory. In that case, it can price its laboratory products competitively and retain the profits instead of allowing them to accrue to the hospital or the commercial laboratory.

For products offered at every level of firm size, such as a simple laboratory test like a white blood count, the production technique may shift from labor-intensive to capital-intensive as the firm grows. This is pure and simple factor substitution, which occurs as the firm is able to take advantage of large capital equipment. But this does not mean that the solo practice physician cannot avail himself of such advantages. It is more than likely he will send the patient or his specimens to a large-scale laboratory that is capital-intensive.

Meanwhile, what is happening to the physician? I submit that there is no apparent shift in factor use as a result of changing firm size. A careful reading of the medical literature confirms this view: there is no discussion of specific cases of capital-for-labor substitution or of significant instances of paramedical man hour-for-physician substitution. Increasing lip service is being paid to the need for training new types of personnel to assist physicians with their various tasks, and many companies are seeking to develop products which will result in similar opportunities to substitute capital for physician labor, but evidence of significant factor substitution for physician time is lacking in the literature.

If paramedical labor could be substituted for physician labor in many routine examinations, the physician would be free to produce what he alone can produce. Total production of the firm would rise because paramedical labor is generally more readily available in most parts of the country than is physician labor. It is not immediately obvious, though, that such an occurrence would result in any change in returns to scale. However, such substitution of paramedical for physician labor could be very meaningful in increasing average physician productivity and lowering unit costs in all firms as the cheaper labor factor is substituted for the more expensive. The substitution of capital for physician labor might result in declining unit costs because of indivisibilities and financial externalities, but its effects on *physician* productivity (more office visits per hour) might be quite indirect. To date, most capital innovations in medicine have affected ancillary, not physician, products. Since these ancillary products come from many firms other than those owned by practicing physicians, all physicians have had access to the benefits derived from increasing the capital intensity of the production process. Of the two substitution possibilities, the former — that of using paramedical personnel increasingly in the production of physician products — offers the most fruitful solution. To repeat, this is a more pressing goal than increasing returns to scale.

THE MEDICAL FIRM IN PERSPECTIVE

Traditionally, most physicians work in somewhat limited physical surroundings. Most medical practices function with minimal capital investment by the physician. The capital-intensive medical institutions are hospitals, commercial laboratories, major teaching centers, and a few large clinics. Physicians usually turn to these organizations for assistance with difficult testing, diagnostic, or treatment procedures. Other institutions which supply the physician with needed goods or services are the pharmacies, certain hospitals providing intensive care, and another group of hospitals specializing in long-term problems such as tuberculosis and mental illness. These other organizations, which often are financed with public funds, make it unnecessary for most physicians to have a more capital-intensive firm to ensure that their patients will have access to the complete range of products that may be essential to good medical care.

Many people today, impressed with the increasingly complex technology of medicine, seem to feel that the physician needs to be in intimate daily contact with the elaborate tools and equipment used in hospitals, laboratories, and the like. These people look to the large multi-specialty groups or clinics as the best setting for the production of medical services. But is this really so? If we observe how many of these existing clinics have developed, technical considerations rarely stand out as the major factor in their formation and growth. In the small midwestern cities where group practice first became popular, there was often an inadequate demand base for competing medical service firms. Physicians, wanting these services, internalized such production within their clinics. Many of these clinics even today sell a broad range of laboratory, X-ray, pharmacy, and optical services and goods. Moreover, as specialism in medicine evolved, the combination of a balanced group of specialists within one firm made it seem natural to offer a nearly complete set of medical products, especially if the sale of these services could also be profitable. Although the medical clinics appear to be vertically integrated, the single-specialty group practices have evolved as single firms offering multiple services (outputs) rather than single outputs. The point to be emphasized here is that there appears to be no medical necessity to incorporate many of these ancillary products into the production process of any large groups. Rather, factors of market size, assurance of availability of certain services, and profitability have probably been more important than technical considerations.

In most large cities multi-specialty groups tend to be rare. The large population base is adequate to support many physicians with wide specialty training, the majority of whom continue to be in solo practice or in single-specialty medical groups of two or three. This large demand base makes it possible for a great number of medical service firms to develop to which patients may be sent for certain services or from which the physicians may purchase services directly. We find many commercial laboratories (usually owned by pathologists) and hospital laboratories that exist by performing laboratory tests for physicians; medical practices which are frequently owned by several radiologists or hospitals which provide extensive X-ray services; pharmacies (owned by pharmacists); eye care specialists (ophthalmologists, optometrists, opticians) who not only examine eyes but dispense glasses; and, of course, the many business service firms mentioned earlier. In the large cities, there often are one or two teaching centers or major hospitals which provide physicians with unusual low-volume tests and procedures. Given the availability of this wide range of medical and business services – produced by firms and institutions which not only specialize in such production but which may be large enough to achieve internal economies that the normal clinic could not – it seems reasonable to assume again that there is no technical necessity for these services to be produced internally in the medical firm. Failure to accept this assumption means that we must argue that physicians do not really know what they need in order to produce medical services, an assumption which I am not yet willing to accept.

SOME EMPIRICAL FINDINGS ON ECONOMIES OF SCALE

Whereas many commentators on medical economics have based their analyses on general postulates of economic theory – and then have proceeded to follow a course of what has appeared to be sound deductive reasoning – most of the insights of this paper, both theoretical and empirical, have come from approximately three years of intimate and often frustrating contact with physicians engaged in private practice. The reasoning applied herein has generally been more inductive than deductive and has necessarily been forged and buffeted by the sheer weight of observation and measurement.

As stated earlier, the "classical view" of the medical services production process envisions a single production function, which implies that larger

Table 1: Average Physician Production, 1966[a]

Production Measure	Firm Size[b]				
	Solo	Two-Man	Three-Man	Four- to Five-Man	Clinics
No. of office visits	2,727	2,653	2,421	2,277	2,561
Dollar value of office visits	$29,298	$29,385	$31,517	$25,064	$34,824
No. of hospital visits	901	677	1,079	782	n.a.
Dollar value of hospital visits	$10,225	$8,039	$13,884	$10,347	$9,040

[a]Based upon data obtained from a selected sample of internists practicing in the San Francisco Bay area.
[b]The number of practices represented in each category of firm size is solo, 12; two-man, 4; three-man, 6; four- to five-man, 5; clinics, 4.

organizations should achieve higher average productivity per physician. The possibility of adding to the quantity of capital equipment and the various specialized human resources available to the physician has, accordingly, been seen as an important factor in increasing returns to scale. Data from my study of San Francisco Bay area internists do not support this line of reasoning. Whether the output measure used was patient visits per hour or simply total production of patient visits in a month or a year, internists in the large multi-specialty groups were found to be no more productive than smaller group or solo physicians. As the production data in Table 1 indicate, very little difference was found in the total production of office (and hospital visits) among forms of various size. However, if dollar measures of output had been used to reflect total production, these conclusions would be quite different because of the inclusion of multi-product sales in clinics.

Data in Table 2, which cover the month of April 1967 and were collected in greater detail as to type of physician product, substantiate this finding. In this table, weighted production of office visits is derived by assigning to the major categories of regular office visits, annual examinations, and complete histories and physical examinations weights based upon the amount of time the physician normally devotes to each service output. On the average, clinic internists produced more patient visits than the physician in smaller organizations only by devoting more of their total work month to such activity. Total production of clinic internists equaled or exceeded that of some of the physicians in smaller practice; however, the average productivity of the clinic physicians was below that of all other physicians. Again, if we were to use dollar measures of production of these physicians in this same month, our conclusions would be reversed. In that period, the average solo internist

Table 2: Average Physician Production and Productivity, April 1967

Production Measure	Firm Size				
	Solo	Two-Man	Three-Man	Four- to Five-Man	Clinics
Weighted production of office visits/physician	286	278	291	243	286
Weighted production of office visits/physician time with patients	3.4	3.0	3.5	3.1	2.9

Source: see notes to Table 1.

grossed $4,777, the average internist in a three-man practice grossed $6,107, and the average clinic internist grossed $6,725. The proportion of revenue derived from sale of physician products and technical products is even more impressive when firm sizes are compared. In April 1967 the average percentage of revenues earned by sale of physician products for solo, three-man, and clinic internists was 85, 66, and 52 per cent, respectively. Conversely, the sale of ancillary products by these same physician firms was 15, 34, and 48 per cent.

There may be several explanations for the apparent constant returns to scale that we have seen in the production of physician products. The one that I find most satisfactory is related to medical education itself. Group as well as non-group physicians receive the same type of training in medical school and in postgraduate internships and residencies, in which the concept of following accepted patterns of health care is instilled in them. Indeed, various surveys of physician work habits have demonstrated that physicians in a given specialty allocate a remarkably similar amount of time to each kind of patient visit. My survey yielded comparable results. Physicians also feel under considerable compulsion to behave like their colleagues because of the implication that deviance from the norm will be equated with poor quality service. Malpractice laws tend to reinforce this conformity. Even in medical practices that are widely known for their innovative economic and organizational structure, such as the Kaiser Foundation Health Plan, a recent report indicates that conventional methods of practice dominate – that no economies are evident in the use of health manpower.[13]

All of these findings support the acceptance of a new model which views the production of physician services as highly separable from the production of ancillary services. The separability argument, if carried to its ultimate conclusion, forces a re-evaluation of traditionally accepted arguments about factor substitutability in the medical firm. It forces us to consider the multi-

Table 3: Physician-Paramedical Hours, April 1967

Hours and Ratios	Firm Size				
	Solo	Two-Man	Three-Man	Four- to Five-Man	Clinics
Average physician hours	218	222	197	200	197
Average paramedical hours/physician	187	181	225	271	499
Average technical hours[a]/physician	7	11	9	44	122
Paramedical hours/ physician hours	0.858	0.817	1.142	1.353	2.531

[a]Technical hours cover time spent by paramedical personnel in the use of EKG machines and tapes and in X-ray and laboratory activities.

Source: see notes to Table 1.

product nature of many of the larger practices and to carefully distinguish between outputs and inputs. With regard to the use of paramedical personnel, group practice advocates frequently maintain that data on ratios of paramedical workers to physicians, or paramedical hours to patient visits, or paramedical hours to physician hours indicate greater personnel substitution in large organizations.[14] In fact, an accurate measure of paramedical substitutability would consider only those personnel who assist in the production of "physician products." Table 3 demonstrates that a considerable proportion of paramedical hours are devoted to ancillary products. At the same time, the data confirm that as the size of the organization increases more paramedical personnel per physician are added. Theorists in the past have deduced that this latter phenomenon points to a substitutability that must directly increase physician productivity. The basic assumption is that certain physician functions lend themselves to a degree of paramedical assistance resulting in direct substitution for physician time. The average physician productivity data in Table 2 contradict this conclusion. Productivity in the large clinics (as measured by patient visits per hour) was found to be lower on the average than in smaller practices. Total production, on the other hand, was about the same at the two extreme sizes. These data suggest that the addition of paramedical personnel does not directly affect physician production rates but may result in the substitution of paramedical time for physician time spent on certain tasks which are extraneous to patient visits. In sum, these data suggest that adding paramedical personnel merely frees more of the physician's total monthly work hours for contact with patients. Since physician time is regarded as the only scarce input and we find that paramedical time is seldom substituted for physician time in the production of physician products, it appears that the marginal physical productivity of paramedical personnel diminishes at an accelerated rate.

Even though the production of physician products is labor-intensive, should we reasonably expect to see increases in physician productivity with additions to capital, as some analysts have noted? The above discussion suggests that the answer is no. The conventional approach to the production function of the medical firm based upon a single product should be abandoned in favor of recognizing the multi-product model. When one does this — focusing upon the separateness of the various production functions — the capital economies argument is effectively eliminated. A simple inventory of equipment vital to the physician's delivery of services reveals that capital is not a relatively scarce or important input. The typical internist requires no more than five thousand dollars' worth of depreciable assets, the most expensive of which are often examining tables and various scopes. The decision to produce a variety of ancillary products internally alters this asset picture considerably, but the efficient delivery of physician services does not appear to be dependent on their internal production.

Although production of physician services can be characterized as devoid of significant possibilities for non-physician labor or capital substitution (in the short run), production of other outputs of the firm can demonstrate more flexibility in factor use and, more important, short-run increasing returns to scale. Laboratory testing at a volume which can efficiently utilize automated equipment and full-time technologists shows clear evidence of increasing returns. Such equipment is justified economically only as part of the diversified product offering of a medical firm in which there are a sufficient number of physicians to generate demand internally. The important point here, however, is that the individual physician's productivity is not affected by possessing such equipment. He can usually obtain laboratory, X-ray, and other technical products from other firms which specialize in them. Thus the decision to produce them internally can be separated from the decision to order the tests at all.

SUMMARY

It is a natural expectation, given the historical development of our economy, to assume that economies of scale should exist in medical practice. Indeed, in a sense they do. But the questions to which this paper is addressed are to what extent and where do such economies exist or not exist, and why or why not? In the solo practice of medicine the issues of physician productivity and economies of scale may be intertwined because the output of such firms is almost exclusively a single product. When we examine larger practices, the introduction of multiple products makes it necessary to consider physician productivity apart from the issue of economies of scale. Most analysts in the past have not made this distinction because they have used financial measures of output, rather than physical measures, and thus the significance of multiple products has been obscured. This approach has also led observers to believe that considerable substitutability of labor or capital factors for physician time occurs in the larger practices. The present analysis and data refute this belief.

It has been noted that by examining the production functions for separate products of the medical firm, certain activities such as laboratory tests or administration and record-keeping may display increasing returns to scale. But I strongly believe that the most basic production process in the medical firm – physician services – does not vary as a result of changing firm size. This rigid production function may have the same effect as the well known "bottleneck constraint" found in linear programming solutions. This reasoning is further encouraged by observation of the scarcity of large, multispecialty clinics in large cities. When a substantial number of firms exist explicitly to serve the demands of physicians for technical and business products or services, most physicians find that they do not need a large, integrated medical firm. These services are not essential components of the physician's production function; they need not be produced jointly with physician services. Rather, they are complementary goods which can be produced apart from the physician's organization – often in firms where increasing returns of scale are clearly recognizable.

Of course, it is not possible to say that the physician's production function will never change. It may be that it is changing considerably but that substantial lags in the adoption of new techniques are inevitable. The process of change may be very difficult, given the obstacles of long lead times in education, the legal posture of malpractice, and the monopolistic structure of the medical service industry and its many components. One thing seems clear, however: many of our present beliefs about economies of scale in medical practice are founded on sand, not rock.

NOTES

1. *General Theory of Employment, Interest and Money* (New York: Harcourt, Brace and Company, 1958), p. 383.

2. *Ibid.*, p. 384.

3. *The Doctor Shortage: An Economic Diagnosis* (Washington, D.C.: The Brookings Institution, 1967), p. 98.

4. Herbert E. Klarman, *The Economics of Health* (New York: Columbia University Press, 1965), p. 128.

5. John Gardner, "A Report to the President on Medical Care Prices," February 28, 1967, p. 4.

6. (Washington, D.C.: U.S. Government Printing Office, 1968), p. 160.

7. *The Doctor Shortage*, p. 97.

8. *Ibid.*, p. 99.

9. G. W. Hunter, M.D., in *The Physician and Group Practice*, ed. E. P. Jordan, M.D. (Chicago: Year Book Publishers, 1958), p. 48.

10. P. 22.

11. See, for example, Donald E. Yett, "An Evaluation of Alternative Methods of Estimating Physicians' Expenses Relative to Output," *Inquiry* 4 (March 1967):3–27.

12. See Paul J. Feldstein, "Research on the Demand for Health Services," *Milbank Memorial Fund Quarterly* 44, no. 3 (July 1966):152–55; J. A. Boan, *Group Practice* (Ottawa: Royal Commission on Health Services, 1966), pp. 23–31.

13. *Report of the National Advisory Commission on Health Manpower*, vol. 2 (Washington, D.C.: U.S. Government Printing Office, 1967), pp. 206–7.

14. See especially Boan, *Group Practice*, pp. 23–28.

Melvin W. Reder
Stanford University

COMMENT

In offering an explicit challenge to the proposition that group practice entails economies of scale, Professor Bailey has rendered a distinct service to students of medical economics. Clearly, it is essential for purposes of public policy as well as those of positive science that we acquire a firm basis for appraising the effect of size of medical firm on cost of patient care and, if economies of scale exist, for identifying their sources. Bailey has made a significant contribution to this task; however, his argument leaves me unconvinced on several important points.

COSTS, PRODUCTION RELATIONS, AND OUTPUT MEASUREMENT

Bailey argues (see pp. 262ff. above) that the outputs of a medical firm may be separated into two classes, physician-generated and laboratory-generated. He alleges that none of the inputs of any physician-generated output (mainly physician time) is also an input of any laboratory-generated output and that no input related to a laboratory output also serves as an input for a physician output. He further contends that such economies of scale as may be found within a medical firm arise solely from the laboratory-generated outputs.*

But this is not an adequate description of the production process of a medical firm. In most cases, a laboratory output should be considered as an input to the process of rendering physician services to a patient. In many cases a laboratory test greatly reduces the amount of physician time needed

---

*Presumably, scale is measured by number of physicians in the firm.

274

to diagnose a particular ailment, and in others it distinctly changes the quality of output by permitting otherwise unobtainable diagnoses. For simplicity, consider only the time-saving case. Here, laboratory tests are an input to the production of physician services, potentially capable of substitution for physician time, and the tests are an intermediate output — even when they are billed separately. In short, the production function of a medical firm is not separable in the manner Bailey describes.[1]

Whether laboratory tests are produced within the firm or purchased from the "outside" depends upon the size of the diseconomies of joint production, if any, of physician services and laboratory services within a single firm relative to the transaction costs between firms (billing, record-keeping, etc.) that result from complete specialization of function. It may be that transaction costs are partly due to monopoloid practices and/or short-run disequilibrium within the "laboratory industry," but to determine this would require a separate investigation. Whatever their source, transaction costs require explicit consideration, which Bailey does not accord them.

If I understand him correctly, Bailey does not deny that there are increasing returns to scale in laboratory production or that, in cases of joint production, such economies are empirically associated with the scale of operations in terms of number of physicians. What he does seek to deny is that such increasing returns are attributable to increases in output per physician. The data in the tables he presents support his contention. However in another paper, his data suggested that there are increasing returns to scale in profit per hour worked but that this is offset by a tendency for physicians (internists) in larger firms to work fewer hours per month.[2] Perhaps Bailey does not consider increasing returns per hour as "genuine" increasing returns, for he remarked in his earlier paper that "physicians in these practices appear to be working fewer hours, having fewer physician-patient contacts and enjoying more leisure time. In the process they are making higher incomes."[3] However, the reduced monthly hours with higher hourly earnings surely represent a preference for such rewards over more hours and lower hourly earnings. *Ceteris paribus*, this should increase the supply of physicians, thereby making hourly compensation (and presumably consumer price per output unit) lower than it otherwise would have been.*

The inference in my last sentence might be challenged: e.g., it might be argued that the supply of physicians is rigidly determined by the number of places in medical schools and is independent of physician reward. To this I would reply (1) that the supply of physicians *to private practice* would be responsive to rewards in such practice even if the argument were valid; i.e., physicians may choose careers in research, public health, teaching, or adminis-

---

*Moreover, increased producers' surplus of physicians should be reflected as increased output.

tration as alternatives to private practice; and (2) that higher rewards will increase the number of applicants for medical schools, thereby improving physician quality (see below). I would further note that an increase in physician supply might increase either quality of care or patient contact with physicians, or both, instead of, or in addition to, decreasing relative price per office call.

MEASUREMENT OF OUTPUT

Taken literally, Bailey's definition of the output unit as an office visit makes it impossible to discuss "quality of care" as an output dimension; I consider this undesirable. It is obviously tempting to ignore quality as an output dimension because doing so permits us to treat the relatively abundant data on "visits," patient-doctor "contacts," etc., as output data. Under certain conditions, and for certain purposes, this may be appropriate. But, consensus or no, under other conditions it is inappropriate.

In general, the production of services involves a personal relation between producer and consumer, a most important aspect of which is time spent per contact. Impatience on either side is felt as an adverse element in the exchange. The variation in doctors' willingness to spend time talking with individual patients is notorious. Even if it were granted that physician training rigidly limits variations in minutes per procedure, which I doubt, variations in physician manner would affect the number of visits per hour. It is not unreasonable to suppose that a more unhurried manner will be reflected in a higher price per visit, which will be accepted in exchange for what is felt to be superior service, even if such service is not "medically superior."[4]

For the purpose of Bailey's cross-sectional analysis, it may be appropriate to measure output in "office visit" units. This could be done if physician time per office visit were uncorrelated with firm size. But if large clinics tend toward an impersonal and curt form of physician service, as is often alleged, it may be that the tendency toward increasing returns per physician hour (reported by Bailey) is spurious and is the result of deteriorating quality with increased firm size. The truth of such an assertion would have to be determined by a detailed time and motion study of procedures, patient satisfaction, etc., but such a study would require, *inter alia*, explicit consideration of the quality of care in different sizes of medical firms; it would not suffice to assume fixed quality.

More generally, the relation of economies of scale and quality of care requires an explicit judgment as to the effect on quality that allegedly results from access to the wide variety of specialists who practice in large clinics. This greater access is presumed to reflect greater willingness of physicians to refer within the firm than outside it.* Variations in the strength of the "anti-outside-referral factor" with the size of the medical firm and the relation of this factor to the quality of care are clearly matters for investigation, but part of the economies of scale *may* lie in superior quality of care at a constant deflated dollar cost to the patient.

NOTES

1. An excellent example of a situation where there would seem to be appreciable substitution of laboratory tests for physician time (as compared with a conventional method of medical practice) arises in the multiphasic screening procedure used by the Kaiser Foundation Health Plan. For a description of this procedure, see M. F. Cullen, "Periodic Health Examinations Using an Automated Multitest Laboratory," *Journal of the American Medical Association* 195, no. 10 (March 1966): 830–33.

2. Richard M. Bailey, "Economies of Scale in Outpatient Medical Practice," Table 9, p. 21, quoted in D. Strope, B. Cohen, and A. Yonkers, "Increasing Productivity in the Delivery of Ambulatory Health Services; a Review of Literature and Ongoing Projects" (Paper prepared for the Department of Health, Education, and Welfare under Contract HEW-OS-68-22, May 1968), p. 63.

3. *Ibid.*, p. 20.

4. I have discussed this and related questions in "Some Problems in the Measurement of Productivity in the Medical Care Industry," in *Production and Productivity in the Service Industries*, ed. Victor R. Fuchs (New York: National Bureau of Economic Research, 1969), pp. 95–131. It should be remarked that it is not easy to separate superior care from better patient attitudes induced by good personal relations with a doctor.

*This boils down to a transaction cost between firms.

Harold A. Cohen
University of Georgia

HOSPITAL COST CURVES WITH EMPHASIS ON MEASURING PATIENT CARE OUTPUT

The purpose of this paper is to develop a partial measure of hospital output in order to construct long-run hospital cost curves. These cost curves would be useful both for the planning and expansion of hospital facilities and for the application of reimbursement formulas. Hospitals, like universities, are involved to different degrees in education, research, and service — three activities which can be expected to have mutual positive externalities. This paper tries to develop cost curves for the patient care segment of hospital output.

It has been persuasively argued that the patient care output of a hospital should be measured in terms of the hospital's final product, expressed as episodes of illness treated, rather than in terms of the intermediate services which produce this output.[1] Nevertheless, for the purpose of planning and reimbursing hospitals, this writer believes it important to find measures of hospital size based upon the numbers of intermediate services performed. This paper, then, will not present a direct measure of episodic care and its effectiveness but will develop a measure of service by a weighting of intermediate services.

MEASURING PATIENT CARE

In an article by Saathoff and Kurtz it was recognized that patient care cannot be measured by adult and pediatric patient days alone.[2] The patient day is not only a partial measure of intermediate care but often is a poor

The author wishes to thank the United Hospital Fund of New York, its member hospitals, and especially Miss Hortense M. Dillon, Supervisor, UHF Department of Distribution, for allowing him reference to their annual reports.

279

proxy for the other services. Berry attempted to solve this problem by treating as a group hospitals offering the same services and then using patient days as a proxy for all services.[3] He then could make generalizations about each such grouping, but because no weighting mechanism existed, there was no way to compare groups. To obtain a sufficient number of observations in each of his forty homogeneous groups, Berry was forced to use a very large sample (15 per cent of all short-term, general and special non-federal hospitals in the United States), thereby including hospitals with vastly different accounting procedures and making it difficult to account for non-patient care costs.

In an earlier study this writer attempted to find a measure of service which weighted each intermediate service included by its estimated average cost in dollars.[4] Certainly, in the non-competitive, non-profit, consumer-ignorance-filled, insurance-influenced world of the demand for hospital services, their value is not proportionate to their price or their average cost. However, in the revenue-constrained world of the supply of these services, relative average cost is an important determinant (along with subjective estimates of benefit) of which services are offered and how much of each. Thus cost is a valid weighting measure for supply purposes. In this study the earlier work is updated and improved upon by the use of a more recent and larger sample that permits the development of a more inclusive measure of service. Findings and conclusions of the two studies then are compared.

Weighting services by average cost requires using a sample composed of hospitals with similar or, even more preferable, identical accounting systems. The forty-six short-term general hospitals which are members of the United Hospital Fund of New York supply such a sample. UHF requires each member hospital to submit detailed cost schedules prior to receiving Fund support. Until calendar year 1966 the cost schedule included a work sheet calling for a stepdown allocation of costs to "basic" and "auxiliary" service cost centers.* The costs (direct plus allocated overhead) and units of basic services and some auxiliary services were then reported to the Fund, but for some auxiliary services only costs were reported. Allocation of overhead was based upon units of service provided. Since 1965, income has been used as the allocative mechanism. Thus, 1965 is the last year for which the Fund has homogeneous cost data allocated according to service units for numerous services.

---

*The "basic" service centers or services for which service units were reported to the fund are routine adult and pediatric "hotel"-type bed care and nursery, out-patient department, emergency room, and ambulance service. Units also were reported for operating rooms, delivery rooms, radiology departments, and laboratories, but only costs were reported for some auxiliary service centers, while neither costs nor service units were reported for others.

In the earlier study, which was based on data from a smaller number of UHF member hospitals, access to records was obtained by visiting half of the hospitals. Records housed at the Fund's main offices were used for the present study, and a questionnaire was sent to all member hospitals asking for units of auxiliary services which were not at the main office. This generated a larger sample, especially for the fully reported services.

UHF MEMBER HOSPITALS COMPARED WITH NATIONAL HOSPITALS

A. Size

In 1965 the composite average UHF member hospital differed in many ways from the average voluntary, non-profit, short-term general hospital. Table 1 gives the percentages of UHF member hospitals reporting various

Table 1: Percentage of Hospitals with Selected Facilities, United States vs. UHF

Service	U.S.	UHF
Blood bank	67.3	88.8
Clinical laboratory	97.9	100.0
Pathology laboratory (with pathologist)	67.1	100.0
Electroencephalography	31.7	84.1
Dental facilities	36.4	77.3
Pharmacy (with registered pharmacist)	66.7	95.5
Occupational therapy	13.4	40.9
Physical therapy	60.2	88.6
Premature nursery	63.7	56.8
Intensive care unit	32.5	63.6
Organized outpatient care	40.9	97.7
Emergency	93.7	100.0
Home care	5.9	36.4
Operating room	97.4	100.0
Obstetrical delivery room	90.9	86.4
Postoperative recovery room	74.9	97.7
Social service department	21.1	95.5
X-rays, diagnostic	98.3	100.0
X-rays, therapeutic	46.4	81.8
Radioactive isotope treatment	38.4	81.8
Psychiatric inpatient care	14.9	22.7
Rehabilitation, inpatient	8.4	27.3
Cobalt therapy	13.1	40.9
Radium therapy	39.9	75.0
Family planning	5.3	52.3
Routine chest X-ray on admission	34.3	68.2

Source: *Hospitals* 40, no. 15 (August 1966):154–58, 466–71.

specific services and the percentages for all voluntary hospitals. Most of the differences stem from size, location, and the presence of many other hospitals in the New York City area. Hospitals within UHF averaged about 400 beds in 1965, whereas the nation's voluntary hospitals averaged about 150.[5]

The UHF hospitals rank below the national average only in provision of nursery care and delivery room services. The prevalence of specialization and the presence of many other hospitals in the area explain this difference. Fewer member hospitals offer psychiatric inpatient care than their size would predict. This is probably the result, at least in part, of the large psychiatric units associated with some of the municipal hospitals and the existence of six psychiatric hospitals in New York City. That more UHF member hospitals offer organized outpatient care, home care, social service workers, family planning assistance, and routine chest X-rays than size would explain can be attributed to the urban milieu in which UHF functions.

B. Quality

There is no doubt that some hospitals are better than others. Presumably, a better hospital is one at which a randomly selected patient is expected to attain better health, either by the time of discharge from the hospital or by the end of his medical treatment.[6] While methods for determining different levels of quality have been suggested (such as impartial medical audits), and relevant variables have been cited, they have not been estimated systematically enough to establish relative qualities for hospitals in a statistically meaningful sample.[7] However, a review of any listing of the "best" hospitals suggests that certain types of approval are positively correlated with given levels of quality. Hospitals can be divided into three quality groups, in each of which the average level of patient care is progressively higher: (1) hospitals not accredited by the Joint Commission on Accreditation, (2) hospitals accredited by the Joint Commission but not affiliated with a medical school, and (3) hospitals affiliated with an approved medical school.

When this grouping is examined, it would appear that UHF hospitals as a group are better than the average voluntary hospital. All but one of the UHF hospitals, or 97.8 per cent, were accredited by the Joint Commission, and almost one-half, or 43.5 per cent, were affiliated with medical schools. Additional evidence of UHF quality is that over 80 per cent of the member hospitals were approved for residency and internship programs (87.0 and 80.4 per cent, respectively) and that a substantial amount of medical research was carried on by member hospitals during 1965.[8] The prevalence of teaching and research activities is the result both of size and of the religious and ethnic sponsorship of the member hospitals.[9] Tunley's listing of the best United States hospitals supports the assertion that UHF hospitals are better than average. His expert panel named four UHF hospitals as among the top fifteen in the nation, with one more in the next fifteen.[10]

The effect of the quality of patient care on the average cost of individual hospital services is not entirely clear on an a priori basis. For example, it may be good patient care to administer chest X-rays or Pap smears as a routine admission procedure, but unless we know something of the economies of scale in administering these tests, we cannot predict their effect on average cost. Quality care might take the form of excellent diagnosis and early ambulation, which would restrict the use of certain services to cases in which expected benefit is highest and would change the relative use of outpatient, inpatient, and home care services. Again, the effect of quality on the average cost of these services is indeterminate on a priori grounds.

In both of the above instances quality care, as measured by expected health gains, is brought about through reorganizing or restructuring the way in which completely homogeneous services are dispensed. In the first instance, expected health gains are increased by "forcing" high benefit-cost services on patients. The chest X-rays and Pap smears in such a hospital are assumed to be the same as in "non-forcing" hospitals. Thus scale determines relative average costs. In the second instance, physicians exercise discrimination in diagnosing and treating patients: it is the use of services that is different, not their quality. For example, if two people take the same medicine but only one needs it, the service input will be the same, but the contribution to health will differ.

Quality care, moreover, may take the form of better individual services. "In a fine hospital everybody functions in a fishbowl. . . everything out in the open."[11] Total service quality is better not only because diagnosis is better but because intermediate services are better. Services may be better because the persons performing them are more highly skilled.* They may be better because more persons are involved in performing them.† They may also be better because equipment is more reliable or extensive.‡ Where qual-

---

*This would result in higher average hospital costs only if the services were performed by hospital employees. It also involves the allocation of cost between the educational and healing aspects of teaching hospitals, a very difficult task that UHF has not satisfactorily accomplished.

†For example, when residents and interns are present at operations or when numerous members of the permanent staff are consulted about a patient. Unfortunately, UHF does not allow its member hospitals to allocate intern and resident cost according to where time is spent. Instead, the cost is carried as "other cost" and is allocated to inpatients (including the nursery), despite resident and intern time spent in ambulatory and auxiliary departments.

‡Again, this should result in higher average service costs, but this added cost will be mainly depreciation, and depreciation is not reported to the UHF on an individual-service basis.

ity care takes the form of better individual services, the expectation is that these services, and hence total output, as defined in this paper, will appear to be more costly. The assumption is that quality and cost will be positively correlated despite the faulty accounting procedures of the Fund, which tend to understate the costs of quality.

This paper examines the relationship between quality and cost in two steps. First a dummy variable (1, if the hospital is affiliated with a medical school; 0, if not) is used to see whether variations in cost unexplained by service units can be explained by quality differences.* The second step is the trial application of three sets of weights to distinguish the services of affiliated from those of non-affiliated hospitals. The first step was performed for the various services because the effects of interhospital quality differences on different services may not be parallel. For example, surgery may be more costly but better in affiliated hospitals, while X-ray films may be of equal cost and quality. If quality differences explain some variations in the costs of individual services, it follows that quality differences also explain part of the difference in total cost. Therefore, the dummy variable was introduced into the regressions to see if it improved the explanation of variations in total cost.

The existence of quality differences also forces us to question the validity of the cross-sectional data. Presumably, the cost curve is valid only if the outputs are homogeneous.[12] This problem is common in economics and is generally solved by using an index number approach. Cadillacs and Volkswagens are weighted in price in determining quantity in an automobile supply curve. For reasons cited by Klarman[13] and in the text above, such a weighting system seems very doubtful in the medical field. In the absence of any definitive set of weights suitable for comparing output in teaching with that in non-teaching hospitals, three sets of weights were chosen to give the reader a choice and to evaluate the effects of these weights on the cost schedules.†

Measure of Output

The services included in the unit of output, their average and relative costs, and the number of observations are shown in Table 2. As can be seen, certain services fairly common in large hospitals, such as occupational therapy and intensive care units, are not included because of the small numbers of observations. The number of observations was lower than the number of UHF hospitals performing the services for several reasons. First, twenty-five usable

---

*Since only one UHF hospital was not accredited by the Joint Commission, this hospital was not used in the samples.

†Just as a Cadillac is "more car" than a Volkswagen and is thus treated as more basic car units on a supply schedule, a high-quality physical therapy visit is "more physical therapy" than a low-quality visit and must be weighted accordingly.

Table 2: Average Cost and Relative Cost for Selected Services in UHF Member Hospitals

Service Units	Average Cost[a]		Relative Cost (Wi)[b]		Number of Observations	
	1962	1965	1962	1965	1962	1965[c]
Physical therapy treatments	$ 3.71	$ 4.59	0.15	0.13	19	22
Electrocardiograms	4.92	5.73	0.20	0.16	20	24
X-ray treatments	9.44	14.96	0.39	0.41	13	15
Blood transfusions (including plasma)	21.74	20.30	0.90	0.56	17	21
Electroencephalograms	17.59	24.78	0.73	0.62	8	12
Radioactive isotope treatments[d]	–	27.19	–	0.75	–	5
Operations, weighted[e]	114.35	143.22	4.75	3.90	22	44
Deliveries	56.92	78.83	2.36	2.15	15	38
X-rays, diagnostic[f]	3.83	4.31	0.16	0.12	23	43
Laboratory examinations	1.66	1.60	0.07	0.04	23	43
Newborn days	12.72	18.11	0.53	0.49	14	38
Outpatient visits	6.72	9.29	0.28	0.25	21	43
Emergency room treatments	3.97	5.73	0.16	0.16	19	42
Ambulance trips	–	12.58	–	0.34	–	24
Adult and pediatric patient days	24.09	36.43	1.0	1.0	22	45

[a]Teaching costs, including costs of interns and residents, are not included.

[b]Average routine cost of service divided by average cost of an adult and pediatric patient day.

[c]Units of the first six services listed were obtained by questionnaire and the remainder from UHF headquarters.

[d]Radioactive isotope treatment is included despite the small number of observations because of the clustering of individual hospital average costs around the average 1965 cost. A $125 mean for cardiopulmonary examinations and a $61 average cost for basal metabolism readings, both based on the same number of observations, were felt to be unreliable due to high dispersions of individual means.

[e]Major operations, plus one-third of all minor operations.

[f]One-twentieth of all dental films plus all other films.

questionnaires were returned of the forty-five sent out (three more were returned saying that all of the data requested were unavailable); second, many of the usable questionnaires listed some data as unavailable; third, most hospitals failed to allocate costs to all service areas; and fourth, some data were reported in unusable form.[14] One hospital did not have a record of major and minor operations, and another lumped therapeutic and diagnostic X-rays together. In addition, some hospitals defined and applied the service unit differently than others.

Using the weights (Wi), the output of any hospital is measured by summing the products of the weights and units of any service performed in that hospital; i.e.,

$$S^k = \sum_i Wi Q_i k$$

where S^k is service output in the kth hospital, Wi is weight of the ith service, and Q_i^k = quantity of the ith service in the kth hospital. This unit of service treats all outputs in all hospitals as homogeneous. In developing the average cost curves which will be presented later, a simple weighting system was introduced to distinguish between the service output of teaching and of non-teaching hospitals. We assumed that the average output unit of an affiliated hospital is composed of 10, 20, or 30 per cent "more care" than that of a non-teaching hospital. Thus, for some regressions, the unit of service is modified to

$$S_d{}^k = d \sum_i WiQ_i{}^k$$

where d is a dummy variable equal to 1 if the kth hospital is unaffiliated and to 1.1, 1.2, or 1.3 if the kth hospital is affiliated.

Table 2, in addition to showing the 1965 data, shows the changes that occurred since 1962. The average cost of all services except laboratory examinations and blood transfusions increased. The later sample may include more hospitals with access to free blood. The laboratory examination cost is not significantly lower, especially when one considers that hospitals are free to decide what is considered a single examination.

The percentage increases have been largest in X-ray treatments, routine adult and pediatric days, and emergency room treatments. The last two are quite likely to have been the result of very high labor intensities, whereas the former may have been the result of the existence of a higher percentage of salaried radiologists in the newer sample.

It appears quite likely that the data for 1965 to the present and in the near future will show routine patient day cost continuing to rise as fast or faster than the other services, so that the weights of the other services will fall over time. This however, could be partly or fully offset by wider use of new elaborate and expensive techniques, such as more operations which in terms of cost might be considered "very major."

REGRESSION AND CORRELATION RESULTS

The quality dummy was a significant explanatory variable for only certain service centers, but these centers made up about 80 per cent of the weighted output. It was significantly and positively correlated with the cost residuals for the operating room, nursery, routine inpatient care, outpatient department, physical therapy department, laboratory, and blood bank (transfusions). It was insignificantly correlated with the cost of deliveries, diagnostic X-rays, X-ray treatments, emergency treatments, ambulance calls, electroencephalograms, and electrocardiograms. When the sample was divided into affiliated and non-affiliated hospitals, it was not large enough to determine the dummy's significance with regard to radioisotopes.*

Since the dummy variable is significant in explaining the cost of some hospital services, it seems permissible to use it in explaining total hospital costs.[†] However, in the sample the respondents' costs determined the weights (Wi), so that a very high correlation could be expected between the respondents' total costs and their units of output (S^k). That correlation was .983. But the second-order equation was the most economically meaningful, and is presented with and without the dummy:

*As an example, the explanatory equations, one with the dummy and one without, for the operating room were:

(1) total operation cost = 60,600 + 84.9 (operations) + .0075 (operations)^2
                                         (27.5)   (.0022)
                                                                                      (R^2 = .8949).

(2) total operation cost = 74,000 + 67.2 (operations) + .0072 (operations)^2 +
                                         (25.9)   (.0020)
        .0023 dummy   (R^2 = .9035).
        (.0006)

The first equation suggests an optimum (major, plus one-third minor) operating scale of about 2,840.

For equation 1,

$$AC = \frac{TC}{Ow} = \frac{60,600}{Ow} + 84.9 + .0075\,Ow$$

$$\frac{dAC}{dOw} = \frac{-60,600}{Ow^2} + .0075 = 0$$

$$Ow^2 = \frac{60,600}{.0075} = 8,080,000$$

$$Ow = 2,843$$

The second equation suggests a scale of 3,200.

All total cost relationships were run as first-, second-, and third-order equations. The cubic coefficient was never significant, and thus no cubic total cost functions are reported in this paper. The coefficients of the first-order equations were frequently negative, and the second-order equations, with or without a first-order term, often produced the most meaningful cost curve. This supports Feldstein's use of U-shaped average cost curves (see note 6 to text), but falling average cost curves were found for several services, including electrocardiograms, electroencephalograms, diagnostic X-rays, physiotherapy, laboratory, ambulance, and emergency room.

[†] Total costs for all equations include only costs associated with services in the unit of output and services routinely offered (though not routinely administered), such as oxygen therapy. All non-patient care costs have been eliminated, as have costs of special services such as psychiatric inpatient care.

(1) $$TC = 4{,}100{,}000 + .000052\,(S^k)^2 \quad (R^2 = .92)$$
$$(.000003)$$

(2) $$TC = 3{,}700{,}000 + .000049\,(S^k)^2 + .013d \quad (R^2 = .93).$$
$$(.000004) \qquad (.006)$$

Using patient days as the independent variable, the cost curves for the questionnaire returners would be

(3) $$TC = 4{,}700{,}000 + .00013\,PD^2 \quad (R^2 = .87)$$
$$(.00001)$$

(4) $$TC = 3{,}900{,}000 + .00012\,PD^2 + .019d \quad (R^2 = .88).$$
$$(.00001) \qquad (.09)$$

The first equation has a low point at 280,000 units of service and the third at 190,000 patient days. Both of these figures would be generated by a hospital of between 560 and 575 beds operating at slightly more than 90 per cent of capacity. The second and fourth equations have low points of about 270,000 units of service and 180,000 patient days, approximately equal to those of a 540- to 555-bed hospital.

When the index number approach is used to compare units in affiliated and in non-affiliated hospitals, the optimum hospital size increases as the premium given teaching hospitals rises. The three equations generated by the respondents' data were:

(5) $$TC_{1.1} = 4{,}300{,}000 + .000042\left[S^k\,(.1d + 1)\right]^2 \quad (R^2 = .92)$$
$$(.000003)$$

(6) $$TC_{1.2} = 4{,}500{,}000 + .000035\left[S^k\,(.2d + 1)\right]^2 \quad (R^2 = .91)$$
$$(.000002)$$

(7) $$TC_{1.3} = 4{,}600{,}000 + .000029\left[S^k\,(.3d + 1)\right]^2 \quad (R^2 = .91)$$
$$(.000002)$$

where $d = 0$ for unaffiliated and 1 for affiliated hospitals.

The low point of each equation is calculated by assuming either that the dummy equals zero or that the cost of quality exhibits constant returns. In equation 5 the minimum point is obtained as follows:

$$AC = \frac{TC}{S^k} = \frac{4{,}300{,}000}{S^k} + .000042 S^k$$

$$\frac{dAC}{dS^k} = \frac{-4,300,000}{(S^k)^2} = .000042 = 0$$

$$(S^k)^2 = \frac{4,300,000}{.000042}$$

$$S^k = 320,000$$

At 500 S^k per bed, the minimum point is 640 beds.

The three equations suggest minimum average cost at approximately 640, 700, and 790 beds, respectively, with average cost for routine inpatient care at \$27, \$25, and \$23 for unaffiliated hospitals. This sample clearly indicates that large hospitals are more efficient than small ones.

Unit of service (S^k) and patient days then were used to explain the costs of the non-responding hospitals. Since exact numbers of certain auxiliary services were not known, it was assumed that all services, where available, were offered in the same ratio to inpatient days as they were offered in the responding hospitals. These ratios are shown in Table 3. For these services, contrary to the basic argument of this paper, it was assumed that patient days are an exact proxy for all individual services. Thus, if the unit-of-service approach explains more of total cost than does patient days, it is not simply the result of a self-fulfilling technique.

The units of service for the nonrespondents were calculated as follows:

$$S^k = \sum_i W_i \frac{\sum_R Q_i R}{\sum_R P_i R} d_i k \; P^k + \sum_J W_j \; Q_j k,$$

Table 3: Ratios of Selected Services to Patient Days in a Sample of UHF Hospitals

Service Units	Relative Cost (W_i)	Units Per Patient Day	Average Cost Per Patient Day (R_i)
Physical therapy treatment	.12	.10	.012
Electrocardiograms	.16	.09	.014
X-ray treatments	.41	.03	.012
Blood transfusions (including plasma)	.56	.05	.028
Electroencephalograms	.62	.007	.004
Radioactive isotope treatments	.75	.01	.008

Source: questionnaire returns from twenty-five UHF hospitals.

where

W_i = weights of services not reported to UHF

$\sum_R Q_i^R$ = units of ith service offered in UHF reporting sample

$\sum_R P_i^R$ = patient days in UHF reporting sample of hospitals offering ith service

d_ik = dummy signifying whether ith service is offered in kth non-responding hospital

Pk = patient days in kth non-responding hospital

W_j = weights of services reported to UHF

Q_jk = units of jth service reported to UHF by kth hospital

From the last column in Table 3 and the last nine figures in column 5 of Table 2 one can find the values used in the simplified formula for estimating the output of hospitals which did not answer the questionnaire:

$$ S^k = \sum_i R_i \, d_ik \, P^k + \sum_j W_j \, Q_jk . $$

The equations for the non-respondents' total costs, with and without the dummy,* were as follows:

(8) $TC = 620{,}000 + 21.2 S^k + .000046\,(S^k)^2 \quad (R^2 = .96)$
                  $(7.6) \qquad (.000019)$

and

(9) $TC = 780{,}000 + 19.1\,S^k + .000049\,(S^k)^2 + .0022D \quad (R^2 = .96).$
              $(8.9) \qquad (.000021) \qquad\quad (.0011)$

---

*It is easy to approximate the marginal cost per unit of service for a hospital of any size or to calculate the size of hospital associated with a particular marginal cost by recalling that 500 units of service is approximately equal to one bed in a full-service hospital. Thus, using equation 8 we can find the hospital size that will keep marginal cost at or below $35:

MC = $21.2 + .000092\,S^k$
35   = $21.2 + .000092\,S^k$
S^k = $150{,}000$
Beds = 300

The first equation has a low point of $32 at about 120,000 units, and the second has a low point of 130,000 units associated with about the same average cost. The earlier study had a low point of about 85,000 units and a cost of $21.25.

Using patient days as the explanatory variable, we get

$$(10) \qquad TC = 6,200,000 + 34.9PD + .00010PD^2 \quad (R^2 = .94),$$
$$ (14.5) \qquad (.00006)$$

and when the dummy is introduced the first-order term drops out, yielding

$$(11) \qquad TC = 2,300,000 + .00021PD^2 + .011D \quad (R^2 = .94).$$
$$ (.00002) \qquad (.0045)$$

The low points suggest 240- and 320-bed hospitals, respectively.

When the weighting system was introduced, the resulting quadratic equations suggested average cost curves to the left and below those just described:

$$(12) \qquad TC_{1.1} = 860,000 + 19.7S^k (.1d + 1) + .000035 \left[S^k (.1d + 1) \right]^2$$
$$\phantom{(12) \qquad TC_{1.1} = 860,000 + } (6.8) \qquad\qquad\qquad (.000016)$$
$$(R^2 = .95)$$

$$(13) \quad TC_{1.2} = 1,130,000 + 17.6S^k (.2d + 1) + .000028 \left[S^k (.2d + 1) \right]^2$$
$$\phantom{(13) \quad TC_{1.2} = 1,130,000 + } (6.4) \qquad\qquad\qquad (.000014)$$
$$(R^2 = .95)$$

$$(14) \quad TC_{1.3} = 1,380,000 + 15.4S^k (.3d + 1) + .000024 \left[S^k (.3d + 1) \right]^2$$
$$\phantom{(14) \quad TC_{1.3} = 1,380,000 + } (6.1) \qquad\qquad\qquad (.000012)$$
$$(R^2 = .94).$$

These results suggest hospitals of about 310, 400, and 480 beds, with lowest average costs of $30.50, $29, and $27, respectively. Since marginal cost is rising fairly slowly along a straight line, there is a fairly wide range of hospital sizes which will have an average cost near the low point. For example, according to the third equation, hospitals producing between 220,000 and 260,000 units of service will have average costs under $28.

SUMMARY AND CONCLUSIONS

The cost curves found in this study suggest that the optimum size for hospitals is one which delivers between 120,000 units and 395,000 units of service (equations 8 and 7, respectively), as service has been measured in this paper.* All curves have very high coefficients of multiple determination, and the curve on which the reader relies should be determined more by his choice of quality weights than by these coefficients.

Quality, as measured by accreditation, is seen to be positively correlated with cost and, along with size, provides a significant explanation for cost variations despite biases in the UHF statistics which tend to underestimate the effects of quality on cost. Note also that only in the slight leftward shift of low points between equations 1 and 2 was the assumption of a larger quality differential, or the introduction of the quality dummy as an explanatory variable, associated with a lowering of optimum hospital scale.

The second series of equations was made when only partial information on the individual hospital outputs was available. This may suggest that the first set of equations with low points of 540 to 790 beds is most reliable. It is also true that for teaching purposes we may want hospitals that are well beyond the optimum scale and have rather high average costs. Equity requires that much of this cost be allocated to education on the basis of causal responsibility. Furthermore, in urban areas depreciation and land costs may well make very large hospitals most economical.

It is clear that much work will be necessary before both the quantity and quality differences in the outputs of hospitals can be fully compared. Perhaps this paper has suggested some fruitful avenues for approaching that goal.

NOTES

1. See Anne A. Scitovsky, "An Index of the Cost of Medical Care – A Proposed New Approach," in *The Economics of Health and Medical Care*, ed. S. J. Axelrod (Ann Arbor: The University of Michigan, 1964), pp. 128–42.

2. Donald E. Saathoff and Richard A. Kurtz, "Cost Per Day Comparisons Don't Do the Job," *The Modern Hospital* 99, no. 4 (October 1962):14, 16, 162.

3. Ralph E. Berry, Jr., "Competition and Efficiency in the Market for Hospital Services, the Structure of the American Hospital Industry" (Ph.D. diss., Harvard University, 1965), pp. 155–58.

4. "Variations in Cost among Hospitals of Different Sizes," *Southern Economic Journal* 33, no. 3 (January 1967):355–66. The unit of service used there can be derived from Table 2, col. 3, above; in the same way the unit in this study is derived from Table 2, col. 4.

5. *Hospitals* 40, no. 15 (August 1966):154–58, 439.

6. See Paul J. Feldstein, "An Analysis of Alternative Incentive Reimbursement Plans," *Federal Programs for the Development of Human Resources* 2 (March 1968):567. Some discounting factor should perhaps be used.

7. See Walter J. McNerney and study staff, *Hospital and Medical Economics* (Chicago: Hospital Research and Educational Trust, 1962), 1:450, for an example of a list of relevant variables.

---

*The mix of individual services which might be used to attain this size will be partly determined by medical practice. For example, the final mix would not include ten newborn days per delivery.

8. See *Hospitals* 40, no. 15 (August 1966):154–58; also Pts. 2 and 3 of United Hospital Fund of New York annual reports for 1965, issued in 1966.

9. James A. Hamilton, R. Bruce Butters, and Elbert E. Gilbertson, *Patterns of Hospital Ownership and Control* (Minneapolis: University of Minnesota Press, 1961), p. 125. The percentage of hospitals within UHF which are church-affiliated follows the national pattern, but an additional quarter are Jewish-sponsored, and "Jewish hospitals in the United States are extremely active in education and research."

10. Roul Tunley, "America's 10 Best Hospitals," *Ladies Home Journal* 34, no. 2 (February 1967):34, 134.

11. *Ibid.*

12. See Caleb Smith, "Survey of the Empirical Evidence on Economies of Scale," in National Bureau of Economic Research, *Business Concentration and Price Policy*, A Conference of the Universities – National Bureau Committee for Economic Research (Princeton, N.J.: Princeton University Press, 1955), pp. 213–30, for other arguments concerning statistical cost curves.

13. Herbert E. Klarman, *The Economics of Health* (New York: Columbia University Press, 1965), p. 28.

14. See Cohen, "Variations in Cost among Hospitals of Different Sizes," pp. 359–60, for certain criticisms of the UHF data. About one-half of the affiliated hospitals returned the 1968 questionnaire. This group had more beds and offered more services than those which did not return the questionnaire.

Paul J. Feldstein
University of Michigan

COMMENT

The present paper extends some of Professor Cohen's earlier work on measuring hospital output. He earlier developed an index of hospital output based upon a system of weighting the various hospital services by their respective costs. In that effort differences in costs that were a result of differences in quality were not considered. The present paper is an attempt to solve this problem.

Measures of the effect of quality on differences in total costs and on the costs of each service center were constructed in two ways. First, the hospitals in the sample were classified as affiliated or non-affiliated with a medical school and this information was used as a dummy variable in a regression equation together with a weighted output measure. The second measure was constructed by assigning three different weights (1.1, 1.2, and 1.3) to hospitals affiliated with medical schools, rather than using the single measure. In addition to showing the influence of these two measures of quality on cost, Professor Cohen also estimated optimum hospital size and how it changed as allowance was made for these measures of "quality."

I have some difficulty in accepting both the weighted output and quality approach which Professor Cohen uses to estimate total cost functions. Weighting outputs by cost is a proxy for differences in patient mix in a hospital, severity of illness, services provided and services available, amenities available (such as number of television sets and proportion of private, semi-private, and ward accommodations), the efficiency with which the hospital is operated, and the amount of research, teaching, and other functions performed by the hospital.

I am not sure for what purpose or decisions the aggregate proxy measure used by Professor Cohen is applicable. I am equally uncertain that it represents an improvement over some other estimates of hospital cost functions in which allowances for the effect of specific services or types of patients have been made. More specific measures of output would be needed if they were to be used for making decisions about reimbursement, budgeting, or long-term investment. The work in this paper on estimating cost functions by service centers is less aggregative and therefore, I believe, is much more promising.

With regard to the measures used for estimating quality, however, I am afraid that I am not too enthusiastic about the prospects for further work along these lines. Again, the main problem appears to be that the measure is too gross. The fact that a hospital is affiliated with a medical school may indicate that care is better than in a small rural proprietary hospital, but it certainly is not a sufficiently discriminating measure for all quality differences among large hospitals in an urban area. What is more important, in the equations in Professor Cohen's study, the measure may be indicating merely the higher costs per unit of output that are associated with medical school affiliation. These would not be costs of increased quality. Other economists have tried to estimate the effect of the medical school on total hospital costs as well as on other facilities and services. Similarly, use of the same measure of quality for the cost functions of service centers could be interpreted to mean that the costs associated with the dummy variables are the costs not of quality but of association with a medical school. To complete this approach, it would be necessary to allow for the effects on cost of all the other affiliations and non-patient care functions of the hospital. However, even were this to be done, the result could not be termed the effect of quality on costs, but merely the costs of these additional functions. For example, if as part of the teaching function interns prescribe more tests, the resulting cost is higher, but it may be unrelated to quality.

The second approach, that of giving progressively larger weights to hospitals affiliated with medical schools, does not satisfy this objection. It appears to be saying that the higher the fixed cost which we attribute to a hospital, the larger will be the hospital at which average costs will be at a minimum. These findings, therefore, are not unexpected.

The empirical findings with regard to the effects on total cost of these two quality approaches are very small, and when larger premiums are given to teaching hospitals, the so-called optimum size appears to increase by the approximate amount of the premium.

I think that future research in the area of hospital cost functions might proceed along the following lines. If we are concerned about reimbursement (and we are), then we must be able to estimate the cost of different types of patients and the services they receive, and must also be able to measure different levels of quality. If we are interested in more efficient operation, then we should estimate cost curves by department or service center, as Professor Cohen has attempted to do, so that decisions such as "make or buy" or sharing services can better be understood by hospital management. We must also determine which departments are interrelated and should therefore be provided for jointly. Finally, in order to plan effectively for a community, we must determine the trade-offs between lower costs that result from economies of scale in the provision of certain services and the increased patient travel time that results if fewer but larger services are provided. We need to think in terms of minimizing the total hospitalization cost of the patient, not just that portion which relates to hospital cost.

Mark V. Pauly
Northwestern University

David F. Drake
American Hospital Association

EFFECT OF THIRD-PARTY METHODS OF REIMBURSEMENT ON HOSPITAL PERFORMANCE

INTRODUCTION

From the very inception of the Medicare program for purchasing institutional health care on a cost-plus basis, economists have been arguing (1) that a cost-plus basis of reimbursement provides an inducement for hospital managers to operate inefficiently and thus maximize the amount of plus factor accruing to the hospital, and (2) that a cost-plus basis of reimbursement does not provide a rational basis for allocating capital to the health industry or among producers in the industry.[1] In what is perhaps a rare instance of immediate public acceptance, the economists' arguments have been translated into a public program of "incentive" reimbursement experiments.[2] Such methods will presumably induce hospital managers to economize in the operating use of health resources and will provide an effective capital allocation system to and within the industry.

Our study bears in part on the presumptions of this program of experimentation. We have examined some of the effects of four different reimbursement methods which have been employed by Blue Cross plans in the relatively homogeneous states of Illinois, Indiana, Michigan, and Wisconsin. The purpose of the study was to discover whether differences in the methods of payment for hospital services would affect the economic behavior of hospitals. The study also was intended to explain the basis for such differences in performance as were found. Basically, we have concluded that differences in the method of payment in these cases did not alter operating behavior, i.e.,

The authors wish to thank Joseph Matisoff, Thomas Mitchell, and Michael Redisch for assistance with the calculations.

297

there were no discernible improvements in short-run production efficiencies in these four states. We did, however, detect different patterns of capital allocation among hospitals which could prove to be important in evaluating system efficiency.

DISCUSSION OF MODELS

Efficiency of Regulating Systems

The purpose of regulation, whether done directly through controls over hospital behavior which are tied to reimbursement, or indirectly through the type of reimbursement scheme used, is to cause some change in the performance of the regulated agents. The effectiveness of a regulatory system may be tested in two ways: (1) by comparing actual performance of regulated agents (firms) against some criterion of optimal performance, and (2) by comparing performance of similar (ideally, identical) firms that are and are not regulated or are regulated in a different way. Since criteria of optimal performance for hospitals are vague and, in many cases, non-existent, we have adopted the second approach.[3]

The regulatory agency presumably desires the system to behave in a particular way. The behavior of the system at any point in time is a result of the performance at that time of the individual agents in the system and the pattern or arrangement of the individual agents, which in turn depends upon the past performance of the individual agents and the regulatory agency, if any. At any point in time the agency can only affect part of the performance of given individual agents; over time, however, it can alter their character and behavior; that is, in the short run, it can affect only some parameters, while others are fixed and can be (or are) altered only over time. System efficiency, as defined by the criteria of the regulatory agency, is thus a result of efficient short-run performance of the regulated agents, efficient long-run performance of the regulated agents, and efficient long-run configuration of the regulatory system. Schemes which achieve desired short-run effects may not necessarily achieve desired long-run effects. We shall show that the regulatory devices used in the four states studied clearly had almost no effect on short-run efficiency. Analysis of comparative behavior in the four states on the basis of short-run indicators shows no differential effect of reimbursement schemes. There is evidence, however, that the regulatory agencies have affected long-run performance and the configuration of the system, which may in turn have affected long-run system efficiency.

What This Study Tests

One purpose of this study is to test the effectiveness of various reimbursement schemes. Refutation of the null hypothesis, which states that the form of the reimbursement scheme makes no difference in hospital behavior, would constitute evidence that these schemes can be used to affect hospital behavior. This study has a second purpose, however. If different reimbursement schemes affect hospital performance in different ways, then the manner in which it is affected provides some information about how hospitals behave. The schemes studied may support some models of the hospital over others, and then those models can be used to generate hypotheses about the effects of other reimbursement schemes on hospital behavior. If, on the other hand, the null hypothesis is confirmed, this would mean that models of the hospital which indicated otherwise may be inappropriate and that other hypotheses based on those models may be incorrect.

Models of the Hospital and of the Hospital System

The distinction between short-run and long-run performance and efficiency can be illustrated by a consideration of the incentive scheme proposed in the Miller report. All of the variants of the scheme discussed there have the following property: "Because of the differential flow of funds among hospitals, those which are most efficient and of the highest quality would prosper and expand under the suggested scheme in the long-run, while the poorest and least desirable hospitals would become a diminishing portion of the total hospital sector."[4] As the report notes, this is a long-run result; the configuration of the hospital system is altered by a differential flow of funds among hospitals, with larger amounts (for capital investment, presumably) going to hospitals with low costs than to those with high costs. (Alternatively, hospitals could be paid only out-of-pocket costs, and distribution of capital funds could be made directly.) But whether such a scheme would be expected to cause hospitals to behave in the short run differently from the way in which they would behave under a cost repayment scheme, and how their behavior would vary, depends on the model of the hospital we assume. The notion implicit in much of the discussion in the literature seems to be that by rewarding excellence and discouraging inefficiency hospitals will be induced to make efforts to lower their per diem cost. This will be true, however, only if they are concerned with the size of the plus they earn – if they desire to "prosper and expand," and hence try to maximize the funds generated for expansion purposes. It will be true only if a growth maximization or a long-run output maximization model of the hospital is appropriate. This model of the hospital, because it is implicit in much of the discussion of incentives, is the one which will be tested in this paper.

Regulatory Agency Models

We also need some models of regulatory agency behavior, since Blue Cross can, by the use of various reimbursement schemes, perform a regulatory function.

Industry-Identification Model

Although agencies may nominally be concerned with the public interest or effectiveness of the system, such goals are too vague to be useful. The agency obtains information from and in the interest of the regulated firm, and persons doing the regulation are ordinarily supposed to be experts, which usually means that they come from regulated firms themselves, so that it may well occur that regulatory agency goals become identified with the goals of the regulated firms. This can lead to a situation in which there is an appearance of regulation, while the actions of firms are no different from what they would be in the absence of the regulatory agency. The function of the agency is only to approve what would be done anyway and, perhaps, act as a clearinghouse for the exchange of information among firms, with no real desire to alter their behavior.

Specific-Goals Model

We can set up a model of regulation in which we assume that the agencies desire specific goals. The effectiveness of the regulation is then indicated by the extent to which those goals are achieved. For example, we might hypothesize that regulatory agencies desire large hospitals to grow relative to smaller ones; this is a potentially testable hypothesis. To test such a model it is not necessary to specify why the agency desires those specific goals.

Optimality Model

We might, on the other hand, assume that the ultimate object of the regulatory agency lies in some notion of optimality or efficiency in the provision of a service. Achievement of efficiency depends on both the effectiveness of the agency in causing industry behavior to change in specific ways and the effectiveness of those changes in producing efficiency. Failure to achieve efficiency may not mean that the agency was ineffective in regulation; it may only mean that it chose the wrong method.

Direct and Indirect Regulation

Regulation can be either direct or indirect. Direct regulation implies the use of directives for specific operations of specific hospitals. Reimbursement schemes can be used for direct regulation in at least two ways. Participation in Blue Cross may be tied to acceptance of specific directives, either from the Blue Cross plan or from areawide planning agencies whose goals Blue Cross endorses. The hospital is faced with an all-or-nothing decision in regard to Blue Cross participation. Planning agency directives are accepted in exchange for the convenience of Blue Cross membership in terms of regularity and certainty of payment. In the second method of direct regulation, only those charges which are associated with activities approved by the planning agency are paid, and charges paid by Blue Cross must be the same as those to non-subscribers. If a hospital were to engage in an unapproved activity, it could not charge for its costs. Indirect regulation, as we have defined it, involves only the choice of the form of Blue Cross reimbursement — whether cost-plus, charges, etc.

REIMBURSEMENT SCHEMES USED IN THE FOUR STATES

Wisconsin

The Wisconsin Blue Cross plan simply pays 97 per cent of billed charges to member hospitals. It also pays 100 per cent of charges by non-member hospitals. (Incentives for participation in Blue Cross derive from the fact that benefits from the regularity and certainty of payment may more than offset the 3 per cent loss in billed charges.) There are no other controls on hospital operation or financing. Blue Cross in Wisconsin is treated like any other purchaser of hospital care, except that it receives a slight quantity and regularity-of-payment discount. Blue Cross is, moreover, not a large purchaser of care in Wisconsin; it covered only 26.8 per cent of the population in the state in 1966. Wisconsin thus provides a good example of a case in which third-party reimbursement exerts no controls, either direct or indirect, over hospital operation.

Illinois

In Illinois payment is made for 105 per cent of costs incurred or for charges, whichever is lower. Charges may be lower than cost because the hospital receives income from non-patient sources, such as philanthropy or local government tax revenues. Costs are costs incurred on behalf of plan members, with apportionment on the basis of patient days. The purpose of the excess over full cost is to provide for improvement (capital investment), community service, and bad debts. Depreciation is permitted at a rate of 2 per cent of historical cost on buildings and 6 per cent on equipment. Costs of educational programs are generally not reimbursable. Interest on borrowed funds is permitted without limit. The thirteen proprietary hospitals registered in the state are treated like other hospitals. In 1966, Blue Cross covered 24.5 per cent of the state's population.

Michigan

The Michigan plan pays 102 per cent of costs or charges, whichever is lower, with per diem apportionment. The extra 2 per cent is to go for improvement and community service, and for a capital contribution. Depreciation is 2 per cent of historical costs on plant or equipment, subject to adjustment in special cases. Medical education costs are reimbursable. Interest on debt is paid on debt which (currently) does not exceed 52 per cent of plant asset value. This limit descends at a rate of about 3 per cent of plant asset value per year. Costs and balance sheets are audited. Proprietary hospitals are generally not eligible for participation. Michigan has controlled, by excluding from participation, some hospitals which have failed to heed areawide planning recommendations. Blue Cross covered 51.1 per cent of the population in 1966.

While both Michigan and Illinois reimburse on the basis of cost plus, Michigan provides a less generous plus than Illinois, as well as a smaller depreciation allowance. In Michigan, Blue Cross participation has been tied to acceptance of areawide planning, while in Illinois there have been no such controls.

Indiana

The plan in Indiana pays 100 per cent of controlled or approved charges. Moreover, charges to Blue Cross patients must be the same as those to non-member patients, so that the rate paid by Blue Cross governs the charge to all patients. Major items and a random sample of smaller items are audited, as are financial statements. The plan has the authority to evaluate charge systems, and capital investment proposals are carefully reviewed. The scheme used in Indiana is one which offers considerable control over hospitals. The requirement of equal charges means that the hospital cannot charge anyone for unapproved items, so the plan has more leverage than its 34.8 per cent enrollment would indicate.

HYPOTHESES TO BE TESTED

The Null Hypothesis

The null hypothesis leads to the prediction that reimbusement schemes will have no differential effect on short-run or long-run indicators of hospital performance. This hypothesis will therefore be tested for every indicator.

Short-Run Indicators

Cost Indicators

Cost comparisons of otherwise identical hospitals at a given point in time provide some information on the short-run behavior of hospitals. We shall consider both direct and indirect controls.

Indirect controls. If payment to hospitals is based on costs, as in Illinois, hospitals clearly have no incentive to keep costs down. Indeed, if hospitals receive a fixed percentage of costs as a plus, and we assume that they wish to maximize that plus in order to attain maximum growth or to treat the maximum number of patients over the long run, then cost-plus reimbursement leads to a perverse result. Hospitals which are striving to increase funds available for capital investment will try to increase costs, since that will increase the absolute amount of the plus they earn. If, however, payment is based on charges, as in Wisconsin, the long-run growth-maximizing hospital has a positive incentive to minimize costs. Effective cost minimization will allow the hospital to earn a larger plus on its operations, and this excess can be put into capital investment to increase the capacity or degree of modernity of the hospital. Hence, we would expect, *ceteris paribus*, that charge-based hospitals would have lower costs, however defined, than cost-based ones. This hypothesis is reinforced if we note that charge-based hospitals are subject to some uncertainty as to loss avoidance or the size of the plus they will eventually earn because they must set charges *ex ante*. They would therefore minimize the risk of loss by striving to keep costs down. This hypothesis is still somewhat tenuous, however, since uncontrolled charge-reimbursed hospitals can also raise charges (up to some undefined limit) as a substitute for reducing costs. (That hospitals minimize short-run costs does not imply that the system is efficient: there is no assurance that either the pattern or the absolute amount of capital investment in hospitals is optimal.)

Direct controls. Direct controls exist in a charge-based scheme in Indiana and in a cost-based scheme in Michigan. We might assume that the regulatory agency would try to get hospitals to reduce their costs – to become more efficient. Hence, we might see whether costs, either measured per patient day or per admission, are lower in controlled than in uncontrolled states. Conformation of this hypothesis provides an indication that regulatory agencies can get hospitals to lower their costs, and that they wish to do so. Refutation of the hypothesis is, however, consistent either with the notion that controls are ineffective or with an industry-identification model of the regulatory agency, in which the agency has no desire to put effective pressure on hospitals to cut costs.

Occupancy

The occupancy rate, which reflects the extent of utilization of fixed inputs, is another short-run indicator of hospital efficiency. Although 100 per cent occupancy is ordinarily not efficient,* up to some limits increases in occupancy rates imply reduction in excess capacity.

---

*In fact, the optimum occupancy rate is probably not uniform in all communities, since it depends on the aversion individuals have to being unable to obtain a hospital bed when they wish or need it. The use of some ideal occupancy rate, e.g., 80 per cent, agreed upon by experts, is invalid, since the strength of this aversion probably varies from community to community.

Indirect controls. Costs and charges are usually computed in different ways. Charges are usually figured *ex ante*; in order to determine the per diem charge for a coming period, the hospital estimates its total costs and the plus it desires and divides this by an estimate of the number of patient days it expects to provide during the period. On the other hand, per diem costs that are reimbursed by Blue Cross are computed after the fact; costs incurred during a period are divided by patient days produced during that period to compute average cost.

Under reimbursement based on charges, the "marginal revenue" from filling an otherwise empty bed is equal to the per diem charge. For cost-reimbursed plans, however, the marginal revenue is equal only to the marginal (incremental) cost of filling one more bed (and also the plus on this incremental cost), which usually will be considerably less than the average cost or charge because of the high fixed costs hospitals incur. Hence, hospitals reimbursed on a cost basis will usually receive less revenue for an additional patient day than those on a charge basis. The marginal revenue and marginal profit obtainable by filling an otherwise empty bed is greater under charge-based plans. With the growth maximization models, we would expect that charge-based hospitals would have a higher occupancy than cost-based hospitals.

Direct controls. Since higher occupancy is usually taken as an indicator of efficiency, we might expect that, under effective regulation, directly controlled states would, *ceteris paribus*, display higher occupancy rates than other states. Effective regulation can take two forms: an efficient scheduling of patients so that higher occupancy results, and an efficient allocation of capital to hospitals so that excess beds are not built. Refutation of this hypothesis is again consistent either with ineffective regulation or lack of a desire to regulate.

Long-Run Indicators of System Change

In addition to altering the way in which hospitals behave in the short run, differences in reimbursement schemes might also alter the composition of the hospital system by altering the size distribution of hospitals. As we indicated above, regulatory agencies might have specific ways in which they would like the hospital system to change. It is generally accepted that, when appropriate adjustments are made for quality differences, large hospitals are more efficient than small ones. Our purpose is not to discuss the validity of this proposition; rather, we wish to suggest that, because of its general acceptance, it seems reasonable to assume that control agencies desire to foster the relative growth of larger hospitals.

Neither indirect scheme would be expected to produce a predictable differential pattern of growth. If all hospitals in Illinois receive 105 per cent of costs from Blue Cross, and if all other sources of funds for investment are assumed to be given, then each hospital will invest and grow proportionately. In Wisconsin the pattern of growth will likewise depend on the pattern of excess earnings, but there is no way to predict what that pattern would be.

We would expect states that are directly controlled to be different. In Indiana and, to a lesser extent, in Michigan, reimbursement schemes can be used to get hospitals to conform to some notions of proper patterns of expansion. If areawide planning agencies wish to foster the growth of larger institutions, and if Blue Cross plans agree with these goals, we would expect to observe differentially greater growth by larger institutions in Indiana, and perhaps Michigan, than in Illinois and Wisconsin.

System Efficiency

Even if regulators do affect the structure of the hospital system, we cannot determine how this affects system efficiency simply by looking at individual hospitals. Instead, we must look at some measures for the system as a whole. Regulation is effective, *ceteris paribus*, if the mean cost per diem is less in regulated states than in unregulated states, or if the occupancy rate is higher in regulated states than in unregulated states. This hypothesis, however, is not tested in the present study.

The hypotheses we wish to test, then, are the following:

1. Cost measures will be lower in Wisconsin than in Illinois.

2. Cost measures will be lower in Indiana than in Wisconsin, and lower in Michigan than in Illinois.

3. Occupancy will be higher in Wisconsin than in Illinois.

4. Occupancy will be higher in Indiana than in Wisconsin, and in Michigan than in Illinois.

5. Large hospitals will grow proportionately more in Indiana (and Michigan) than in Illinois and Wisconsin.

6. The method of reimbursement will not affect indicators of hospital performance (the null hypothesis).

EMPIRICAL RESULTS

Costs

Means of several cost indicators are shown in Table 1. Although there appear to be significant differences, they do not support any of our hypotheses. In addition, we compared the means of various production indicators from Hospital Administrative Services (HAS) hospitals, stratified by bed size,

Table 1: Means of Two Cost Indicators

State	Average Cost	
	Per Diem	Per Admission
Illinois	$49.63	$421.66
Indiana	43.07	340.25
Michigan	52.56	436.25
Wisconsin	42.47	327.02

Source: *Hospitals* 41, no. 15 (August 1967).

and conducted chi square tests on the observations. There were no statistical differences in the way these hospitals produced health care services.* Comparison of means is misleading, however, since hospital costs could be affected by many things other than the reimbursement scheme.

Factors which are commonly believed to affect hospital costs are number of beds, income, range of services offered, and quality of care. One possible solution would be to stratify the data, but a more powerful test is suggested by Stigler and Friedland's work on regulation of electric public utilities.[5] In order to find out whether or not regulation affects the level of electrical rates, they ran a multiple regression with electrical rates as the dependent variable. Independent variables included a number of possible determinants of the level of rates, and among them was a dummy variable indicating the presence or absence of regulation. The effect of regulation is then indicated by the regression coefficient of the dummy variable and the change in the coefficient of multiple determination (R^2) caused by running the regression with and without the dummy variable for regulation.

We have used a similar technique in this study. To data for individual hospitals from pairs of states, we fitted the following equation:

$$X_1 = a + bX_2 + cX_3 + dX_4 + eX_5 + fX_6 + gX_7 + hX_8 + iX_9$$

where X_1 is log of cost per patient day; X_2 is number of facilities; X_3 is number of approvals; X_4 is denomination 0 if non-Catholic, 1 if Catholic; X_5 is support 0 if public, 1 if nonpublic; X_6 is log of number of beds; X_7 is log

---

*The sample consisted of six months of HAS data for the period from January through June 1966 (the last period prior to Medicare), with forty-five observations from Illinois, thirty-four from Indiana, fifty-three from Michigan, and thirty-three from Wisconsin. We compared nursing with total expense, payroll with total expense, employees per inpatient day, nursing hours per inpatient day, nursing hours with total employee hours, hourly wage rate for indirect employees, hourly wage rate for nurses, and total hourly wage rate for all four states. There were no discernible differences in either means or standard deviations.

of county population density; X_8 is log of average county family income; and X_9 is dummy variable for type of reimbursement scheme (e.g., 0 if charge-based, 1 if cost-based). The logarithmic form of the equation was chosen because it provided a much better fit (higher R^2, with or without the regulation variable) than did the same equation using arithmetic values. Data were obtained from the 1967 *Hospitals* Guide Issue for all hospitals providing complete responses. Variable X_3 was used as a proxy for quality of patient care, and variables X_4 and X_5 were included to see whether denomination or the presence of tax support affected hospital costs.

Results of these regressions for several possible binary comparisons are shown in Table 2. (Data for all four states were run together with the following values for the reimbursement scheme variable assigned to reflect the degree of strictness of regulation: Wisconsin, 0; Illinois, 0.333; Michigan, 0.667; Indiana, 1.0.) The most important and significant variable in all the regressions was family income; other coefficients which were usually significant were those associated with number of approvals, support, number of beds, and population density.

In no case was the coefficient of the variable for reimbursement scheme either large or significant. Moreover, the value of R^2 was almost unaltered by addition of the variable.* This test provides powerful evidence that at least those reimbursement schemes in use in the four states do not affect cost per patient day. Similar results are shown for cost per admission in Table 3. Denomination and support, which were always insignificant, are excluded here, but number of physicians per square mile is included. Population density and physician density turned out to be consistently significant; income was significant in only one case.

The dummy variable was statistically significant in three cases — Wisconsin-Illinois, Wisconsin-Michigan, and Indiana-Illinois. Both Illinois and Michigan — cost-based states — displayed significantly higher costs than those in charge-based Wisconsin, and costs in Illinois were also higher than those of controlled charge-based Indiana. There do appear to be significant differences in cost per admission, but there is no apparent explanation for these differences. In any case, even when the regulation coefficient was statistically significant, it was always numerically small. Costs would have been less than 5 per cent higher in Illinois than in Wisconsin, and they were only affected by 2 to 3 per cent in the Illinois-Indiana and Michigan-Wisconsin cases. The changes in R^2 were correspondingly small.

In sum, whether hospitals are paid on the basis of costs or of charges does not seem to affect cost per patient day, the most commonly used indicator.

---

*A similar regression run for a subsample of hospitals with more than a hundred beds provided higher R^2s in the neighborhood of 0.5, but regulation in this case also had no effect.

Table 2: Coefficients of Independent Variables
(Dependent Variable: Log of Cost per Patient Day)

Constant Term	No. of Facilities	No. of Approvals	Denomination (1 if Catholic, 0 if not)	Support (1 if public, 0 if not)	Log of Bed Size	Log of County Population Density	Log of Average County Family Income	Reimbursement Scheme	R^2 without Regulation and with Regulation
Wisconsin (0) – Illinois (1)								
.856* (.171)ᵃ	.004 (.005)	.010* (.003)	-.013 (.014)	-.049* (.017)	-.078* (.033)	.041* (.012)	.406* (.107)	.010 (.014)	.384 .384
Wisconsin (0) – Indiana (1)								
.897* (.258)	.012 (.008)	.005 (.004)	-.007 (.019)	-.025 (.019)	-.090* (.046)	.065* (.021)	.357* (.163)	-.001 (.006)	.320 .320
Wisconsin (0) – Michigan (1)								
.485* (.258)	.021* (.008)	.007 (.005)	-.007 (.018)	-.011 (.021)	-.042 (.042)	.005 (.016)	.583* (.154)	.011 (.211)	.299 .299
Illinois (0) – Michigan (1)								
.774* (.183)	.010 (.006)	.007* (.003)	-.003 (.015)	-.033* (.015)	-.030 (.030)	.018 (.011)	.423* (.107)	-.001 (.012)	.256 .256
All Four States								
.718* (.139)	.012* (.004)	.006 (.002)	-.006 (.012)	-.029* (.012)	-.048* (.024)	.025* (.010)	.459* (.084)	-.006 (.015)	.382 .383

ᵃValue in parenthesis represents standard error.
*Significant at the .99 level.
Source: *Hospitals* 41, no. 15 (August 1967).

Table 3: Coefficients of Independent Variables
(Dependent Variable: Log of Average Cost per Admission)

Constant Term	No. of Facilities	No. of Approvals	Log of Bed Size	Log of Average County Family Income	Log of Physician Density	Log of Population Density	Reimbursement Scheme	R^2 without Regulation and with Regulation
Wisconsin (0) – Indiana (1)								
2.11* (.246)	.016* (.008)	.005 (.004)	.016 (.042)	.047 (.153)	.077* (.033)	.066* (.020)	.001 (.002)	.469 .470
Wisconsin (0) – Illinois (1)								
2.01* (.196)	.009 (.006)	.004 (.013)	.049 (.034)	.044 (.119)	.070* (.029)	.055* (.013)	.046* (.015)	.443 .458
Wisconsin (0) – Michigan (1)								
1.85* (.254)	.012 (.008)	.003 (.004)	.057 (.040)	.190 (.153)	.047 (.030)	.031* (.015)	.015* (.005)	.381 .404
Illinois (0) – Indiana (1)								
2.20* (.215)	.009 (.006)	.006 (.004)	.047 (.035)	.011 (.123)	.060* (.035)	.061* (.014)	-.028* (.011)	.426 .438
Illinois (0) – Michigan (1)								
2.00* (.216)	.009 (.006)	.004 (.004)	.064* (.033)	.103 (.125)	.041 (.029)	.043* (.012)	.019 (.013)	.319 .322
All Four States								
1.80* (.157)	.017* (.005)	.003 (.003)	.040 (.026)	.235* (.093)	.047* (.022)	.042* (.010)	.014 (.015)	.399 .399

*Significant at the .99 level.
Source: *Hospitals* 41, no. 15 (August 1967).

Payment on a cost-plus basis, however, does seem to cause costs per admission to increase slightly. Direct regulation through control on charges or through restrictions on allowable cost does not appear to affect short-run costs, either cost per day or cost per admission, at all; thus hypothesis 2 is disproved.

Occupancy

This indicator provides information on short-run efficiency, but it also is affected by the long-run pattern of allocation of capital. Data on average occupancy is given in Table 4. These results seem to disprove the growth maximization hypothesis, since Wisconsin has a lower occupancy rate than Illinois. They also appear to suggest that there is less excess capacity in directly controlled states than in indirectly controlled ones.

Table 4: Average of Occupancy

State	Percentage
Illinois	79.1
Indiana	83.6
Michigan	82.1
Wisconsin	74.4

Source: *Hospitals* 41, no. 15 (August 1967).

As a more rigorous test, average occupancy (average daily census in a hospital as a percentage of total beds) was regressed on the logs of bed size, county population density, average county family income, and physician density, with and without the dummy variable for regulation. The results for the Illinois-Michigan and Illinois-Indiana combinations are shown in the first two lines of Table 5. Apparently, direct control, either by encouraging the use of beds or (more likely) by discouraging the construction of additional ones, brings about high occupancy rates. Even after adjustment for population density, bed size, and the other variables, Indiana and Michigan displayed higher occupancy rates than did Illinois.*

Long-Run Indicators

It was suggested above that a reasonable model of the regulatory agency was one in which it tried to foster the growth of larger hospitals. Data bearing on this problem are presented in Tables 6 and 7. Table 6 presents rates of change in several indicators for hospitals in the AHA Guide Issue. In Indiana and Michigan average hospital size and total beds increased more than in

*It should be noted, however, that inclusion of bed size does raise some identification problems, as it may be related to regulation.

Table 5: Coefficients of Independent Variables (Dependent Variable: Occupancy)

| Constant Term | Log of Bed Size | Log of Population Density | Variable | | Reimbursement Scheme | R^2 without Reimbursement Variable | R^2 with Reimbursement Variable |
			Log of Average County Family Income	Log of Physician Density			
Illinois (0) – Michigan (1)							
40.0* (17.3)	12.8* (1.67)	1.71 (1.00)	-.369 (10.1)	3.28 (2.41)	4.58* (1.10)	.234	.265
Illinois (0) – Indiana (1)							
25.8 (21.6)	12.0* (2.40)	1.92 (1.42)	8.70 (12.86)	2.59 (3.54)	1.24* (1.365)	.208	.236
Wisconsin (0) – Indiana (1)							
179 (111)	8.64 (11.8)	6.52 (8.90)	-74.2 (69.8)	-3.14 (14.8)	1.90 (2.26)	.005	.009
Wisconsin (0) – Illinois (1)							
111** (59.4)	11.3 (7.18)	4.33 (4.13)	-36.9 (36.8)	.170 (9.01)	-1.00 (4.47)	.015	.015

*Significant at the .99 level.
**Significant at the .9 level.

Source: *Hospitals* 41, no. 15 (August 1967).

Table 6: Hospital Efficiency Indices

	Illinois	Indiana	Michigan	Wisconsin	U.S.
Rates of change[a]					
Average total expense					
per patient day	6.1%	6.0%	6.3%	7.5%	7.1%
Average total expense					
per case	7.5%	7.8%	8.7%	8.7%	8.6%
Average hospital size	1.9%	2.8%	2.1%	1.5%	1.9%
Total beds	2.6%	3.2%	2.8%	2.2%	2.9%
Growth attributed to					
average size increase	73.1%	87.5%	75.0%	68.2%	65.5%
Absolute change in					
average occupancy	3.0%	6.8%	3.0%	1.9%	2.8%
Beds per 1,000 population	4.4	3.6	3.7	4.6	3.9

[a]Average rate of increase for the nine-year period 1957 to 1966 for non-federal, short-term general hospitals.

Source: hospital data are derived from *Hospitals* 32–41 (August 1958–1967); population data are derived from *Survey of Buying Power* (New York: Sales Management, Inc., 1966).

Illinois and Wisconsin. Moreover, the percentage of growth in size attributable to average size increase was significantly higher for Indiana than for Illinois and Wisconsin, and for Michigan it was slightly higher.

A second measure is shown in Table 7, with data taken from the HAS sample. The ratio of capital charges to current charges, which provides an indication of the extent of growth, is significantly higher for larger hospitals

Table 7: Ratio of Capital to Current Payments,[a] HAS Hospitals

Bed Size	Illinois		Indiana		Michigan		Wisconsin	
	No.	%	No.	%	No.	%	No.	%
500+	5	3.7	2	10.6	2	7.3	0	0
300–499	5	18.5	6	11.8	5	7.1	5	11.4
200–299	5	14.3	4	7.4	10	10.1	5	9.0
100–199	17	12.3	9	3.4	14	10.4	7	12.7
50–99	12	8.9	12	6.8	18	10.4	12	10.8
31–49	1	0	1	(1.1)	4	5.4	4	8.3
Total	45	11.1	34	6.8	53	9.5	33	10.7
Standard deviation		8.5%		8.4%		6.3%		6.6%
Coefficient of variation		76.6%		123.5%		66.3%		61.7%

[a]Capital/current payments = depreciation + net income/total expense − depreciation.

Source: Hospital Administrative Services, January–June 1966.

Table 8: Growth in Bed Strata, 1957–1966

| Bed Size | Illinois | | Indiana | | Michigan | | Wisconsin | |
	Beds	% of Growth	Beds	% of Growth	Beds	% of Growth	Beds	% of Growth
500+	(165)	(2.0)	86	2.1	153	3.3	(107)	(3.3)
300–499	1,089	13.4	937	22.8	621	13.3	128	4.0
200–299	1,564	19.3	1,197	29.2	1,696	36.5	1,494	47.0
100–199	3,664	45.1	938	22.8	958	20.6	450	14.2
50–99	1,292	15.9	567	13.8	504	10.8	617	19.4
Below 50	673	8.3	384	9.3	721	15.5	595	18.7
Total	8,117	100.0	4,109	100.0	4,653	100.0	3,177	100.0

Source: *Hospitals* 32, no. 1 (August 1958), 41, no. 15 (1958, 1967).

in Indiana. In none of the other states did there appear to be a perceptible pattern. The Indiana measure may, however, be misleading, since a significant number of small hospitals there are publicly owned and charge no depreciation on publicly provided investment.

In addition, we compared the growth of hospitals, stratified by bed size in 1957, during the 1957–1966 period. These results appear to confirm, at least partially, our capital flow analysis. The results appear in Table 8 and are especially significant with regard to the Illinois pattern of growth. It is possible that variables other than differential regulation in Indiana might have produced these results. Until such variables are identified and tested, however, one can conclude from these data that the presence of direct regulation through a reimbursement scheme in Indiana did alter the pattern of hospital growth from that in Illinois and Wisconsin, where there was no direct regulation.

CONCLUSION

Three conclusions can be drawn from this analysis. The first is that the growth cum "plus"-maximization model, as tested by the Illinois-Wisconsin comparison, received little support. Cost per patient day was not higher in Illinois than in Wisconsin, and the hypothesis that cost-plus schemes balloon costs was not supported. Incentive schemes depend in part for their effectiveness on surplus-maximizing or surplus-increasing behavior by hospitals, and this behavior was not observed, at least, not when the incentives covered one-fourth to one-half of potential patients. The second conclusion is that the existence of direct controls in the reimbursement scheme does not affect either cost per patient day or cost per admission. The third conclusion is that reimbursement schemes involving direct controls do seem to affect the pattern of allocation of capital to hospitals. They caused large hospitals to grow more than proportionately, and they may have contributed to higher occupancy rates. In sum, direct controls appear to have affected long-run system performance.

Our general conclusion is that it is important, both for purposes of investigation and for policy, to evaluate the effects of various devices in terms of both their short-run and long-run effects. Current period accounting costs are a poor indicator of hospital performance, since they reflect past experience and indicate nothing about the over-all configuration of the system.

NOTES

1. See William Gorham, *A Report to the President: Medical Care Prices* (Washington, D.C.: Department of Health, Education, and Welfare, 1967); and *Report of the National Advisory Commission on Health Manpower* (frequently referred to as the Miller Commission report) (Washington, D.C.: U.S. Government Printing Office, 1967).

2. Public Law 90-248, sec. 402 (Social Security Amendment of 1967), contains the description of the program.

3. Richard Caves, "Direct Regulation and Market Performance in the American Economy" (with comments by R. Coase), *American Economic Review Papers and Proceedings*, May 1967.

4. *Report of the National Advisory Commission on Health Manpower*, p. 58.

5. George J. Stigler and Claire Friedland, "What Can Regulators Regulate? The Case of Electricity," *Journal of Law and Economics* 5 (October 1962):1–16.

Herbert E. Klarman
The Johns Hopkins University

COMMENT

The paper by Pauly and Drake is noteworthy for several reasons. It is a first attempt to measure the third-party effect quantitatively – to go beyond inferences from basic propositions. It draws on the standard economic literature for its theorizing and approach to measurement. It makes a distinction between short-run and long-run effects, a distinction which is not prominent in the discussion of this subject to date or in the official *Guidelines for Incentive Reimbursement Experiments.*[1] Finally, and not least important, both sets of findings – the absence of short-run effects and the apparent presence of a long-run effect – are surprising.

I see the discussant's task as twofold: to analyze the findings reported and to suggest some next steps.

EFFECT ON PER DIEM COST

The core of the paper is the analysis of short-term effects, especially the effect of regulation on hospital cost per patient day. The finding is negative. Regulation is entered as a dummy variable in a nine-variable equation, along the lines of Stigler-Friedland. For the most part, the comparison is performed for hospitals in two states at a time. Let us focus on the variable regulation. In the Stigler-Friedland article regulation is defined simply as the presence of a state electric utility commission.[2] Pauly-Drake appear to define it in various ways. In the definition of variables, the example given is that of reimbursement at charges vs. cost. From the description of the four Blue Cross plans it appears that regulation entails denial of reimbursement for services rendered in facilities not approved by the given Blue Cross plan. It is possible that regulation refers to a reimbursement policy that is less liberal than in the

315

unregulated states or one in which the elements of cost are scrutinized more closely and increases in the reimbursement rate are restricted. (Apparently, both the Indiana and Michigan plans follow the former policy, while only Indiana follows the latter to a marked degree.) Regulation is likely to affect behavior differently depending upon its nature. If it amounts to not paying for certain services, it will affect expenditures for hospital care through limitation of hospital use by subscribers, but not through the price (or cost) per unit. Conversely, a reimbursement scheme aimed at limiting cost per unit need not be associated with a reduction in use.

How pervasive is regulation? In the Stigler-Friedland article, the state commission sets rates for all customers. Since Blue Cross plans pay only for their subscribers, their payment policies affect only a share of the hospital's patient revenues except in a state like Indiana, where the Blue Cross plan's controlled charges are said to apply to all patients. Only in Indiana, therefore, can regulation be said to apply to all patients. In the other states the influence of the Blue Cross plan must be weighted by its relative importance in the hospitals' income statements.

What weights, then, are appropriate? Pauly-Drake present figures on the percentage of the population subscribing to Blue Cross in each of the four states. For Indiana, as suggested above, it seems warranted to discard the enrollment percentage of 35 per cent and to apply a weight of 100 per cent. In the other states the percentage of enrollment may or may not accurately reflect the role of the Blue Cross plan in hospital finances. Some data for New York City will throw light on this problem. In 1957, 50 per cent of the population was enrolled in Blue Cross. However, the Blue Cross plan accounted for only 44 per cent of all hospital patients, 37 per cent of all patient days, and 27 per cent of all operating income. When the hospitals were disaggregated and examined separately by ownership category, the municipal hospitals showed very low percentages of Blue Cross participation, whereas participation in the voluntary hospitals approached the enrollment proportion of 50 per cent for patients and patient days.[3] The figures are likely to vary with time and place, but two points emerge. The percentage of the population enrolled may not accurately gauge the degree of financial influence of a Blue Cross plan. Furthermore, it may be desirable to examine such influence separately, by hospital ownership category.

So far the discussion has had no time reference. Pauly-Drake analyze data for 1966 (officially, for the year ending September 1966 but more likely, on the average, for the year ending June 1966). July 1, 1966 marks the inauguration of Medicare, which covers a sizable percentage of all hospital patients and an even larger percentage of all patient days. The authors characterize Medicare reimbursement policy as cost plus. Although the statute talks about "reasonable cost," in actuality a plus factor of 2 per cent is applied to capture those items of cost which may escape the elements that are explicitly paid for. (Note that the plus factor was deleted in 1969.) However, what is important about the Medicare reimbursement policy is the cost component, not the plus. There would be little change in the nature of the reimbursement problem if the plus factor were eliminated while reimbursement at cost remained. If the plus factor were of predominant importance, it would make sense to discuss the hospitals' behavior in terms of accumulating funds for expansion, and the like. Conversely, if the cost component is the important factor, it is more useful to focus on the possibility that reimbursing at the cost to the individual hospital may constitute a disincentive to efficient operation.

Obviously, a hospital's management is not likely to be influenced by cost reimbursement if only 5 or 10 per cent of its income is derived in this manner. It is almost certain to be influenced if the proportion is 90 or 95 percent. The percentage point at which such influence becomes manifest is not known. There is good reason to believe, however, that in some hospitals this point has already been reached or even passed. It has been estimated that with the advent of Medicare there took place an over-all increase in the proportion of patient days reimbursed at the individual hospital's cost on the order of 75 per cent or more.[4] Medicaid will have contributed an additional increase. What is needed are data on the distribution of hospitals by the percentage of all patient days reimbursed at, or in relation to, cost.

Let me offer a small piece of evidence, which is illustrative but not conclusive, on what has happened to hospital cost recently in the four states under study. The following percentage increases in patient day cost[5] occurred between 1966 and 1967 in all short-term hospitals and in the voluntary hospitals:

State	All Hospitals	Voluntary Hospitals
Illinois	10.2%	10.8%
Indiana	6.6%	7.9%
Michigan	12.7%	13.3%
Wisconsin	11.7%	11.1%

Evidently, Indiana has been more successful in curtailing cost increases than the other three states.

The finding leads to another point. Is it possible that research on this problem will prove more fruitful if comparisons are made before and after a major event, such as Medicare, rather than through attempts to explain differences in behavior cross-sectionally? Can one formulate guidelines for research strategy — when and where the one approach can be said to be more promising than the other? Does a trade-off perhaps exist between gaining a better understanding of a process and developing a mechanism for cost control?

OTHER POSSIBLE EFFECTS

My remarks on the other effects of reimbursement that are analyzed in the paper are shorter.

Cost per Admission

The study of cost per admission also yields negative findings, and so it should. Cost per admission equals cost per patient day times average duration of patient stay. In a given locale the latter tends to be a fixed aspect of medical practice, which is not likely to change readily in response to changes in reimbursement policy.

Rate of Occupancy

The study of cost per admission also yields results that Pauly-Drake regard as unexpected or disappointing. It may be that their expectations were based on an incomplete or mistaken theory. That would clearly be true if the supply of beds were the major determinant of hospital use in an area, as some students have argued. In that case, rates of occupancy (standardized in some fashion) would tend toward equality among areas. I appreciate that this proposition does not command universal assent; witness the papers by Carr and, an even better example, by Stevens presented at this conference. But the evidence on the other side is at least as strong.[6]

The optimum rate of occupancy is affected by factors other than average daily census and available bed capacity. The size of the facility, the extent to which facilities are segregated for whatever reason, and the average duration of stay are also important. The last factor has to do with the frequency of vacant beds and the lag in filling them or the cost of overcoming the lag; it has not yet been quantified. Data on the segregated or distinctive use of facilities are not easy to come by. Rosenthal has, however, adjusted occupancy rates for differences in average size of hospital by calculating "pressure points," which are ratios of observed occupancy to maximum occupancy for the entire bed capacity, estimated on the basis of the Poisson distribution.[7]

Size of Hospital

For the long run Pauly-Drake focus on the changes in average hospital size. The findings are interesting in themselves. One should be cautious in interpreting them for two reasons, however. The paper does not say what the regulatory mechanism was that accomplished this result and how long it has been operative, nor is this effect linked to changes in cost. The fact is that from a base line in 1947, presumably prior to the advent of the regulatory mechanism, the four states have not changed in the rank order of patient day cost; this is particularly true of the voluntary hospitals when examined separately. Moreover, even if large hospitals were less costly than small ones, when all other factors are held constant, they might not be able to achieve the lower cost in actuality, given the tendency for the range of services and teaching programs to expand with hospital size.

I am impressed with two other figures presented in Table 6 of the paper. The ratio of beds to population is 20 per cent lower in Indiana and Michigan than in Illinois or Wisconsin. The rank order of the states in hospital cost per capita is more strongly favorable to Indiana and Michigan than is Table 1 on patient day cost. The problem is in trying to explain how these results were achieved, in view of the limited information on mechanisms and institutions.

CONCLUSIONS

This first attempt to look at the problem of hospital reimbursement quantitatively is welcome. I have raised several questions concerning the Pauly-Drake findings. The concept of regulation requires clarification and the mechanism of regulation requires greater specification. A measure is needed of the pervasiveness of regulation. Owing to Medicare, results in 1968 are likely to differ from those in 1966. Finally, is a before-and-after comparison likely to be more fruitful, when a major event takes place, than an analysis of cross-sectional data?

NOTES

1. Department of Health, Education, and Welfare, *Guidelines for Incentive Reimbursement Experiments* (Washington, D.C.: U.S. Government Printing Office, 1968).

2. George J. Stigler and Claire Friedland, "What Can Regulators Regulate? The Case of Electricity," *Journal of Law and Economics* 5 (October 1962):1–16.

3. Herbert E. Klarman, *Hospital Care in New York City* (New York: Columbia University Press, 1963), pp. 420–22.

4. Herbert E. Klarman, "Reimbursing the Hospitals – The Differences the Third Party Makes," *Journal of Risk and Insurance* 36, no. 5 (December 1969):553–66.

5. Data are from *Hospitals* 41, no. 15 (August 1967):462–63, and *ibid.*, 42, no. 15 (August 1968):448–49.

6. Herbert E. Klarman, "Approaches to Moderating the Increases in Medical Care Costs," *Medical Care* 7, no. 3 (May–June 1969):175–90.

7. See Gerald D. Rosenthal, *The Demand for General Hospital Facilities*, American Hospital Association Monograph 14 (Chicago: By the Association, 1964), pp. 48–49, 57.

Edgar W. Francisco
Yale University School of Medicine

ANALYSIS OF COST VARIATIONS AMONG SHORT-TERM GENERAL HOSPITALS

Presented in this paper is an analysis of hospital cost per patient day, taking into account various hospital characteristics. The cost data and the "patient day" service unit have the inadequacies recently summarized by Thompson.[1] There have been at least three approaches to these various hospital "mix" problems. One, that of Saathoff and Kurtz[2] and Cohen,[3] has been the development of weighted output indices to overcome the inadequacy of patient days as a measure of the multiple outputs of a hospital. A second approach, used by Feldstein,[4] focuses on the problem of case mix. The variation in hospital facilities and services, a confusing factor in the study of the size-cost relationship, has been studied by Ingbar using multiple regression analysis[5] and by Berry, using homogeneous grouping, with separate analysis of each group.[6] For a review of these and other research methods, see Lave.[7] The present study reports the similarity in results obtained by either separate analysis of homogeneous groups of hospitals or by multiple regression analysis of all hospitals, using an index of facilities and services.

A tape of the American Hospital Association's annual survey for 1966 was sorted to obtain data for short-term general hospitals with full and complete cost, utilization, and personnel information. Extensive checks on the data were devised and run for over a year. For example, comparison of the data reported in each of several years revealed numerous gross deviations for one or more years, each of which was checked and corrected where necessary.

This paper summarizes a portion of the research toward a doctoral dissertation at Yale University Department of Economics. The author is a Research Associate in the Department of Epidemiology and Public Health, United States Public Health Service. The research was supported in part by Public Health Service Grant CH00037-06.

321

The discrepancies in the code for control were caused, in some cases, by use of incorrect identity codes by hospital administrators, and, in other cases, by errors in reporting or key punching. Discrepancies between the hospital code on one of the first identification cards and the following data cards revealed several errors: for example, in one case data were interchanged for two large hospitals after being punched and before being taped. None of these errors would have been discovered except by extensive sort and compare programs. After all the test programs were completed, the records of 4,710 hospitals were accepted for analysis.

CURVILINEAR ANALYSIS OF GROUPS OF HOSPITALS
HOMOGENEOUS WITH RESPECT TO A COMBINATION OF FACILITIES

Curvilinear analyses of total cost and of average cost per patient day as a function of output (total patient days) were undertaken for each sizable group of hospitals found to be homogeneous with regard to the number of facilities and services available (out of the sixteen now reported to the AHA) and with regard to a specific combination of those facilities and services. The groups were obtained by sorting the 4,710 short-term general hospitals into the 2^{16} possible combinations of the sixteen facilities and services. A statistical package was developed for this analysis which sorts (in this case by all possible combinations of facilities and services), counts the number of hospitals having each combination, stores on another tape or disk those combinations represented by a predetermined number of hospitals, and uses these sets of data as inputs to the regression program. Of the 65,536 possible combinations, 64,378 were not represented by a single hospital. The distribution is summarized below:

No. of Hospitals Having Each Combination of Facilities and Services	No. of Combinations
0	64,378
1–9	1,060
10–19	58
20–29	15
30–39	10
40–49	5
50 and over	10

Only those combinations represented by thirty or more hospitals were included in the regression analysis. Twenty-five groups of hospitals were therefore analyzed.

Presented in Table 1 are some of the findings of the curvilinear analysis of total hospital costs as a function of total patient days. While twenty-one of the twenty-five groups have positive intercepts (not shown in the table) for

Table 1: Curvilinear Regression Analysis of the Relationship between
Total Cost and Output in Short-Term General Hospitals

Group No.	No. of Hospitals in Group	No. of Facilities and Services	Available Beds $\bar{X}$	σ	Maximum Degree of Curve Fitted
1	125	1	30	15	1
2	40	2	28	10	1
3	150	2	34	12	2
4	77	2	41	18	1
5*	41	2	48	22	1
6	39	3	33	18	1
7	31	3	36	18	1
8*	68	3	39	16	1
9	30	3	46	24	1
10	66	3	51	28	1
11	37	3	56	27	1
12*	34	4	34	19	3
13	69	4	54	21	1
14	32	5	76	28	2
15*	41	6	100	39	2
16	53	6	103	46	2
17	59	7	106	40	1
18	32	8	130	54	1
19	35	8	159	56	1
20	59	9	208	87	1
21	47	10	201	64	1
22	49	12	318	102	3
23	30	13	372	116	1
24	30	14	543	229	3
25	54	16	952	670	1
Total	1,328				

*Groups for which the intercept is positive and significant at the .05 level in the degree
1 curves.

the degree 1 curves, only four have intercepts that are significantly different
from zero. Four out of twenty-five does not constitute an impressive case for
decreasing average cost. As for the linearity of the curves, Table 1 shows that
the total cost-total output relationship is best explained by a second-degree or
third-degree curve for seven of the twenty-five groups. Of these seven, five
reflect costs increasing at an increasing rate (convex from below), and the
other two are increasing at a decreasing rate. For the other eighteen groups,
the higher degree curves have coefficients which are not significantly different
from zero. Two of these have significantly positive intercepts. That leaves
sixteen which fit a constant returns to scale hypothesis, with only one of the
other nine, Group 12, departing impressively from constant returns to scale.
However, additional information is provided by the average cost curves discussed below.

Table 2: Curvilinear Regression Analysis of the Relationship between
Average Cost and Output in Short-Term General Hospitals

Group No.	ΣF	Average Annual Patient Day Output	Average Cost per Patient Day	Maximum Degree of Curve Fitted	Degree 1 curve (Y = average cost, X = patient days)
		(hundreds)			(hundreds)
1	1	7.02	30.69	0	$33.51 - 0.40X$
2	2	6.23	38.12	2	$48.26 - 1.63X*$
3	2	7.66	31.83	1	$36.03 - 0.55X*$
4	2	9.00	30.67	0	$33.17 - 0.28X$
5	2	11.81	33.79	0	$41.27 - 0.63X$
6	3	8.37	30.00	0	$35.44 - 0.65X$
7	3	8.65	32.32	1	$38.69 - 0.74X*$
8	3	8.97	32.08	1	$36.97 - 0.55X*$
9	3	11.48	30.98	0	$31.93 - 0.08X$
10	3	12.14	34.50	2	$40.11 - 0.46X*$
11	3	14.00	32.95	1	$41.39 - 0.60X*$
12	4	7.52	29.97	1	$36.80 - 0.91X*$
13	4	12.88	35.18	0	$40.16 - 0.39X$
14	5	19.20	39.58	0	$45.42 - 0.30X$
15	6	27.41	44.23	2	$55.64 - 0.42X$
16	6	28.53	43.29	0	$50.32 - 0.25X$
17	7	28.49	47.94	0	$52.46 - 0.16X$
18	8	34.20	39.77	0	$43.40 - 0.11X$
19	8	43.66	45.52	0	$57.56 - 0.28X$
20	9	60.77	44.22	0	$48.91 - 0.08X$
21	10	55.23	42.79	0	$41.76 + 0.02X$
22	12	96.11	45.51	0	$39.98 + 0.06X$
23	13	109.36	43.50	0	$49.51 - 0.05X$
24	14	152.91	48.95	0	$41.71 + 0.05X$
25	16	276.34	50.91	0	$56.45 - 0.02X$

*Groups for which the regression coefficient is significantly different from zero at the .05 level in the degree 1 curves.

Presented in Table 2 are some curvilinear relationships between average hospital cost per patient day and output (patient days) for the same twenty-five groups. For twenty-two of the twenty-five groups, average cost is less for the large hospitals in each group. This corresponds with the study of forty groups by Berry, who emphasized his finding of thirty-six negative coefficients out of the forty, with twenty-six of the thirty-six making some contribution (T-ratio greater than 1). However, only seven of his regression coefficients were significantly negative and one was significantly positive. Had he emphasized the latter finding, we would be in close agreement, since the present study finds seven of the twenty-five regression coefficients to be significant.

These very similar results are obviously subject to varying interpretations. While the results hint at the presence of economies of scale, this writer is uncomfortable with the paucity of groups meeting tests of significance. However, if this analysis is carried one further step, the proper interpretation of these results becomes clear. The twenty-five groups should not be thought of as twenty-five votes on the question of economies of scale. They represent very different hospital populations, as may be seen when they are arrayed, as they are in Tables 1 and 2, by number of facilities and services (and, where numbers of facilities are equal, by output). If the results are re-examined, it can be seen from Table 1 that all four of the groups with significantly positive intercepts for the total cost degree 1 curves have average bed capacity of 100 or less. In Table 2 it is indicated that only seven groups have significantly negative regression coefficients for the average cost degree 1 curves, and all seven have average bed capacities of 56 or less. Since the next group has an average of 76 beds, it could be stated that in groups with, on the average, 70 beds or less, seven out of twelve show significant economies of scale. None of the thirteen groups of larger hospitals show significant economies of scale. Finally, for groups with ten or more facilities and services and, on the average, over 200 beds, three out of five show increasing costs, though not significantly so. None of the twenty groups of smaller hospitals show increasing costs. Finding significant coefficients in seven out of twelve of the small hospital groups is sufficiently beyond chance for this writer to believe that there are economies of scale for the types of hospitals represented by those groups (that is, for hospitals with relatively few facilities and services and which range in size up to about 100 beds). This analysis finds little evidence to challenge a constant returns to scale model for the larger hospitals, with fuller components of services.

GROUPS HOMOGENEOUS WITH REGARD ONLY TO THE NUMBER OF FACILITIES AND SERVICES

An analysis identical to the one reported above was made for groups homogeneous with respect to only one of the two characteristics used above, that is, homogeneous with regard to the total number of facilities and services but not with regard to a specific combination of facilities and services. For comparison of the results, the average cost curves for the seventeen groups (with none through sixteen facilities and services) are presented in Table 3. Fifteen of the seventeen groups show decreasing average hospital cost, eight of the regression coefficients being significant. Again, the important point is which groups show significantly decreasing costs. Of the nine groups composed of hospitals with an average of 135 beds or less, seven show significantly decreasing costs over the range of hospitals in the group. (One could justify omitting Group 0, in which case seven of eight groups show significantly decreasing costs.) For the eight groups having an average of 185 or more beds, only one shows significantly decreasing average cost.

For almost all of the groups presented in Tables 2 and 3, the degree 2 average cost curves are properly U-shaped. As expected, the minimum average

Table 3: Curvilinear Regression Analysis of the Relationship between Average
Cost and Output in Short-Term General Hospitals (Homogeneous with Respect to ΣF)

Group No. (ΣF)	No. of Hospitals in Group	Available Beds		Average Cost per Patient Day	Maximum Degree of Curve Fitted	Degree 1 Curve (Y = average cost, X = patient days)
		$\bar{X}$	σ			(hundreds)
0	28	26	12	28.70	0	27.01 + 0.28X
1	167	32	18	30.46	0	32.36 − 0.26X
2	391	38	19	32.91	1	37.28 − 0.48X*
3	457	44	24	34.60	2	40.07 − 0.51X*
4	474	54	27	37.35	1	41.54 − 0.32X*
5	464	68	36	38.93	2	42.14 − 0.19X*
6	421	86	43	40.75	2	44.47 − 0.16X*
7	375	102	50	41.74	1	44.18 − 0.09X*
8	370	135	64	43.30	2	46.75 − 0.09X*
9	310	185	89	43.16	0	45.57 − 0.05X
10	318	220	97	44.13	0	46.24 − 0.03X
11	258	258	116	44.98	0	48.50 − 0.05X
12	204	342	147	44.34	0	48.82 − 0.04X
13	202	402	192	46.83	1	54.82 − 0.07X*
14	136	514	287	48.12	0	53.46 − 0.03X
15	81	606	289	51.35	0	49.05 + 0.01X
16	54	952	670	50.91	0	56.45 − 0.02X

*Groups for which the regression coefficient is significantly different from zero at
the .05 level in the degree 1 curves.

cost points increase with the average size and the average number of facilities
in the group. As expected, in the groups of small hospitals there are a larger
proportion of institutions operating on the decreasing side of the curves.
None of these figures are presented because most of the degree 2 curve
coefficients are not significant. The few which are significant are so indicated
in the tables under the heading "Maximum Degree of Curve Fitted."

REGRESSION ANALYSIS WITH DUMMY VARIABLES

An alternative method to the one used above should be noted briefly.
Rather than run twenty-five sets of regressions, as discussed on p. 322 above,
dummy variables could be used, one for each of the twenty-five groups. Thus,
fifty variables were needed for the degree 1 curves. Similarly, a model with
thirty-four dummy variables was used for analysis of the seventeen groups
homogeneous with respect to number of facilities and services, as discussed
above. Of course, the resulting regression equations were identical to those
obtained above, but required less work. The saving is only the difference
between one and twenty-five sets of printouts, since the sorting must be done
in both cases to identify the specific groups. However, to obtain the results
from the thirty-four dummy variables it is not necessary to have a sort sub-
routine, the dummy variables being added as part of the one-regression run.

While the dummy variables yield identical equations to those obtained above, the two methods are different in their emphasis. In the analysis of each homogeneous group the proportion of variation in cost within a group explained by output is obtained without any indication of how much of the total variation in cost is being investigated. The strength and weakness of the method is that the relationship between cost and facilities available is held in the background. In contrast, the analysis with dummy variables brings facilities back into competition with patient day output as an explanatory variable and emphasizes the close correlation between facilities and output, with the dummy variables for facilities being highly significant compared with the relatively small contribution indicated for variations in output. However, dummy variable analysis would not point up the difference between the groups of large hospitals and the groups of small hospitals with regard to economies of scale unless the dummy variables for facilities had been assigned to groups already arrayed by size.

MULTIPLE REGRESSION ANALYSIS, INCLUDING AN INDEX OF FACILITIES AND SERVICES

Multiple regression analysis of hospital costs was undertaken, with one of the variables being ΣF, an unweighted index of facilities and services. Thus, the influence of facilities and services on average cost was represented by one variable, in contrast to the thirty-four or fifty required in the analysis involving dummy variables discussed above. A comparison of the methods is aided by seeing the correlations between average cost and some of these measures of facilities and services.

1. Using dummy variables for the number of facilities and services:

   $R = .32$ with seventeen dummy variables for the seventeen groups homogeneous by number of facilities and services

   $R = .34$ with eighteen variables: patient days plus seventeen dummy variables

   $R = .36$ with thirty-four variables: seventeen each for intercepts and betas

II. Multiple regression analysis:

   $R = .31$ one variable, ΣF

   $R = .33$ two variables, ΣF plus patient days

   —   no equivalence to the thirty-four-variable case

For the data being analyzed the index, ΣF, is shown to approximate the performance of the more matrix-consuming dummy variable methods reported above. The correlation between average cost and ΣF is .31, in comparison with .32 using seventeen dummy variables to represent the seventeen groups by number of facilities and services. (A weighted ΣF would, of course, yield the correlation .32.) When the variable patient days is added to each analysis, the correlations increase to .33 and .34. Note that the additional contribution of the variable patient days is .02 in both methods. Finally, from the equations for average cost as a function of patient days and of some representation of facilities and services, the regression coefficient for patient days is -.039 when seventeen dummy variables are in the equation as compared with -.037 when only the index, ΣF, is in the equation.

In summary, for these data an unweighted index, ΣF, is shown to be a very good substitute for the use of dummy variables in measuring the influence of facilities and services on average cost and in taking that influence into account while other factors are studied. Since the dummy variable method is identical with the separate analysis of each of a set of homogeneous groups as far as the regression equations obtained are concerned, the three methods should produce the same results for these data, and it can be shown that they do.

Equation 3 in Table 4 is the equation cited above to show the similarity between the results of multiple regression analysis, including ΣF, and the results of the separate analysis of each of the groups. The regression coefficient for patient days is negative and significant but is small compared with that of ΣF. Actually, the impact on average cost of a 1 per cent change in ΣF is over seven times that of a 1 per cent change in output. The addition of patient days adds .02 to the multiple correlation (equations 2 to 3), but R more than doubles when ΣF is added to patient days (equations 1 to 3). This corresponds to the finding of eight significant regression coefficients out of seventeen groups used in the first method, a method that yielded no information about the variance between groups due to ΣF. If predicting, or accounting for, variation in average cost is the objective, then the multiple regression analysis shows that a measure of output makes little contribution once facilities are taken into account and no contribution once one or two other factors are added. If the objective is only to see the cost-output relationship with other factors held constant, regardless of whether it makes any noticeable change in cost, then on the basis of the multiple regression analysis one can say that there is a statistically significant negative relationship. The separate analysis of the groups shows a significant negative relationship for some groups, but not for most.

Equation 5 shows the importance of percentage occupancy relative to output, once location and facilities have been determined. Notice in equation

Table 4: Estimates from Multiple Regression Analysis of the Relationship between Average Cost/Patient Day and Output (Patient Days), 4,710 Short-Term General Hospitals, 1966

Equation No.	R	a	(1) % Occupancy	(2) Patient Days	(3) ΣF	(4) Urban	(5) (1) × (4)	(6) (2) × (4)	(7) (3) × (4)
1	.15	39		0.04 (10.0)					
2	.31	32			1.25 (22.6)				
3	.33	30		-0.04 (-5.6)	1.67 (21.5)				
4	.48	46	-0.25 (-17.4)[a]		0.98 (15.6)	10.62 (23.2)			
5	.49	44	-0.23 (-16.0)	-0.04 (-8.6)	1.36 (17.8)	11.06 (24.4)			
6	.49	40	-0.19 (-10.1)	-0.09 (-5.9)	1.90 (15.6)	22.20 (10.3)	-0.10 (-3.3)	0.07 (4.2)	-0.92 (-5.6)
7	.49	42	-0.22 (-12.3)		1.41 (15.6)	22.00 (10.7)	-0.08 (-2.8)		-0.77 (-6.1)

[a]Figures in parentheses represent T-ratios.

4 how little difference it makes to omit patient days from equation 5. This relationship may be carried one step further, as shown in equation 6, where percentage occupancy and urbanization (dummy variable for SMSA) are added, with urbanization interacted with percentage occupancy, patient days, and ΣF. As expected, the equation for urban hospitals is shifted up (as seen by the coefficient for independent variable 4). Average cost decreases with higher occupancy rates in both urban and non-urban areas, but more so in urban areas (independent variables 1 and 5). The ΣF-urban interaction (independent variable 7) is in the opposite direction from the variable ΣF, but ΣF remains highly significant for both urban and non-urban hospitals. However, the addition of the patient days-urban interaction (independent variable 6) results in an insignificant relationship between patient days and average cost in urban hospitals (independent variables 2 and 6). Since size and urbanization are closely correlated, this is another way of stating that above a certain size there are no additional economies of scale.

Finally, the lack of contribution to the variations in cost accounted for by output may be seen in a comparison of equation 6 with 7, where removing the output variables has no effect on the correlation coefficient; of equation 5 with 4, where the drop is .01; and of equation 3 with 2, where the drop is .02.

The markedly different distribution of economies of scale among large and small hospitals was noted in the first method of analysis discussed at the beginning of this paper and again in the multiple regression analysis presented in Table 4. Finally, the twenty-five groups (1,328 hospitals) were combined into two groups, the first fourteen of which were treated as a group of small hospitals and the last eleven of which were combined into one large group. Equation 9 in Table 5 shows the familiar relationship for the total – a negative, significant patient day regression coefficient, but one which makes almost no impact on cost for a hospital with given facilities (equations 9 and 8). The contrast between the two groups of hospitals is striking. The coefficient for the large hospitals is not different from zero. The coefficient for the small hospitals is not only significant but is many times larger, and for the first time makes a large contribution to the correlation coefficient.

SUMMARY

Three seemingly different methods of analysis of the cost-output relationship, designed to take into account variations in facilities and services, were shown to yield either identical or similar results. The methods were analysis of the cost-output relationship for each homogeneous grouping of hospitals, using simple linear and curvilinear regression, the use of dummy variables to represent each of the facility-service combinations studied, and the use of multiple regression analysis with an unweighted index to represent facilities and services.

Table 5: Estimates from Multiple Regression Analysis of the Relationship between
Average Cost/Patient Day and Output (Patient Days), 1,328 Hospitals

Equation No.	R	a	Regression Coefficients	
			Patient Days	ΣF
Small hospitals (N = 839)				
1	.13	35.11	-0.26 (-3.9)[a]	
2	.10	29.62		1.19 (3.0)
3	.21	31.21	-0.37 (-5.5)	1.97 (4.8)
Large hospitals (N = 489)				
4	.04	44.91	0.005 (0.99)	
5	.14	40.38		0.51 (3.0)
6	.15	39.03	-0.01 (-1.4)	0.74 (3.2)
Total (N = 1,328)				
7	.24	35.67	0.04 (9.1)	
8	.45	29.81		1.44 (18.0)
9	.46	29.04	-0.3 (-3.3)	1.78 (15.8)

[a]Figures in parentheses represent T-ratios.

In all three analyses the over-all cost-output (total patient days) relationship was shown to be negative but weak. The first method yielded generally negative regression coefficients, the majority of them insignificant. The second and third methods showed the partial regression coefficient for patient days, holding facilities and services constant, to be negative and significantly different from zero, but indicated that this factor made little or no contribution to the explanation of variations in average cost.

While significant economies of scale were found to be questionable in the over-all analysis of both a set of 4,710 hospitals and a set of 1,328 hospitals, when groups of large hospitals and groups of small hospitals were studied separately, significant economies of scale for the small hospitals became clear. In contrast, the large hospitals did not exhibit any significant departure from constant returns to scale.

Maintaining the homogeneity of the groups with respect to facilities but treating the groups of small and large hospitals separately, multiple regression analysis confirmed the findings of the first method. The partial regression coefficient for output, showing a significant negative relationship with average cost in the small groups, had a substantial influence on average cost. For the larger hospitals the coefficient lacked significance and had little or no influence on average cost.

It was not the purpose of this paper to determine the best estimate of the cutting point for economies of scale, given the composition of facilities. The paper does show that whether analyzed separately or combined for multiple regression analysis, groups of homogeneous hospitals having four or less of sixteen facilities and having an average size of under 70 beds exhibit economies of scale. (Some hospitals in these groups have over 150 beds.) The groups of large hospitals do not exhibit economies of scale. In the less homogeneous grouping (by number of facilities only) of 4,710 hospitals, groups having eight or less facilities and an average of 135 or less beds were shown to have significant economies of scale while the groups of larger hospitals did not.

NOTES

1. John D. Thompson, "On Reasonable Costs of Hospital Services," *Milbank Memorial Fund Quarterly* 46, no. 1 (January 1968):33–51.

2. Donald E. Saathoff and Richard A. Kurtz, "Cost per Day Comparisons Don't Do the Job," *The Modern Hospital* 99, no. 4 (October 1962):14–16.

3. See his article in the present volume.

4. Martin S. Feldstein, "Hospital Cost Variations and Case Mix Differences," *Medical Care* 3, no. 2 (April–June 1965):95–103.

5. Mary Lee Ingbar, "A Statistical Study of Differences in Hospital Costs: Cost Functions for 72 Massachusetts Hospitals" (Paper presented to the Econometric Society, Chicago, Ill., 1965).

6. Ralph E. Berry, "Competition and Efficiency in the Market for Hospital Services, the Structure of the American Hospital Industry" (Ph.D diss., Harvard University, 1965).

7. Judith R. Lave, "Review of Methods Used To Study Hospital Costs," *Inquiry* 3, no. 2 (May 1966):57–81.

PART VI

FACTORS OF PRODUCTION

Stuart H. Altman
Brown University

THE STRUCTURE OF NURSING EDUCATION AND ITS IMPACT ON SUPPLY

The nursing labor market is faced today with what some consider to be a paradox. Many experts acknowledge that the nation faces a severe shortage of trained professional nurses, yet many schools of nursing have been forced to close. In this paper a comprehensive theory of the economic forces that influence nursing education will be developed, with a view toward understanding what has motivated the dramatic changes in the structure of nursing education and what impact these changes are likely to have on the future supply of professional nurses. I hope to show that the structure of the nursing educational system has had an important bearing on the type of labor market in which nursing services are provided and has played a major role in influencing individuals to enter nursing.

BRIEF HISTORY OF NURSING EDUCATION

The establishment of hospital schools of nursing in the early 1870s resulted neither from legal action by government nor from public concern over the quality of nursing care, but rather because their existence added to the operating efficiency of hospitals. The wisdom of this action was quickly verified, and between 1873 and 1910 the number of hospital schools of nursing grew from 3 to 1,069.[1]

The author wishes to express his appreciation to Linda Mansfield for her assistance throughout the project. The research reported in this paper is part of a study of the supply of nurses, supported by Contract PH108-67-204, Division of Nursing, United States Public Health Service. The views expressed here are the author's and do not in any way reflect those of the Division of Nursing.

Although significant unemployment among nurses existed in the United States and Canada in the 1930s, hospital schools of nursing continued to function at almost pre-Depression levels. When asked why, a number of superintendents stated that while the schools improved the tone and intellectual atmosphere of the hospital in general, the main reason for their existence — especially in the minds of hospital trustees — was the supply of cheap labor which they provided.[2]

Each new student in a typical early hospital school was given a preparatory course of instruction of from three to four weeks, during which time she also worked twenty-five to thirty hours per week in the hospital.[3] For a period of about three years thereafter she continued in a training status but with almost all of the training taking place in a work setting. By and large, the size of the student class and the subjects taught were dictated by the work needs of the hospital.[4] It therefore appears that almost all, if not all, of the benefits during these early years of nursing training were received by hospitals while the nurse was in training. As a matter of fact, most nursing graduates left hospital nursing altogether to pursue other aspects of nursing.[5]

In hospitals without schools of nursing such services were provided by practical nurses and attendants; in hospitals with schools almost all nursing services were provided by student nurses. It is estimated that in the late 1920s not a single graduate nurse was employed in 73 per cent of hospitals with nursing schools.[6] The student nurse paid no tuition and in most instances received a salary of from ten to twelve dollars per month plus maintenance[7] (as compared with ninety-six dollars per month paid to a graduate professional nurse[8]). With the onset of the Depression, significant unemployment developed among nurses, and a reduction in salaries followed. Hospitals for the first time found it profitable to employ graduate nurses, and by the end of World War II most hospitals no longer relied on student nurses as their main source of nursing services.[9]

Until the mid-1950s only a relatively select group of nurses had a college education. Such training was geared primarily to public health nurses and those seeking executive positions. As late as 1949, only 7.5 per cent of all student nurses were enrolled in collegiate schools of nursing.[10] The introduction of the two-year associate degree collegiate program in 1952 marked the turn from the traditional mode of training. Although shorter than the baccalaureate program, the associate degree program followed the goals of the four-year college in stressing general education and classroom learning. From 1952 to 1966 students in programs offering these two forms of college education for nurses grew from eleven thousand to more than forty-eight thousand.[11] By 1966 enrollment in hospital-operated schools had declined to slightly over 65 per cent of total student nurse enrollment; four-year baccalaureate programs accounted for almost 24 per cent, and associate degree programs for 11 per cent.[12]

The trend away from on-the-job instruction and hospital training for nurses is clear. What is not so well understood is the reason for this trend, and what import it has for the future of nursing education and the supply of nursing personnel. In the next two sections I hope to provide a framework to help answer these questions by analyzing the original motivation behind the establishment of nursing training outside the main stream of higher education and the changes which have occurred in recent years that have tended to reverse this situation. An attempt will also be made to determine what impact these changes have had and will have on the prospective nursing student. Finally, estimates will be presented of what the supply and composition of nursing students is likely to be in the early 1970s.

A THEORY OF NURSING EDUCATION

The Training Establishment

Most hospitals are either non-profit corporations or are controlled by some governmental unit. As such, their decisions are likely to differ from those of the more traditional profit-maximizing firm. Recognition of these differences, however, does not rule out the use of traditional economic theory as a tool for explaining the behavior of the non-profit corporation. Once the goals of the institution are established, it is reasonable to assume that it will operate to attain them in the most efficient manner.[13] Furthermore, although the demand for nursing services includes factors other than revenue production, a demand function can be derived, and we can speak of the "marginal product" of an additional nurse, regardless of what is included in the concept of product.

Using this undefined concept of marginal product and the assumption that hospitals will attempt to produce that level of output (service) in such a manner as to equate, on the margin, the benefits derived from the last unit produced with the costs of producing that last unit, we can establish the equilibrium conditions under which a training establishment will be operated.

From the historical sketch above it is clear that student nurses performed a valuable service to the training institution, the value of which was enough to repay the cost of their training plus the wage paid to them during training. We can formally state the equilibrium condition for these early schools of nursing (prior to 1930) as follows:

$$(1) \qquad B_s^h = C^h$$

where

$$B_s^h = \sum_{t=0}^{n-1} \frac{(MP_t^s - W_t^s)}{(1 + i)^t}$$

$$C^h = \sum_{t=0}^{n-1} \frac{C_t^h}{(1+i)^t}$$

B_s^h is present value of the benefits to the hospital of employing a student nurse; C^h is present value of costs to the hospital of providing professional nursing training (other than wages paid to the student nurse); MP_t^s is value to the hospital of the marginal product of the student nurse during the tth period of her training; W_t^s is wage paid to the student nurse during the tth period of her training; C_t^h is cost to the hospital of providing nursing training during the tth period (other than the wages paid to the student nurse); i is discount rate; and n is number of years of training.

With the employment of large numbers of graduate professional nurses in the hospitals, it became possible to extend the benefits past the training period. Benefits could continue to accrue to the training institution provided the student nurse continued to work for it after graduation and the marginal product of the graduate nurse exceeded her wage.

(2) $$B_g^h = \sum_{t=n}^{m-1} \frac{(MP_t^g - W_t^g)}{(1+i)^t} > 0$$

where B_g^h is benefit to the hospital of employing a graduate nurse; MP_t^g is marginal product of the graduate nurse in the tth period; W_t^g is wage of the graduate nurse in the tth period; and m is number of years of training plus employment in the hospital.

If we continue to assume that all costs are borne during the training period, but that hospitals can charge tuition (T), the new equilibrium equation becomes

(3) $$B_s^h + T + B_g^h = C^h.$$

Traditional economic theory requires only that labor be hired in a competitive labor market in order for the wage of the worker to be equal to his marginal product. Recent modifications in this theory, however, have shown that in situations where a firm provides specific on-the-job training, i.e., training which raises the student's productivity only in the firm providing it, the firm can recoup part or all of the expenses of such training.[14] This can be accomplished by paying the worker his lower opportunity marginal product after training, while at the same time receiving the value of his raised marginal product.[15]

In a competitive labor market it is irrelevant whether the training is specific or general to the industry as a whole, since competition within the industry will bring about equality between a worker's marginal product and his wage. Once the labor market takes on some of the characteristics of a monopsony market, however, a gap develops between a worker's marginal product and his wage, regardless of the type of training he receives. The more insulated the industry from competitive pressures of other industries, the larger the gap; that is, if the training, although common to all firms in a given industry (increases the worker's productivity an equal amount in all firms), is specific to the industry as a whole (does not increase the worker's productivity at all in other industries), then the supply curve to the industry will be relatively inelastic, and the gap between the marginal product and the wage will be larger.[16]

However, because the cost of hiring an additional worker is larger than the wage paid to him, it may be incorrect to interpret the value of the gap as a benefit. In the more normal monopsony situation equation 2 should be modified by substituting marginal factor cost (*MFC*) for the wage. But, as will be explained below, by providing nursing training a hospital may be able to secure part or all of the gap as a return for operating the training program.

The Nursing Labor Market

Although professional nurses are employed by a variety of industries and firms, the dominant industry is health service and the dominant employer is the hospital. In 1964, 93 per cent of all active professional registered nurses in the United States were employed in the health service industry, and 65 per cent were employed in hospitals or similar institutions.[17] In addition, more than 98 per cent of all professional nurses were women, and over 70 per cent were married.[18]

The combination of these two factors produces a situation in which one or a few employers in a community dominate the labor market, and the employee has very limited economically directed geographical mobility. Donald Yett has studied the nursing labor market in great detail and has concluded that it can best be described as an oligopsonistic market with a kinked supply curve.[19] He has shown that employers are conscious of the difference between the wage necessary to attract additional nurses and the marginal factor cost of paying that wage to all members of the staff. Furthermore, they are also conscious of the impact their wage decisions will have on the decision of other institutions in their area.[20]

Whether or not Yett's model is the most appropriate for explaining the nursing labor market, the evidence strongly suggests that it is not perfectly competitive. For graphic simplicity we will use a monopsony model, although the implications of the analysis would be similar if a more complicated oligopsonistic model were used.

Benefits of a Training Program

It is often suggested that because of loyalty, inertia, or other factors institutions providing nurse training are able to retain a substantial portion of their student nurses without paying an above-the-market wage. The importance of this factor can be seen by referring to Figure 1. We can assume that a hospital without a training program would hire nurses up to the point where *MFC* = *MRP*. At this equilibrium position the hospitals would be earning a producer surplus equal to the trapezoid w_0ABC. Let us further assume that by operating a training program, recruitment at w_0 could be increased; the larger the program, the larger the number of additional nurses. While the supply curve beyond q_0 can be thought of as being perfectly horizontal for an institution with a training program (S_1), the hospital would have to consider the additional costs of operating such a program $(C^h > B_g^h)$; that is, the marginal factor cost would have to include both the wage offered to the graduate nurse and the cost of training her. Assuming training costs to

Fig. 1. Importance to hospitals of benefits from nurse training programs.

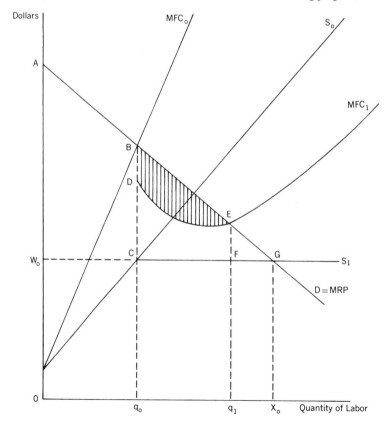

be positive, MFC_1 will be above S_1 at every point, but for those institutions which operate a training program MFC_1 will be below MRP for a certain range; that is, a benefit or surplus will accrue to the training institution equal to the value

$$(4) \qquad B_s^h = \sum_{t=n}^{m-1} \frac{(MRP - MFC_1)}{(1 + i)^t}.$$

The equilibrium position for the training institution would then be at q_1, and the increase in benefits over costs, or increase in the producer surplus, would be equal to the shaded area BDE. The number of budgeted vacancies would be reduced from CG to FG.[21] The more expensive the training program – i.e., the larger the deficit between C^h and B_s^h, the higher MFC_1 is above S_1. For those institutions where MFC_1 is above MRP at all levels, it would not pay to establish a training program.

The operation of a training program, therefore, depends on whether it is more profitable to maintain such a program or to rely on other institutions to produce new nurses. Given that only 11 per cent of hospitals operate nursing schools,[22] it is clear that such an operation is not profitable for all. The question is why such an operation is profitable for some institutions and not for others.

If we assume that within a labor market w^g is the same for all nurses with comparable experience in the same position, then differences in B_g^h will depend on variations in MP^g. It is not unreasonable to assume that, as the size and complexity of a hospital grows, the number of rules and procedures specific to the hospital also grows. In a large, complex institution it is necessary for all personnel to become familiar with these special rules and procedures, either through orientation courses or on-the-job instruction. It is clearly to the advantage of the hospital to provide this orientation while the nurse is a student as opposed to being on the payroll as a registered professional. We can, therefore, differentiate for these large hospitals, at least for the first six months to a year, the higher value of a nurse trained by them as compared with one trained in another program. The more specific the functions in the hospital, the greater the difference in value between the two groups and the larger B_g^h.

In the absence of salary differentials between institutions, the retention rate of the ith institution will in part be related to its proportion of total employment in the area. Therefore, large institutions will benefit by having larger retention rates than could be accounted for purely on the basis of loyalty and inertia.

Finally, there is also strong evidence to indicate that the per student cost of training (C^h) is negatively related to the size of the institution. In a study of the cost of nursing education, it was found that when each hospital school was ranked for the number of student-weeks accumulated during the year and for the cost of educational functions per student-week, the relationship between the two ranks was -.495.*[23] The relationship appeared even stronger when the institutions were divided into three subgroups by size of enrollment – small (less than 70 students), medium (from 70 to 120 students), and large (120 studer   r more). The average rank of schools in terms of cost of education was 101.60 for small schools, 61.58 for medium-size schools, and 47.78 for large schools.[24]

In summary, there are three reasons why we would hypothesize that the size of an institution is a critical factor in determining whether or not it operates a training program: (1) a positive correlation exists between the size of a hospital and the value of the firm-specific portion of its training; (2) retention rates will be larger for large institutions; (3) economies of scale tend to reduce training costs per student.

To test this hypothesis, all general private and governmental non-federal hospitals in the United States were placed in seven categories based on number of beds in the institution. Within each category the proportion of hospitals with schools of nursing was calculated. As can be seen in Table 1, the correlation between bed-size category and presence of a nursing school was almost perfect. In hospitals with less than 100 beds, only .0025 had a nursing school. At the other end of the spectrum, in hospitals with 750 beds or more the proportion reached .6452.

Our hypothesis would also predict that if C_t^h is going up and MP_t^s is going down proportionately for all hospitals, those programs which would feel the

Table 1: Location of Hospital Schools of Nursing[a]

Bed Category	No. of Hospitals	No. of Schools	Proportion of Hospitals with Schools	Proportion of Schools That Intend To Close
1–99	3,192	8	.0025	–
100–199	1,070	139	.1299	.1367
200–299	541	196	.3623	.0918
300–399	294	153	.5204	.0784
400–499	145	98	.6322	.0612
500–749	117	70	.5983	.0857
750+	62	40	.6452	.0999
Total	5,421	704		

[a]Includes all general voluntary (non-profit), governmental (non-federal), and proprietary (profit-making) hospitals in 1965.

Source: *Hospitals* 41, no. 15 (August 1967).

*A high correlation exists between the size of an institution and the number of students enrolled in its training program.

pressure most strongly would be located in smaller hospitals (administering smaller programs). Consequently, the closing rate among small schools would be greater than among large schools. This relationship was less clear-cut than in the first instance, but the data still suggest a higher proportion of closings among the smaller schools. Of the schools in the 100- to 199-bed category, .1367 were expected to close, while those in the 400- to 499-bed category reached a low of .0612. In the two largest bed categories, however, the proportion rose again. Although this result appears to contradict the implications of our theory, it may not actually do so. Schools in these larger institutions are more likely to have merged with some type of collegiate program where general education would be provided at the college and clinical subjects at the hospital. By freeing itself of all general education courses the hospital greatly reduces the cost of training, and by continuing to offer clinical instruction it can still provide some hospital-specific instruction.

Costs and Benefits to the Student

The most obvious benefit of undertaking nurse training to the student is that without it she cannot become licensed as a registered professional nurse. To the extent that the earnings of a registered nurse plus the non-pecuniary benefits of nursing provide a "surplus" or "quasi-rent" above the most attractive alternative occupation, a student would be willing to pay the cost for part or all of her training. As one moves from the truly dedicated nurse to those whose attachment to the profession is more marginal, the amount of the surplus falls and the amount she is willing to invest in her own training declines. For the truly marginal student the capitalized value of the future benefits of nursing just compensates her for the costs (including foregone alternative earnings and tuition payments) associated with selecting nursing as an occupation.

If we define

$$(5) \qquad B^s = \sum_{t=n}^{m-1} \frac{(W_t^g - W_t^a)}{(1+i)^t} + N$$

$$(6) \qquad C^s = \sum_{t=0}^{n-1} \frac{(W_t^a - W_t^s) + (T_t^n - T_t^a)}{(1+i)^t}$$

where B^s is benefit to the student of selecting nursing as an occupation; C^s is cost to the student of selecting nursing as an occupation; W_t^g is wage paid to a graduate nurse in the tth period; W_t^a is wage paid in the best alternative occupation in the tth period; N is non-pecuniary benefits of nursing relative to the best alternative occupation; W_t^s is wage, if any, paid to the student during training; T_t^n is tuition charges for nursing education in the tth period; and T_t^a is tuition charges for training in the best alternative occupation; then for the marginal student

$$(7) \qquad\qquad B^s = C^s.$$

Factors which increase B^s will tend to move out the area under the total benefit function and increase the number of individuals who find nursing a "profitable" occupation. Likewise, factors which increase C^s will have the opposite effect, tending to reduce the flow of individuals into nursing.

We can now return to the different components of nurses' training and see to what extent each influences these cost and benefit equations. The benefits of orientation-type courses (higher productivity of the worker) accrue only to the institution, since the nurse continues to receive at most her opportunity marginal product, which has not risen. Nursing education courses are somewhat different in that the student's future productivity is raised in all firms which employ her as a nurse. However, part of this increase in productivity goes into an increase in the exploitation gap. Hence the benefits of such training are shared by the student, in the form of higher wages, and the institutions, in the form of an increase in the exploitation gap. The relative proportion going to each depends on the slope of the supply and demand functions.[25]

General education courses, on the other hand, will primarily be of benefit to the student (and to society). To the extent that these courses provide the student with meaningful occupational alternatives to nursing, the supply curve facing all employers of nursing services will shift to the left (less nursing service available at each wage). It will also give the individual greater flexibility to leave nursing if wages and working conditions lose their competitive attractiveness. Thus the nursing supply function will become more elastic at each wage; the more elastic the supply function becomes, the smaller the divergence between the nurse's marginal product and her wage.[26] Thus general education courses will tend to reduce the exploitation gap and for any given value of the nurse's marginal product will increase her wage.

It is clear that if all other things are equal a student would prefer to be trained in a program which emphasizes general education. All other things, however, are not equal. General education courses add to the expense of operating a training program and must either be added to the previous work load or substituted for part of it. If the first alternative is taken, the length of the training program will be increased, adding to the student's opportunity costs (higher ΣW_t^a). If some orientation and nursing education courses are dropped, the benefits of operating a training program to the training institutions are reduced. In both situations an increase in tuition charges would be likely.

It is possible, therefore, that the increased costs of entering a training program with a larger number of general education courses could counterbalance the increased benefits that such training would have for the student. Were it possible to enter a program which tended to stress general education without requiring any increase in training time or in tuition, such a program would clearly be very attractive to a student, and in general it would make nursing a more attractive occupation; i.e., it would shift the entire B^s function without increasing C^s. It is just these factors which have made the associate degree nursing program so popular in recent years.

ANALYSIS OF RECENT EXPERIENCE

As we indicated in the last section, considerable differences exist among the various training curricula respecting benefits to the training institution or ultimate employer, as compared with the student or professional nurse. With hospitals dictating the type of training being offered and few alternatives open to students seeking nursing training prior to the mid-1950s, it is understandable that the curriculum would be heavily weighted in favor of institution-specific and occupation-specific subjects. A major conclusion of a 1949 study on the quality of nursing education in hospital schools was that "the major share of the nursing school program was regarded as not being predominantly focused on education and that to most schools, service to the hospital was as important an objective as was the education of the students."[27]

For the career nurse, however, such a training program had severe limitations. It assured the industry a source of relatively inexpensive labor while providing the career professional with very limited occupational flexibility. With the increased influence of the career professional through the professional nursing associations, one could predict that the structure of nursing education would change. These associations, the American Nurses' Association (ANA) and the National League for Nursing (NLN), made it clear which direction they thought nursing education should follow. In a position paper published in 1965 the ANA stated that "the education for all those who are licensed to practice should take place in institutions of higher learning."[28] Recognizing that a transition to a collegiate program of nursing education would take time, the associations were also interested in reshaping the curriculum of the diploma schools. A major vehicle used to alter diploma education was the accreditation program of the NLN. Its major goals were to reduce substantially, if not eliminate, the hospital-service portion of the training and to greatly enlarge courses geared to general education.

The accreditation program received a major boost in 1953, when the ANA voted to acknowledge it and to support its recommendations. Although nursing schools are permitted to function without NLN accreditation, an unaccredited school faces the burden of trying to recruit faculty and students without the endorsement of the most powerful and prestigious professional nursing association. Also, an unaccredited school in most instances is ineligible for federal funds allocated under the 1964 Nurse Training Act as amended.[29] As a result, the percentage of accredited diploma programs rose from 53 to 72 between 1959 and 1966.[30]

The impact on hospital training programs of curriculum changes necessary to receive accreditation were substantial. By minimizing in-hospital service, MP^s and therefore $B_s{}^h$ were reduced (see equations 1 to 3). The addition of more general education courses substantially increased C^h, and by providing the graduate nurse with greater occupational flexibility reduced the number of nurses who were prepared to work at low wages. Hence the supply function for nursing services became more elastic. Furthermore, to the extent that general education courses were substituted for institution-specific instruction, the hospitals were forced to provide such training after the nurse was officially hired as a registered professional. Thus MP^g was somewhat reduced, at least for the first three to six months.

With benefits reduced and costs increased, there was little most diploma schools could do except increase tuition or close their doors. Furthermore, considering the short working life of many graduate nurses and the promotional path of career nurses, which often takes them away from bedside patient care within a few years, there is even some doubt that the increased emphasis on general education actually added to the long-run productivity of the professional nurse in a hospital setting. It is not surprising, therefore, that many hospital administrators have strongly criticized these curriculum changes as leading to the destruction of nursing education in hospitals[31] and that over two hundred hospital schools have in fact closed since the end of World War II, with more expected to follow in the next few years.

It would be incorrect to place responsibility either for the decline in hospital schools or the shift toward more general education solely on the professional nursing associations. There have also been significant changes in the occupational outlook of female workers. Increased family income, greater availability of scholarship funds and educational loans, and the greater likelihood of spending a significant portion of one's working life in the labor force have made such occupations as nursing far less attractive. Free tuition and relatively high starting salaries but a low lifetime earnings potential, a package which nursing successfully offered up to the 1950s, became increasingly less salable in the postwar period. Whereas almost 7 per cent of female high school graduates entered nursing schools in 1952, the percentage declined to about 4.5 per cent by 1966 (see Fig. 2). Furthermore, even though more than two hundred hospital schools closed during this period, only about 85 per cent of the openings for the incoming class of 1966 in hospital schools were filled.[32]

Fig. 2. Percentage of female high school graduates entering professional nursing schools, by type of program.

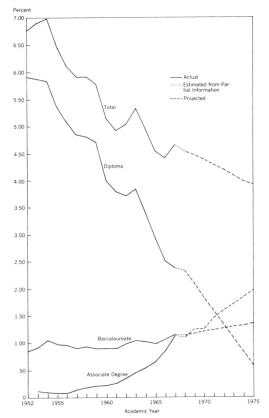

The relative decline in new entrants has not yet reached the point where the outflow from nursing exceeds the inflow. The supply of active nursing personnel increased by over two hundred thousand in the last ten years.* Nevertheless, as can be seen in Table 2, the marginal addition to the supply of nurses is approaching the average per capita level. Should this trend continue, the number of nurses per hundred thousand population eventually will level off and then decline.

To counter this trend, many state and local governments have established schools of nursing as part of their general programs of higher education. Whereas hospitals must consider costs and benefits primarily on an internal

*In absolute numbers, graduations from initial programs of nursing education increased from thirty to thirty-five thousand between 1956 and 1966.

Table 2: Nursing Supply as a Proportion of the Adult Female Population

Year	Marginal Rate[a]	Average Rate[b]
1950	2.11	1.85
1960	2.75	2.21
1965	2.55	2.33

[a]New nursing licenses per hundred thousand female population in a single age cohort of age group 20–24.

[b]Total stock of living professional nurses per hundred thousand female population aged 20–64.

Source: Stuart H. Altman, "An Economic Analysis of the Supply of Nurses" (unpublished study prepared for the Division of Nursing, United States Public Health Service).

basis, the community can justify expenditures by including the social benefits of a greater supply of trained professional nurses. In 1966 alone, fifty-four new associate degree programs and twelve new baccalaureate degree programs were instituted throughout the country.

With collegiate programs offering an alternative source of supply, hospitals were compelled to rethink the long-term benefits of continuing to operate generally unprofitable training programs; that is, assuming that $B_s{}^h < C_s$, a hospital would be in a more favorable position if it could increase its supply of nurses at the market wage without the net cost of training. While a hospital might lose that part of the training benefit which results from the institution-specific instruction and from the greater likelihood of recruiting its own graduates, it could minimize this loss by affiliating with a college program.

We can see what impact the opening of collegiate schools of nursing has had on the relative decline of diploma programs and the over-all flow of admissions to nursing school by referring to Figure 2. If the theory is correct, admissions to college schools should be negatively related to admissions to diploma schools but positively related to over-all admissions.

Between 1952 and 1960 the proportion of female high school graduates entering a hospital school declined from .059 to .040, about 3.6 per cent per year. From 1960 to 1967, during a time when collegiate enrollment increased rapidly, the proportion fell from .040 to .024, a relative decline of 5.7 per cent per year. Over-all admissions, on the other hand, declined by 3 per cent per year between 1952 and 1960, but the rate of descent was reduced to less than 1.5 per cent per year in the 1960–1967 period. In other words, the experience between 1952 and 1967 tends to support the hypothesis that the introduction of collegiate education for nurses has accentuated the decline of diploma programs but has had a positive influence on over-all admission to schools of nursing.

To determine what is likely to happen in the future if these current trends continue, the future entrance rate of female high school graduates into nursing education and the various programs was projected, using the experience of the period 1960-1967.* The following regression equations were estimated:

(8) E_d = 4.4197 - .2463T ; R^2: .95; $S^2_{y \cdot x}$: .2204

(9) E_a = -0.0065 + .1232T ; R^2: .96; $S^2_{y \cdot x}$: .9644

(10) E_b = 0.8636 + .0306T ; R^2: .88; $S^2_{y \cdot x}$: .0435

where E_d is proportion of female high school graduates entering a diploma program; E_a is proportion of female high school graduates entering an associate degree program; E_b is proportion of female high school graduates entering a baccalaureate degree program; and T is a monotonically increasing time or trend variable.

Using equations 8 to 10, the admissions rate was calculated through 1975 and appears in Figure 3. These estimates indicate that admissions to associate and baccalaureate degree programs will actually exceed diploma admissions before 1975. Furthermore, the trend in the proportion of female high school graduates entering nursing schools will continue to fall, but at a rate lower than the over-all 1952-1967 experience.

On the basis of these projected rates and estimated female high school graduates, the number of admissions was also projected through 1975. Although the proportion of female high school graduates entering nursing school will decline at a lower rate in the future than in the past, the number of female high school graduates will grow at a slower pace. Hence total admissions will reach a peak of about 65,900 in 1972-1973 and will decline slightly to 65,600 by 1975-1976.

Unfortunately, the retention rate among those admitted to collegiate schools has not been encouraging. During the period 1963-1966 the completion rate for those in baccalaureate programs averaged 58.3 per cent; for the associate degree program the rate was even lower, 55.6 per cent.[33] In comparison, the completion rate among entrants to diploma programs averaged 72.2 per cent. If this experience continues, the relative increase in new admissions to nursing schools will not lead to a larger supply of practicing nurses.

Using these completion rates, the projected admissions figures were adjusted to arrive at estimates of nursing school graduates during the next nine

*The estimated rates are based entirely on the regression equations and are not adjusted to the actual 1967-1968 rates. The fall in rates from 1967-1968 to 1968-1969 is therefore somewhat steeper for diploma programs, and the increase is somewhat less steep for associate and baccalaureate degree programs.

Fig. 3. Admissions to professional nursing schools, by type of program.

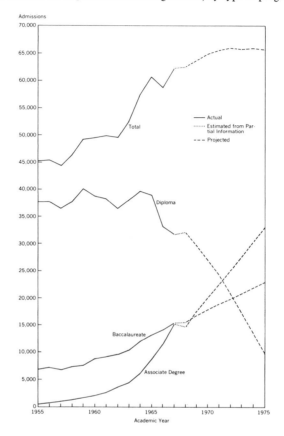

years. By adding new entrants to the estimated stock of all living nurses in different age categories in 1970 and 1975 and adjusting these estimates for expected participation rates of nurses in each age group, we arrived at estimates of the supply of active nurses in 1970 and 1975 (Table 3).[34]

In 1963 a study of a nursing labor market was prepared by a special consulting group to the Surgeon General.[35] In this report it was estimated that the most realistic goal for the supply of active nurses by 1970 was 680,000. As can be seen in Table 3, all but one of the estimates suggest that actual supply will be in excess of this goal.* According to the consultant group, however, even if this goal is attained, there would still be a "need" for 170,000 additional nurses.† Even with the more favorable trend in admissions, supply in 1970 would fall far short of 850,000.

---

*By 1967 there were already 640,000 professional nurses in practice throughout the United States.

Table 3: Projected Supply of Active Professional Nurses

	Census Definition[a]		Adjusted Census[b]	
	1970	1975	1970	1975
1960 labor participation rate applied to living nurses, 1970 and 1975	714,000	776,000	652,000	715,000
1950-1960 growth rate continued and applied to living nurses, 1970 and 1975	778,000	859,000	704,000	800,000

[a]Estimated number of active professional nurses was taken directly from the 1950 and 1960 censuses (see *U.S. Census of Population 1960, Characteristics of Professional Workers; U.S. Census of Population 1950, Characteristics of Professional Workers*).

[b]See U.S., Department of Health, Education, and Welfare, Public Health Service, *Health Manpower Source Book*, sec. 2, Nursing Personnel (Washington, D.C.: By the Department, 1966), Table 1, p. 9.

Source: see Table 2.

CONCLUSION

The projections of future supply which were discussed in the last section were for the most part based on wage conditions that prevailed in nursing during the first half of the 1960s. In the last few years, however, wage increases have been far in excess of those of the preceding five years. Regardless of whether the entire credit for these salary advances is due to changes in the structure of nursing education, it is clear that this behavior is consistent with our expectations and that the likely effect will be to make nursing a more attractive occupation in the future. There is, therefore, some hope that the market is generating the correct signals to bring about a future supply of professional nurses more in line with what experts believe is the minimum amount needed to provide an adequate level of medical care.

NOTES

1. Margaret Bridgman, *Collegiate Education for Nursing* (New York: Russell Sage Foundation, 1953), p. 42.
2. Quoted in G. M. Weir, *Survey of Nursing Education in Canada* (Toronto: University of Toronto Press, 1932), p. 282.
3. Committee on the Grading of Nursing Schools, *Nursing Schools Today and Tomorrow* (New York: By the Committee, 1934), pp. 82–84.
4. *Ibid.*, p. 86.
5. *Ibid.*, p. 102.

---

†This estimate was based on the number of active professional nurses which these experts believed would be necessary to provide the country with "safe, therapeutically effective and efficient nursing service." No attempt was made to estimate what in fact the "market demand" for nursing services will be.

6. *Ibid.*

7. *Ibid.*, p. 91.

8. *Ibid.*

9. *Ibid.*, pp. 103–16.

10. U.S., Department of Health, Education, and Welfare, Public Health Service, *Health Manpower Source Book*, sec. 2, Nursing Personnel (Washington, D.C.: By the Department, 1966), p. 57.

11. *Ibid.*

12. *Ibid.*

13. Armen A. Alchian and William R. Allen, *University Economics*, 2d ed. (Belmont, Calif.: Wadsworth Publishing Co., 1967), chap. 9.

14. Gary S. Becker, *Human Capital* (New York: National Bureau of Economic Research, 1964).

15. *Ibid.*, pp. 18–23.

16. Stuart H. Altman and Linda Mansfield, "The Use of Vacancy Statistics as a Measure of Labor Shortages in Monopsony Markets" (unpublished manuscript, Department of Economics, Brown University).

17. *Health Manpower Source Book*, p. 37.

18. *Ibid.*, Pt. 2.

19. Donald E. Yett, "The Causes and Consequences of Salary Differentials in Nursing" (Paper presented to the annual meeting of the Western Economic Association, Berkeley, Calif., August 26, 1966).

20. *Ibid.*

21. Altman and Mansfield, "Vacancy Statistics."

22. Derived from American Hospital Association, *Hospitals* 41, no. 15 (August 1967).

23. National League for Nursing, *Study on Cost of Nursing Education*, Pt. 1 (New York: By the League, 1965), p. 16.

24. *Ibid.*, p. 17.

25. Altman and Mansfield, "Vacancy Statistics."

26. *Ibid.*

27. Cited in Elizabeth V. Cunningham, *Today's Diploma Schools of Nursing* (New York: National League for Nursing, 1963), p. 3.

28. American Nurses' Association, "A Position Paper," 1965.

29. U.S., Department of Health, Education, and Welfare, Public Health Service, *Nurse Training Act of 1964*, Public Health Service Publication 1740 (Washington, D.C.: U.S. Government Printing Office, 1967).

30. American Nurses' Association, *Facts About Nursing* (New York: By the Association, 1967), p. 118.

31. Thomas Hale, M.D., "Problems of Supply and Demand in the Education of Nurses," *New England Journal of Medicine* 275 (November 1966).

32. Special nursing school vacancy study conducted by the National League for Nursing in June 1967.

33. Derived from American Nurses' Association, *Facts About Nursing*.

34. For a complete description of the estimating techniques, see Stuart H. Altman, "An Economic Analysis of the Supply of Nurses" (unpublished manuscript, Division of Nursing, United States Public Health Service).

35. U.S., Department of Health, Education, and Welfare, Public Health Service, *Toward Quality in Nursing: Needs and Goals, Report of the Surgeon General's Consultant Group on Nursing*, Public Health Service Publication 992 (Washington, D.C.: U.S. Government Printing Office, 1963).

W. Lee Hansen
University of Wisconsin

COMMENT

Stuart Altman's paper, while ostensibly directed toward explaining one phenomenon, actually discusses two distinctly different ones. The first is the shift in the training of nurses from hospitals to colleges, while the second is the monopsonistic structure of the labor market for nurses. Since Sherwin Rosen takes up in detail the monopsony issue in his comments on the Yett paper, the bulk of my comments are directed to the analysis of the shift in the site of training. This is followed by a brief comment on monopsony and on some of the broader implications of the shift in the training of nurses.

What I find most appealing in this paper is its effort to examine the changing structure of the training-education program in nursing within the framework of the human capital model set forth by Becker. In essence, this method calls for viewing hospitals as producing two different outputs, medical services of the traditional variety and trained nurses. We can think of these as joint products, although this is not necessary for the analysis. Given, however, the primacy of the first function – indeed, this is the reason why hospitals exist – the second function is likely to be scrutinized more carefully at all times to determine whether it yields an economic return on the resources used in training which is commensurate with the return on resources used for medical services. (Since hospitals with training programs are non-profit operations, this implies the maintenance of a zero profit rate in each of the two operations.) Of importance, then, are the factors which affect the relationship between the costs and benefits of hospital training programs. This human capital framework is a very useful one in sharpening our understanding of the costs and benefits in this rather unique industry.

In light of the attention given to the monopsony model, the reasons for the shift in nurses' training from hospitals to colleges are less well developed.

353

Therefore, I wish to try to sketch some of the forces and comment on some of the groups which appear to have played a part in the shift. In the 1920s, for example, the hospital training function was presumably seen as an ideal one from all vantage points. Hospitals were provided with a cheap and abundant supply of labor, in a market that was not particularly extensive for female high school graduates. Patients received much "tender, loving care" because of the relative abundance of trainees. Parents of young girls viewed nurses' training as a virtually costless means for their daughters to obtain some highly useful training and to enter a respected profession, and potential nurses no doubt saw training as offering a means of escaping the restrictions of home, facilitating finding a mate, and providing an interesting and valuable work experience. Given the fact that the vast majority of nurse trainees quickly married, dropped out of the labor force, and then remained outside the labor force, the stock of working nurses in hospitals at any one time was not much different from the number of nurses enrolled in the nurse training programs.

What was the nature of the forces which affected the costs and benefits of providing nurse training in hospitals? The tremendous growth in real income after World War II and continuing to the present caused more and more older and younger males to drop out of the labor force, giving rise to a significant expansion in the demand for female labor of all kinds. The expansion in the demand for nurses was even greater than that for labor as a whole. The obvious response was to begin hiring more already-trained nurses by luring them back into the labor force. (Of course, the supply of already-trained nurses was reduced somewhat as other opportunities opened up for these women.) The hiring of already-trained nurses was accelerated by the fact that, as college training became more attractive to female high school graduates, because of the increased opportunity to use such training, the relative, if not the absolute, supply of trainees for nursing schools declined. Thus we can visualize rapid shifts to the right in the demand curve for nurses and for all women workers, a shift to the right in the supply curve of trained nurses, an increasingly elastic supply curve for the stock of already-trained nurses, and a possible shift to the left in the supply curve of nursing trainees.

The net effect of these several forces was to raise the cost of recruiting new trainees and to force the hiring of many already-trained nurses. As a result, nurse training became less profitable for hospitals, and a sizable group of professional nurses were regularly employed in hospitals. To compound an already complex situation, the increased sophistication of surgery and hospital care no doubt led to an even sharper increase in the demand for highly trained nurses, but with the declining percentage of female high school graduates entering nurse training, and with the more able girls going on to college, the average ability of nursing trainees probably began to decline.

What one would like to see is an unraveling of these various forces and, one might hope, a more systematic quantification of them. To gain some insight into the rise in training costs, it would be useful to know how the net benefits received by nursing trainees varied over time and how they compared with alternative opportunities open to them. When did the queue for nurse training programs begin to drop and then decline to zero, and when did vacancies in training programs begin to appear? In understanding the role of larger market forces, it would be helpful to know how the ratio of graduate nurses to all nurses (including students) in hospitals changed over time. To what extent were changes in this ratio associated with changes in the relative earnings of nurses and changes in the mix of nurses, e.g., practical nurses, nurses' aides, etc.? Were skill requirements changing or not? Was the average quality of trainees and of nurses in general changing? Such questions need to be answered if we hope to attach weights to the various forces which were at work.

While one can accept the view that costs were rising much more rapidly than benefits in the hospital-nurse-training industry, the shift to college training of nurses is still not explained. One explanation is that increased professionalization of the occupation gave rise to a desire to tighten standards, to provide more sophisticated training, and the like, all of which might be done most effectively in colleges. Another possibility is that the hospitals themselves urged the transfer, in part because of an awareness of a less favorable benefit-cost ratio in the training operation and in part because of their recognition of a decline in the quality of their trainees. While this may explain why there was an "offer" to shift the locus of training, it does not explain why the colleges accepted the offer. Just as self-interest may have motivated the nurses' group and the hospital organizations, I suspect that self-interest also loomed large in the decision-making of the colleges. They saw an opportunity to complement their medical school and hospital operations, to bolster their claims of service to society, and simply to expand, given the fact that funds are provided largely on a per-student basis, at least in state-supported schools. There is some evidence that universities have long sought to anticipate demands for their services and, more important, that they have gone out of their way to help generate greater demand for them. Thus, before attempting to place responsibility on the professional nursing groups, as Altman comes close to doing, some examination of the role of the other parties involved should be provided.

One is forced to conclude that there may have been several major actors in this drama. Exactly who were they? What roles did they play? When did they come into the act, and so on? These are questions that I hope Altman will take up in his larger study. By so doing, I think that he will give us a much better understanding of the industry and, as a consequence, a better understanding of recent and prospective developments in the supply and demand for nursing manpower.

Now a brief comment on the monopsony model. If there has been monopsony in the labor market for nurses, there has also been monopsony in the nurses' training market, and this latter monopsony power may have been more pervasive in, say, the 1920s than now, and more pervasive than monopsony in the present-day nursing labor market itself. This would suggest that nursing trainees were paid less during their training period than Altman's formulation would indicate. In short, an "excess" return would have been earned by hospitals on a combination of their activities, with the result they were able to generate their own funds for expansion, new equipment, and the like, more readily and that, as a consequence, they may not have had to work so hard at fund-raising. Today's counterpart would be the monopsonist's return earned by hospitals without training functions, but how large is this return, and who gets it? Is it used simply to hold down prices of hospital services? If so, why should hospitals behave in this way? Or does it go into higher earnings or other amenities for staff doctors? Is there any evidence that this happens? Unless we can squeeze some broader implications out of the monopsony model, it is not clear just how useful it is.

Finally, I wish to touch upon some of the implications of the shift in the training of nurses from hospitals to colleges. First, the hospitals have shifted an increasingly costly training operation to the public sector, with the result that nurse training is now subsidized on a scale that is more nearly equivalent to that for other occupations which require college training. This means that recipients of hospital services pay a smaller share of the resources costs; taxpayers in general now contribute also. Second, since the capital market barrier to college attendance is greater than that to nurse training within hospitals, it would appear that opportunities for girls from lower income families are now more restricted than they were previously. Thus we would expect to see a changed distribution in the socioeconomic background of nursing students and to find marked differences between trainees in hospitals and those in colleges.

This raises the whole question of the role of government in subsidizing training of various sorts, in particular, the advisability of concentrating ever larger amounts of vocation-specific training in an environment which is probably most efficient in the provision of general education and research skills. What the consequences of this concentration will be for the medical care industry and for the people attracted to it are difficult to forecast, but an attempt should be made to foresee what they might be.

Donald E. Yett
University of Southern California

THE CHRONIC "SHORTAGE" OF NURSES: A PUBLIC POLICY DILEMMA

For thirty years there have been complaints of a shortage of professional nurses. Hundreds of articles concerning the problem have been published in scholarly journals and popular magazines. Although much attention has been given this issue, surprisingly few attempts have been made to specify what the term nurse "shortage" means. The few authorities who have attempted to do so usually have defined it as the number of "active" nurses relative to the number "required" to provide the desired level of patient care.

A chronological review of the attempts to estimate the size of the shortage in this sense indicates the following trend: before World War II, nurse employment levels were considered adequate; during the war a shortage developed, estimated at approximately 75,000 in 1943 and 110,000 by the end of the war; despite predictions to the contrary, the shortage declined dramati-

The material for this article, which was originally titled "Yes, Virginia, There Is a Shortage of Nurses, But It's Not Quite As Simple As All That," was drawn from my *An Economic Analysis of the Nurse Shortage* (Washington, D.C.: U.S. Government Printing Office, 1970). The author would like to express his appreciation to George Break, Robert Deane, Jack Hirshleifer, and Judith Mann for their suggestions in connection with an earlier draft of the paper. Editorial assistance was provided by Elizabeth Early and Robert Michaels. This research was supported in part by Grants GN-W-4784, GN-09712, NU-00054, and NU-00277, Bureau of Health Manpower, Division of Nursing, United States Public Health Service, and Grant CH-0024 from the Community Health Facilities Branch of the Bureau of State Services-Community Health, United States Public Health Service. Additional support was provided by the Health Information Foundation through its Research Development Grant from the Ford Foundation, and from Contract PH-108-67-146, Division of Nursing, United States Public Health Service. Computer services were provided by the Washington University (St. Louis) Computer Facilities through Grant G22296, National Science Foundation, the UCLA Health Sciences Computing Facility, and the USC Computer Sciences Laboratory.

cally until 1949, when it was approximately 50,000, a level which was maintained throughout the Korean War; by the mid-1950s the shortage numbered 70,000, and subsequent estimates climbed to a new high of 125,000 in 1966; by 1970, according to a 1963 forecast, the shortage will be between 170,000 and 200,000.

Despite some discussion of whether there has been a misuse of professional nursing skills rather than an actual shortage, most experts remain convinced that the situation has deteriorated since the 1950s. They agree that there has been a large increase in the *supply* of nurses but emphasize that there has been a greater increase in the nation's *need* for nurses. This is the sense in which we must take the statements of hospital and nursing leaders that we have had a chronic nurse shortage for almost thirty years. And it is in this same sense that the existence of the "shortage" has become part of the "conventional wisdom."

DEFINITIONS OF ECONOMIC SHORTAGE

To an economist, a labor shortage does not generally mean that additional manpower is "needed" to satisfy a certain public policy goal. Simply described, an economic shortage exists when the amount of something demanded by the public exceeds the amount supplied at the existing market price. Demand is negatively related to price, whereas need is generally construed to be independent of price; thus there is no necessary relationship between an economic and a "need" shortage. However, if both types of shortage exist, the market adjustment process would normally lead to an increase in nurse employment, which, *ceteris paribus*, would reduce each type of shortage simultaneously. Thus it should be interesting to compare the available evidence concerning the probable size of any economic shortage(s) of nurses that may have existed in recent years with the figures based upon "need" given above. To do so, it will first be necessary to specify more rigorously what is meant by an economic shortage.

Few economists have expressed opinions on market conditions in nursing. Although certain occupations said to be experiencing serious "shortages" have been analyzed, no general model has been developed which is directly applicable to the market for nurses. In fact, the literature reveals several disconcerting instances in which "shortage" studies based on virtually identical data resulted in different conclusions. Two economic analyses of the "shortage of engineers" illustrate how opposite conclusions can be reached by applying different models to the same facts. A critical summary of both is given in sections following, and their applications to relevant nurse data are discussed.

The Blank-Stigler Model of a Shortage

David M. Blank and George J. Stigler specify that a shortage "exists when the number of workers available (the supply) increases less rapidly than the number demanded *at the salaries paid in the recent past*. Then salaries will rise [relative to those for other occupations] and activities which once were performed by (say) engineers must now be performed by a class of workers who are less well trained and less expensive."[1]

Figure 1 illustrates their definition. Functions D_1 and S_1 are initially in equilibrium at relative wage W_1 and employment L_1. If demand and supply shift to D_2 and S_2, a shortage of X_1 is indicated. Subsequent shifts to $D_3 S_3$ and $D_4 S_4$ would produce shortages of X_2 and X_4. However, since theirs is a comparative equilibrium approach, they do not expect to observe any X_i, but must rely on relative wage trends to indicate *ex post* whether a shortage exists. Thus the upward-sloping T line indicates the existence of a "shortage."*

Fig. 1. The Blank-Stigler shortage model.

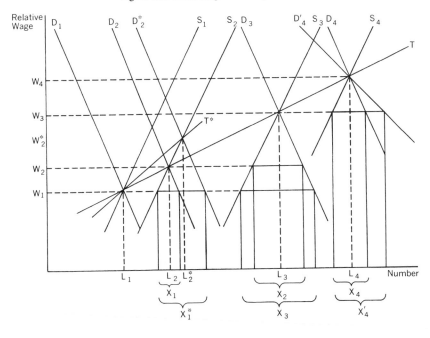

*Blank and Stigler implicitly assumed that, in the absence of disequilibrium, wages for the occupation would rise at the same rate as those of the reference group; that is, in

Data on median nurse salaries relative to those for other workers suggest, in Blank-Stigler terms, a shortage of nurses during World War II* but no postwar shortage until after 1962; in fact, there appears to have been a "surplus" relative to teachers.† Between 1962 and 1966 the situation changed, with evidence of an economic shortage according to the relative wage increase criterion.

The expected rate of return on an investment in training was also studied as an alternative measure of remuneration.[2] Specifically, the following equation was solved for the internal rate of return r:[3]

$$(1) \qquad \int_0^T \left[R_i(t) - O_i(t) - C_i(t) \right] e^{-rt} \, dt = 0,$$

where, for option i, $R_i(t)$ is the receipts stream, $O_i(t)$ is the opportunity cost stream, and $C_i(t)$ is the direct cost stream. Ideally, the returns stream should include the value of the consumption aspects of education, options to increase training, non-monetary rewards, etc., with adjustments at the margin for individual ability differences, motivation, family status, on-the-job training, prior experience, market discrimination, the "quality" of the training, and amount spent on "human capital" improvement (e.g., health care). In practice, such factors are assumed to average out.

---

the absence of a disturbance all workers will benefit equally from productivity gains and/or product price increases. However, if the reference group selected were all workers, it is entirely possible that no occupation would have the same wage trend as the deflator, so that a strict application of their definition would imply that about half of all occupations had experienced a "shortage" and the other half a "surplus." Even if their approach is accepted as an adequate approximation to *ceteris paribus*, the most that could be inferred from a relative wage increase is a "relative shortage" in comparison to other occupations. In times of widespread unemployment such a finding would clearly be meaningless, but even in prosperous times this might be the case. For example, assume that there are shortages in both the general and specific labor markets, that "excess demand" is proportionately larger in the general market, and that the demand and supply curves are steeper in the specific than in the general labor market. As both markets adjust toward equilibrium, the wage for the specific occupation may rise relative to the average of all wages. This would clearly represent a definitional contradiction, as a larger wage increase would have been required to regain equilibrium in the specific than in the general market – even though the specific "shortage" was smaller than the general "shortage."

*This trend may not be reliable in view of the existence and differential administration of wartime wage controls.

†Another possibility is, of course, that there were shortages in both fields, but that the "shortage" of teachers was more severe.

To test the sensitivity of these results to the measure of remuneration employed, estimates were made of overtime pay and of the cash value of maintenance provided nurses, plus salary supplements received by all earners, as well as annual hours worked. Switching from wages and salaries to total compensation, and from monthly to hourly data, gave nurses an absolute advantage over workers in general, but relative trends were little affected.

Table 1: Professional Nurse Salaries Relative to the Earnings
of All Workers, All Female Workers, and Teachers

Year	All Workers	All Female Workers	Teachers
1939	.83	1.18	.72
1946	.89	1.25	.99
1949	.89	–	.86
1959	.85	1.21	.77
1962	.86	1.28	.76
1966	.91	1.37	.79

It was assumed that the receipts streams for nurses and female college graduates are best estimated by their average survivor-adjusted, after-tax earnings (including expected values for scholarships, stipends, and maintenance during training), from the beginning of training (age eighteen) to retirement. Opportunity costs are taken to be the similarly weighted earnings of female high school graduates. Costs of both forms of training include fees and other educational expenses but not living expenses unrelated to training. The first set of estimates assumes 100 per cent employment from graduation to age sixty-five; the second is actuarial, in that the age-specific labor force participation rates for nurses and for female college and high school graduates are applied to their receipts streams up to age eighty.

The estimates based upon 100 per cent labor force participation yield essentially the same results, in Blank-Stigler terms, as did relative wages. The estimates based upon group-specific labor force participation rates diverge from this pattern only with respect to the wartime period, during which they

Table 2: Internal Rates of Return for Nurses Compared with
All Females with Four or More Years of College

Year	Nurses	Female College Graduates	Ratio
100 Per Cent Labor Force Participation Rates Applied			
1939	negative	10.2	negative
1946	8.5	9.4	0.90
1949	9.8	9.3	1.05
1959	2.9	9.0	0.32
1966	7.6	8.6	0.88
Occupational Education-Specific Labor Force Participation Rates Applied			
1939	18.1	15.2	1.19
1946	10.2	14.3	0.71
1949	18.4	14.0	1.31
1959	13.5	14.4	0.94
1966	12.7	12.6	1.01

indicate that there may have been a surplus rather than a shortage.* Thus, it would appear that there was an economic shortage of nurses during and shortly after World War II, a surplus during the 1950s, but a shortage again in the 1960s.

However, this interpretation disregards the second component of the Blank-Stigler definition — that activities formerly performed by professionals would then be performed by cheaper and less experienced workers. Surprisingly few data exist on the substitution of non-professional for professional nurses, and those that are available pertain exclusively to hospitals. What is known is that there has been a fairly steady increase in the ratios of practical nurses and non-professional nursing personnel to hospital-employed registered nurses and, even more dramatically, to general duty nurses.

In Blank-Stigler terms, the conclusions concerning personnel substitution indicate a shortage during the 1950s, whereas the data on relative remuneration imply a surplus. This apparent inconsistency is easily explained. The substitution of non-professionals for registered nurses should be based on their relative costs and productivities. If registered nurse salaries declined compared with those of all workers yet increased relative to those of non-

Table 3: Ratio of Non-Professional to Professional Nurses in Hospitals, 1946–1966

Year	Ratio to Registered Nurses of		Ratio to General Duty Nurses of	
	Non-Professional Nurses	Practical Nurses	Non-Professional Nurses	Practical Nurses
1946	0.997	–	1.723	–
1949	1.178	.167	1.878	.266
1959	1.449	.314	2.426	.527
1962	1.467	.336	2.401	.551
1966	1.677	.372	3.152	.590

*There is a reasonable explanation for this difference. Prior to the war, nursing was one of the few areas open to career-oriented women, and, since most training was in hospitals which typically provided maintenance and small stipends, it represented one of the most highly skilled careers open to women unable to finance a college education. The war brought expanded job opportunities, rising wages, and an increase in employment rates for all women. However, employment rates for nurses somewhat declined, and came to resemble more closely those for other females. The higher employment rates for high school graduates meant higher opportunity costs for all post-high school training. The lower group-specific rates of return for nurses were a consequence of both shifts. Concomitantly, the group-specific rates of return for college graduates declined only slightly, owing to the rise in their employment rates. A strict application of the Blank-Stigler definition would seem to imply a wartime surplus of nurses. Such an interpretation not only lacks intuitive appeal but also ignores the second element of their definition, namely, the substitution of less skilled personnel for those in short supply.

professionals,* the first relative salary decline would still indicate a surplus, although the second would encourage substitution, indicating a shortage.

The evidence thus supports the initial application of the Blank-Stigler definition. The size of the shortages during the 1940s and 1960s still must be determined. Unfortunately, since Blank and Stigler found no shortage (of engineers), they did not explain how to measure one, but certain inferences can be drawn from their model. Given an upward-sloping T curve, three factors will determine, *ceteris paribus*, the size of the shortage.

1. The larger the increase in demand relative to supply, the steeper will be the slope and, hence, the greater the indicated shortage. Thus, if demand shifts from D_1 to D^*_2 (instead of D_2), the steeper curve T^* (not T) and the larger shortage X^*_1 (rather than X_1) are indicated (Fig. 1).

2. Moving along a single linear T curve, the larger the absolute shifts in demand and supply, the greater will be the implied shortage. If, for example, demand and supply shift in one year from D_1, S_1 to D_3, S_3 (rather than D_2, S_2), a larger shortage X_3 (not X_2) will ensue.

3. Changes in demand and supply slopes can also affect the size of the shortage after a shift. The flatter the curves, the larger will be the implied shortage (e.g., a movement from D_3, S_3 to D'_4, S_4, rather than D_4, S_4, results in a shortage of X'_4, rather than X_4).

Since their approach precludes our observing X_i, the "size" of a Blank-Stigler shortage can be measured only by its effect on relative remuneration. This would not be difficult if one could estimate the initial equilibrium and the slopes of the relevant demand and supply curves. Some crude estimates of the short-run supply curve are given below, but it has not yet been possible to make the other required estimates. One may conclude only that, given the elasticities of the demand and supply curves, the larger the relative wage increase the bigger the shortage. But if the curves are steep, a large relative wage increase might indicate a trivial Blank-Stigler "shortage."

Although Blank and Stigler admitted that the situation depicted by their definition "is not necessarily objectionable from a social viewpoint," they nevertheless maintained that it "is a well-defined and significant meaning of the word 'shortage.' "[4] If, in fact, this is so, then any relative wage increase in a freely adjusting market must be evidence of a "shortage." Likewise, if a "significant" definition is one which calls attention to a "problem" that warrants policy consideration, then all relative wage increases should be a source of public concern.

---

*This occurred between 1946 and 1959, when the ratios of general duty nurse starting salaries to those of practical nurses and untrained female and male hospital workers were, respectively, 1.37, 1.69, and 1.47 in 1946 and 1.39, 1.79, and 1.59 in 1959.

Wartime experience proved that a conclusion based on relative rates of return may be the opposite of one based on relative wage trends if an increase occurs in training costs (including foregone earnings) for an occupation relative to the reference group. This implies that "short-run" and "long-run" market conditions differed for that occupation.[5] By basing their analysis on salary trends, Blank and Stigler appear to be concerned mainly with testing a "shortage" in the short-run sense. However, they claim that the study of long-run determinants of supply and demand is their real subject.[6] It is surprising that they paid so little attention to relative training costs* especially because, as W. Lee Hansen demonstrated, these effects can be easily incorporated into their model.

Figure 2 summarizes Hansen's reformulation of the Blank-Stigler model. Starting from equilibrium at $W_1 L_1$, demand shifts from D_1 to D_2. As em-

Fig. 2. Lee Hansen's reformulation of the Blank-Stigler model.

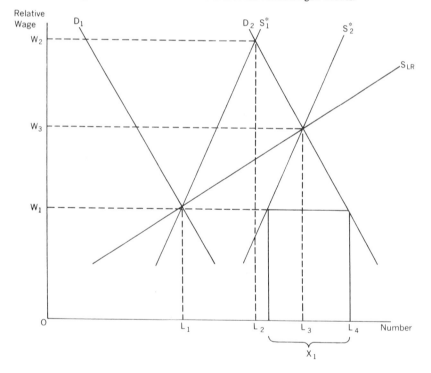

*All they say on the subject is that "since the differentials of engineers' earnings above those of the academically untrained labor force are still in excess of the costs of obtaining an engineering degree, we may expect this trend to continue in the future."[7]

ployers bid against one another for the existing supply of labor, the average wage rises to W_2. The rate of return on training increases, attracting entrants, the short-run supply curve shifts from S^*_1 to S^*_2, and wages fall to W_3. The flow of entrants stabilizes at W_3, since the relative wage advantage and training costs are now equal at the new equilibrium rate of return.[8]

In this situation, Blank and Stigler expected to observe only W_1 and W_3, from which they would have inferred the "shortage" X_1. Yet Hansen argues that a movement from W_1 to W_2 to W_3 might occur,* and with no shortage at W_1 he would consider this sequence to mean the development of a shortage and its elimination. If Blank and Stigler encountered W_2, they would interpret the wage decline to W_3 as indicating a surplus rather than a correction of a shortage.†

Extending Hansen's analysis, assume that as the wage approaches W_3 there is another increase in demand. The T curve will then rise again, and, if this process is repeated, a virtually uninterpretable cyclic T curve will be traced out, indicating, in Blank-Stigler terms, alternating periods of shortage and surplus. However, before the T curve can be interpreted unambiguously in Hansen's terms, additional evidence is needed about equilibrium somewhere along the T curve;‡ otherwise, an upward movement could mean either a declining surplus or a developing shortage. Since the reverse is true of a downward movement along a cyclic T curve, no T curve which does not continuously rise or fall from a known equilibrium can be unambiguously interpreted.

In the nurse market, rates of return based on continuous employment after graduation could be interpreted as indicating a developing shortage or adjustment to a previous surplus between 1939 and 1949 and recovery from a shortage or a developing surplus during 1949–59. Yet the group-specific rate of return estimates indicate recovery from a shortage or a developing surplus during the war, a developing shortage or recovery from a postwar surplus, and an adjustment to the shortage or a developing surplus during the 1950s. (Both sets of estimates indicate either recovery from a surplus or a developing

---

*In order to simplify the argument, it was assumed that D_1 and D_2 represent long-run demand curves. If, in moving between the long-run equilibrium points W_1, L_1 and W_3, L_3, the short-run demand curves always increase much faster than the short-run supply curves, beyond some point the market wage must decline to the new long-run supply price (W_3).

†Since Blank and Stigler assumed that all historically observed combinations of wages and employment were equilibrium levels, they must have had in mind short-run conditions.

‡As Hansen explained, "the choice of one base date over another for comparison can give quite different results; there is no logical basis for determining the beginning of a shortage."[9]

shortage in the mid-1960s.) Measured in these terms, a change in relative remuneration proves neither a shortage nor a surplus in the Blank-Stigler sense.

If relative wage increases do indicate a shortage, is it significant for policy? Blank and Stigler considered all wage-employment combinations to be short-run equilibria; thus no "excess demand" would occur unless wages were prevented from rising. If relative wage increases do not provide evidence of excess demand, what type of shortage do they indicate? Although Blank and Stigler never directly answered this question, two possibilities can be inferred from their analysis.*

1. Even if observed wage-employment combinations indicate short-run equilibria, they may not represent long-run equilibria. Thus short-run wages may exceed long-run supply prices, which certainly is true if the short-run supply curve is steeper than the long-run curve. Under these conditions increased demand might indicate a shortage in the sense that the short-run employment level would be less than the long-run level. If this is their meaning, it may serve to reconcile the fact that Blank and Stigler expressed their model in short-run terms with their claim of primary interest in the study of long-run factors, but it still does not represent a *significant* shortage, in the sense of a manpower problem worthy of serious policy consideration.

2. It is more likely that they considered a "shortage" as a measure of unfulfilled employer expectations, i.e., the difference between *ex ante* and *ex post* hiring decisions. When an employer's demand for labor increases, he expects to hire additional workers at the prevailing wage, but if many employers have demand increases at the same time, the prevailing wage must rise. Each employer discovers that market conditions have changed when he is unsuccessful in expanding employment at the "going wage." Before raising his wage offers, the typical employer will complain of job "vacancies" and of the fact that he is losing some of his older workers. As the new market wage is gradually accepted, hiring expectations will be revised. Whether there will be a "significant" shortage will depend upon the difference between supply and demand at the previous wage and upon the speed at which employer expectations are brought into line with changed market realities. Although Blank and Stigler could not have assumed instant market adjustments and still

---

*Still another possibility has been suggested. During World War II alternative opportunities for employment developed for those who had previously been servants; the higher wages in alternative lines of employment lured many to these occupations, so that "*at the price they had been paying for household help,* many families found they could no longer find such people. Rather than admit that they could not pay the higher wages necessary to keep help, many individuals found it more felicitous to speak of a 'shortage.' "[10]

maintained that theirs was a "significant" definition, they did not incorporate into their model the determinants of a market's adjustment speed. Fortunately, Kenneth J. Arrow and William M. Capron included this refinement in their subsequent analysis of the engineer "shortage."

The Arrow-Capron Model of a "Dynamic" Shortage

In contrast to Blank and Stigler, Arrow and Capron sought to explain "not only the direction of price adjustment (i.e., toward equilibrium) but [also] the rate of adjustment in the face of continued shifts in the short-run functions."[11] Their model is dynamic. It recognizes time lags in responses to demand or supply shifts and applies to situations in which demand for an occupation is continuously increasing. They define a "shortage" as the excess of demand over supply at the prevailing market wage. Further, they specify the "market reaction speed" as the ratio of the rate of increase in the market wage to the excess demand. This ratio depends upon "the time it takes the firm to recognize the existence of a shortage at the current salary level, the time it takes to decide upon the need for higher salaries, and either the time it takes employees to recognize the salary alternatives available and to act upon this information or the time it takes the firm to equalize salaries without outside offers."[12] The slower the market reaction speed and the more inelastic short-run demand and supply, the longer it will take the market to adjust. If demand continuously increases, and the reaction speed is finite, wages will increase without ever becoming high enough to clear the market. The shortage will continue to grow, but it will approach a limit which "is greater the greater the rate of increase of demand and the slower the speed of adjustment."[13]

Arrow and Capron's unusual definitions of supply and demand pose a problem which must be resolved before their model can be applied to the market for nurses. To them, "demand" (supply) means the amount of labor which would be hired (offered) in a particular labor market, in equilibrium at the prevailing wage, "*after complete rational calculation*" of the alternatives. In this sense few firms are likely to know, immediately following an increase in demand, what their demand is. Moreover, an increase in perfect-knowledge demand is not automatically equivalent to an increase in effective demand, which occurs when management suspects a change in product demand or labor productivity. In the presence of such a change, a typical firm will decide to increase employment but, in trying to do so at the going rate, will find little or no labor available. Realizing that it must pay more, the firm eventually will do so, but ordinarily this process takes time, and must be repeated.

Even when the firm has hired the desired number of workers at the new salary, the market will not be in equilibrium, since some firms now pay lower salaries to old employees than to the new ones. Established workers notice they are no longer in equilibrium situations; some change jobs, and management comes to realize that higher starting salaries eventually mean higher salaries for all. Equilibrium is restored only when each firm's effective demand is consistent with its perfect information demand, and when *ex ante* and *ex post* employment levels are equal at the existing market wage.

Blank and Stigler's definition implies that observed wage-employment combinations represent equilibria, but Arrow and Capron's leads to the opposite conclusion. It is almost impossible for the market to return to an Arrow-Capron equilibrium immediately following a general increase in demand because to do so requires *all firms* to be in equilibrium. Since each firm must discover the new market wage and its own true demand individually whenever market demand increases, it follows that every firm "will not, *by definition*, be on its demand . . . curve."* This disequilibrium is what Arrow and Capron call a "shortage." Its existence is indicated by job "vacancies," but because vacancy statistics do not measure the difference between perfect-information demand and supply, they cannot reliably measure the shortage.

Thus the Arrow-Capron definition is no better than Blank and Stigler's in two critical respects: it fails to measure the size of the shortage, and the "problem" it identifies is the difference between behavior under conditions of imperfect and of perfect knowledge. Arrow and Capron also fail to explain why wages will approach equilibrium in their sense if firms are able to hire the amount of labor desired, utilizing only imperfect information.

One may eliminate the latter problem by adding an equation specifying the relation between the firm's actual and its perfect-information demand curves.† This approach is not operational, however, because identification of the latter curve requires perfect information. Alternatively, one might redefine demand and supply in a manner more consistent with traditional economic theory. If "demand" is redefined as each firm's best *estimate* of the labor it wants at the existing wage, then market demand would represent the sum of their desired employment goals. Such an "effective" demand curve would lie to the left of the Arrow-Capron curve. When effective demand increases, the resulting adjustment will be the same as that described by

---

*The analytical problem suggested by this quotation is further compounded if it is explicitly recognized that there is not a single market wage during the adjustment process and that observed wage-employment combinations are not necessarily points on the perfect-information market supply curve.[14]

†As shown above, Arrow and Capron define the market reaction speed (k) as the rate of change in wages relative to the difference between perfect information demand and supply. Obviously, k could be allowed to vary in relation to the difference between the two types of demand. The form of the function would depend, of course, upon the institutional arrangements which determine costs of search, information, etc.

Arrow and Capron, except that each firm will know how many workers it wants at a given wage — but will not know the relation between its demand and over-all market conditions (which can be discovered only by trial and error). In summary, a "dynamic shortage" can be measured at any time by reported job vacancies, which depend upon the rate of increase in demand, the slopes of the short-run market supply and demand curves, and the market reaction speed.

In recent years, 10 to 20 per cent of all budgeted positions for hospital registered nurses, but only 4 to 8 per cent of public health nurse and 1 to 2 per cent of school nurse positions, have been reported vacant. Although there are no data on openings in the industrial and office nurse fields, there is indirect evidence that such vacancies are extremely low.* Further, it appears that there are half again as many unfilled jobs in private duty as in hospitals. The figures for the early 1950s indicate an average "frictional" vacancy rate of approximately 30 per cent in this field.† The slight upward trend since the mid-1950s suggests an increase in either "frictional" vacancies or demand.

Reported hospital vacancies were higher for general duty nurses than for directors, supervisors, and head nurses; vacancy rates for general duty nurses also exceeded those for public health nurses and nurse educators. This seems to conflict with the opinion of many experts that the "shortage" is greatest in the most highly skilled areas of nursing.[15] However, the experts have never claimed merely a shortage of bodies but rather a lack of qualified nurses to fill high-level positions. Nursing and hospital leaders agree that teaching and supervisory positions should be filled by college-trained nurses, but the existing supply is not sufficient.‡ Consequently, many of these positions have been filled by nurses who otherwise would have been assigned to general duty, an area in which, as a result, the shortage appears to be concentrated.

The foregoing analysis assumes, of course, that reliable comparisons can be made among the vacancy series, which is unlikely, except in broad terms.

---

*In industrial and office nursing the typical firm employs only a few nurses. Since there are few opportunities to "stretch out" existing staff, the urgency in filling a vacancy is pronounced. Therefore, the fact that less than 0.1 per cent of the calls received by professional nurse registries are for even temporary placements in these fields suggests that such vacancies do not constitute a serious problem.

†The transitory nature of private duty employment implies a high frictional vacancy rate even in the absence of a "shortage." Moreover, the reported figures are biased upward because they include canceled as well as unfilled calls.

‡There have, however, been sharp differences of opinion as to the relative importance of master's and bachelor's degrees and as to whether the position of head nurse should be included as one of the supervisory levels requiring advanced training. In 1963 it was reported that one-fourth of nurse educators, two-thirds of public health nurses, and nine-tenths of nurses in hospitals and other fields lack degrees. By contrast, almost 30 per cent of hospital nurses have administrative or supervisory responsibilities.[16]

Interpreting the year-to-year pattern for a given field is even more difficult.* The most consistent data are provided by seven American Nurses' Association surveys of hospitals. They suggest that vacancies rose during the 1950s, then declined between 1962 and 1968.† Although the 1958 and 1966 U.S. Public Health Service figures imply a continuously increasing shortage, the absence of an observation for an early year in the 1960s prevents a meaningful comparison with the trend in the ANA data. (The figures are, however, consistently higher in the former than in the latter series.)

While no definitive statement can be made concerning vacancy trends, it is apparent that hospitals have long been reporting relatively high rates. These figures indicate a "shortage" in the Arrow-Capron sense during the 1950s, when the Blank-Stigler approach suggested the opposite. The probable decline in vacancies between 1962 and 1968 implies a declining shortage at the very time when the Blank-Stigler approach suggests a developing shortage. In view of this conflict, it must be determined whether the other Arrow-Capron criteria are met. According to their model, a "dynamic shortage" will occur whenever "(1) there has been a rapid and steady increase in demand, (2) the elasticity of supply [or demand] is low, especially for short periods, and (3) the reaction speed . . . may, for several reasons, be expected to be slow."[17]

Throughout the period 1930 to 1960 census data provide evidence of a strong upward trend in the demand for nurses. The number of employed registered nurses consistently rose faster than the size of the population or the total labor force. However, during the depression decade of 1930 to 1940 the "stock" of living graduate nurses[18] increased faster than the number employed – 55 per cent compared with 33 per cent. Hospital nurse salaries declined in relation to the over-all average and in absolute terms. Nevertheless, serious unemployment was reported during the Depression and was probably still widespread in 1940.

*In 1966, for example, the U.S. Employment Service reported approximately thirty-five thousand nursing vacancies, which is about 5 per cent of total or 7 per cent of hospital registered nursing positions. In the same year an American Hospital Association survey reported a vacancy rate of 13.5 per cent for all hospital nurses. Both figures represent a tremendous decline from the 1962 figure of 20.7 per cent reported by the American Nurses' Association. In turn, the latter figure suggests a large increase in hospital vacancies at the end of the 1950s. Conceptual differences, as well as differences in definitions, survey design, non-response rates, and possibly even seasonal factors are largely responsible for the size of the fluctuations observed. A detailed analysis of these differences will be given in my forthcoming book, *An Economic Analysis of the Nurse Shortage*, chap. 3.

†Even this pattern is suspect. The 1967 and 1968 ANA samples included only large, non-federal general hospitals (which tend to report above average vacancy rates), and positions were quoted in "full-time equivalent" terms. While the selection of hospitals undoubtedly contributed an upward bias and the definition of positions a downward bias, their net effect is uncertain. The present author implicitly assumes that they cancel each other out.

Table 4: Vacancy Rates by Nursing Field and Hospital Position, 1951–1968

Field and Position	1951	1953	1954	1956	1958	1959	1961	1962	1963	1964	1965	1966	1967	1968
Hospitals														
All RNs	11.9	13.6	11.1	12.9	9.3	—	20.1	20.7	—	—	—	13.5	—	—
General duty	—	14.6	13.0	14.5	10.0	—	23.2	23.0	—	—	—	—	18.1	15.0
Directors	—	—	—	6.0	7.3	—	12.0	13.4	—	—	—	—	—	—
Supervisors	—	—	—	7.5	5.3	—	13.1	15.3	—	—	—	—	—	—
Head nurses	—	—	—	10.0	9.3	—	14.0	17.0	—	—	—	—	—	—
Other														
Private duty	28.7	31.8	27.6	34.2	31.6	34.2	32.9	37.3	38.3	37.8	40.0	40.5	41.1	—
Public health														
Total	—	—	—	—	—	3.7	4.9	—	5.5	—	5.6	7.2	8.0	—
Schools	—	—	—	—	—	0.9	0.8	—	—	—	1.8	1.4	2.6	—
Nurse educators	—	—	—	7.3	—	—	—	10.1	—	7.8	—	9.4	—	6.8

Between 1940 and 1950 the total stock of nurses increased by almost 50 per cent, but the number of active nurses by only one-third. The implication that supply increased relative to demand during and following World War II is unlikely, especially with rising wages and the alleged wartime shortage. This apparent paradox is easily resolved by noting that only employed nurses were counted as "active" in the 1930 and 1950 figures. However, the 1940 "active" figure included all nurses in the labor force, including a substantial number of unemployed. The 1940-1950 trend in active nurses thus understates the growth in demand because the unemployed were included in the 1940 figure for active nurses.

The evidence concerning the 1950-1960 period is more difficult to explain. On the one hand, the slower increase in the stock than in the number of "active" registered nurses (30 versus 40 per cent) and the steady increase in hospital nurse vacancies would seem to imply that demand grew faster than supply. However, as we have seen, the relative decline in nurse remuneration would lead Blank and Stigler to the opposite conclusion.

Like the census figures, my estimates of postwar employment by field of nursing are generally indicative of a strong upward demand trend. Total nurse employment grew by 129 per cent from 1946 to 1966. However, the rate of increase appears to have diminished since the late 1940s, possibly because in twenty years the stock expanded by only 72 per cent. (Again, the widening gap between the increase in employment and the stock is indirect evidence that the vacancy data shown in Table 4 might have resulted from the type of market behavior posited by Arrow and Capron.) Over three-fourths of the increase in total active registered nurses is attributable to the 178 per cent growth in hospital nurse employment during this period, as a result of which the proportion of hospital to total active registered nurses rose from 55 to 67 per cent.

Although it accounted for only about 8 per cent of the increase in all active registered nurses, employment grew even more rapidly in the nurse educator and school nurse than in the hospital field. The increase in school nurses paralleled the postwar expansion of the school-age population. The situation with respect to nurse educators is more complex and reflects the shift from diploma to baccalaureate and associate degree programs, with their typically higher faculty-student ratios.

Of the remaining fields, the fastest-growing was office nursing (140 per cent), followed by industrial nursing (94 per cent), and public health nursing (63 per cent). Private duty nursing, the second largest field, showed the lowest postwar growth (5 per cent) and actually declined after 1954.

It is interesting to compare the foregoing employment trends with the salaries paid in different fields of nursing. Although salaries were quite similar for all fields in 1946, their postwar growth trends have exhibited a marked dichotomy. One group, composed of school nurses, nurse educators, public

Fig. 3. Estimated number of professional nurses, by field of practice.

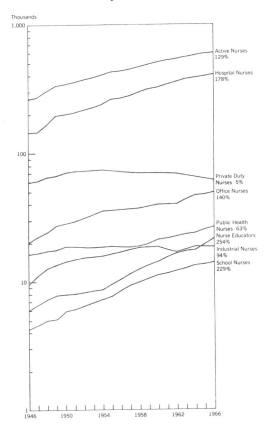

health and industrial nurses, gained substantial wage increases of about 60 to 90 per cent from 1946 to 1966. The other group, which constitutes over 85 per cent of all active nurses and is composed of office, hospital, and private duty nurses, had salary increases of less than 50 per cent. Moreover, the latter group displayed much less dispersion than the former. Surprisingly, all but one of the low-paid fields was among the faster-growing in terms of employment. Taken together, these facts raise two significant questions: what common factor links the three fields with the lowest salaries, and why have their salaries increased so slowly?

Differences in educational preparation are not sufficient to explain the observed groupings. For example, most school and industrial nurses are diploma-school graduates, and lack of a baccalaureate degree does not automatically preclude employment of a registered nurse in public health, or even as a nurse educator. With its high salary scale, the nurse educator field has expanded over 300 per cent without a marked rise in its low vacancies. The

Fig. 4. Monthly salaries of professional nurses, by field of practice (1966 dollars).

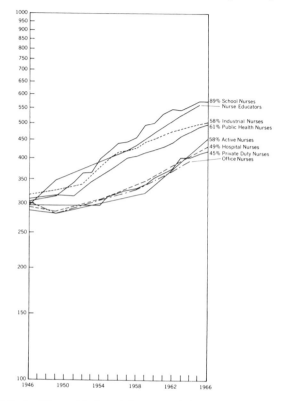

school, public health, and industrial nursing fields also expanded rapidly without experiencing vacancy increases. According to the Arrow-Capron model, these areas would appear to have relatively elastic supply and demand curves and/or rapid market reaction speeds. To test both hypotheses, the salary-setting process for these markets should be examined.

Given the trend in hospital salaries, the rapid gains by nurse educators are surprising in view of the large proportion of them employed in hospital-affiliated schools. The pressure for higher salaries undoubtedly stems from the expanding baccalaureate programs and reflects the general salary rise of other academicians. The growing demand for college degrees may also explain the belief that there is a more acute "shortage" of nurse educators than of hospital nurses, although reported vacancies for the former are lower. Requirements that teachers in baccalaureate programs have terminal degrees have intensified the sense of urgency associated with this problem and have boosted the salaries of nurses holding such degrees. Doubtless competition in this market has also resulted in higher salaries for hospital-affiliated faculty.

The correspondence between the salaries of nurse educators and other academic salaries illustrates a general rule: that nurses employed in an industry where nursing is a minority occupation receive compensation more representative of that industry than of the nursing profession. This principle is further supported by data on school and industrial nurses. In both instances personnel policies are set on the basis of market conditions for typical workers in the industry; management finds it worth a substantial salary premium to hire and retain a few well-qualified registered nurses. This premium is easy to establish where the average salary of other employees with similar training is higher than the going salary for nurses.

The foregoing hypothesis implies that the ratios of the average salaries of school nurses to teachers and of industrial nurses to manufacturing workers should tend toward unity. As a test, both ratios were calculated, and it was found that the former fluctuated from 0.98 to 1.11 and the latter from 0.98 to 1.07. Moreover, since the policy of paying a premium for not having to worry about nursing services would not be continued if it were unsuccessful, low turnover rates for these fields would be expected. No figure for industrial nurses is available, but a 1956 study of New Jersey school nurses disclosed that only 11 per cent were newly appointed that year (compared with turnover rates of 66.9 and 57.5 per cent for general duty nurses and female manufacturing workers, respectively).[19]

Market conditions in the public health field also support the above hypothesis. Salaries are commonly regulated by civil service and tend to be based upon years of training and seniority. However, unlike school nurses, public health nurses have not received higher salaries because of the rapid expansion of their "parent" industry. This may partly explain why the vacancy rates for public health nurses are higher than those of school nurses even though employment in the former field rose more slowly than in the latter.

It is significant that the high-salaried fields account for under 15 per cent of total active registered nurses and that this employment level is determined by demand. At the prevailing salaries, employers in these fields face a virtually horizontal supply curve. They could pay lower wages without losing their recruiting advantage but choose not to do so because the convenience outweighs the cost. In Arrow-Capron terms, the market reaction speed is inconsequential.

Nurses who cannot find jobs in the top-paying fields must choose among hospitals, private duty, and doctors' offices. It is tempting to ascribe the clustering of the salaries paid in these fields to competition, but in reality the pay scales for both private duty and office nurses are largely determined by salaries of hospital nurses. The basic eight-hour fees for private duty nurses hired through registries (which place most of them) are generally set in conformity with local hospital salary levels.* It is therefore unlikely that private duty earnings would diverge from general duty salaries except in areas where individual bargaining is common or where there is a deliberate attempt by the state nurses' association to upset the traditional pattern. For their part, physicians commonly recruit office staff from among the nurses who make the best impression in the hospital. Moreover, since many physicians have some hospital affiliation, they are undoubtedly familiar with hospital salary scales. By offering shorter hours and better working conditions, doctors are able to recruit nurses from the hospitals without open salary competition.

Clearly, hospital employment conditions set the scale for private duty and office nurses, and these three fields employ almost all nurses with salaries not administratively set above the "going wage." If hospitals can be shown to have inelastic demand and supply curves and/or slow market reaction speeds, it would appear that the Arrow-Capron model provides a reasonable economic explanation of the nurse "shortage." Superficially, the small salary rise accompanying the large expansion of hospital employment might seem to indicate a high short-run supply elasticity. The data necessary to test this proposition directly are unavailable, but rough calculations were made of the average short-run supply elasticity for all nurses, which suggest the opposite. In "real" wage terms, the average supply elasticity was low, between 0.25 and 0.34 (or from 0.11 to 0.17 in money-wage terms).[20] Since those fields paying "above scale" do not represent a large source of additional nurses, the figures indicate that the short-run supply elasticities are indeed low in hospital-related fields.

Less is known about the average short-run elasticity of demand. The demand for nurses is a derived demand, determined by the demand for different medical services and by all the factors affecting the productivity of nurses in each of the health fields. It would be necessary to know both the demand and production functions for each health service (in addition to achieving econometric identification) before nurse demand elasticities could be estimated. The notion that short-run demand is inelastic is implicit in the views of the experts who have established nurse-patient ratios as "requirements" for adequate care.† On the other hand, it appears that non-professional personnel are

---

*I am indebted to Elizabeth C. Carroll, State Section Advisor of the California Nurses' Association, for explaining the process by which basic eight-hour fees are determined.

†Actually, the "typical" hospital's demand for nurses depends not only upon its demand and production functions but also upon the supply-price relationships of the other factors it employs. The hypothesis that demand is relatively elastic depends upon the production function implications of the observed substitution of non-professional for professional nurses and the conviction of hospital administrators that while the nurse supply curve is upward-sloping, the supply of non-professionals is essentially horizontal. The implication of the latter is that the ratio of professional to non-professional wages will increase if the hospital attempts to hire more of both.

often substituted for registered nurses (albeit reluctantly), suggesting that the typical market demand curve for hospital nurses may not be as inelastic as the supply.*

Although the probability that vacancies evidence a "dynamic shortage" is reduced if demand is elastic, it must be noted that such a shortage depends upon the net effect of the interaction between relative demand increases, the slopes of the supply and demand curves, and the market reaction speed. Given a stable and inelastic supply curve, there is a good possibility that the increased demand for nurses may have caused such a shortage if the market reaction speed was slow.

Arrow and Capron gave three reasons to expect the reaction in a market for professional personnel to be "slower than that in the markets for other commodities, such as manufactured goods, or even in other labor markets. They are the prevalence of long-term contracts, the influence of the hetero-geneity of the market in slowing the diffusion of information, and the domi-nance of a relatively small number of firms."[22] Long-term hospital employ-ment contracts still are the exception,† and, aside from administrative and supervisory staff, few hospital registered nurses accumulate the type of seniority or tenure-related benefits that would slow the market adjustment mechanism. However, most hospitals are non-profit institutions constrained by annually fixed budgets, which would have the same effect as long-term contracts on the market reaction speed.

Although not all registered nurses are "eligible" to be administrators or supervisors, the qualifications for such positions are not independent of the availability of applicants – i.e., lacking "qualified" applicants, management will reluctantly hire less skilled personnel. Since hospitals do not publicize such practices, information on these job opportunities may be limited, and in Arrow and Capron's terms this factor would slow the market reaction speed. Dispersion of local markets may also hinder spread of information about opportunities elsewhere. However, this fact may not be too important, as over 60 per cent of the nurses are married and are constrained by their husbands' locations. Unmarried nurses may be in a better position to move

---

*On the other hand, it is known that the elasticity of demand for a factor is posi-tively related to the elasticity of the product demand, as well as to the proportion of total cost attributable to the factor. The results of several studies show that the demand for hospital services is quite inelastic.[21] It was estimated that compensation to registered nurses amounted to approximately 14 per cent of total hospital expenses in 1963. Both factors will reduce the elasticity, but their net effect is uncertain.

†The only collective bargaining contracts which cover registered nurses are those negotiated by unions in enterprises employing few nurses (e.g., industrial nurses) or by the ANA's Economic Security Program. As of January 1, 1967, the various state nurses' associations had obtained only 121 contracts, covering 245 employers and approxi-mately 16,850 nurses. In all, less than 5 per cent of active nurses are covered by collective bargaining agreements.

elsewhere in response to higher wage offers, but it appears that their mobility is not great,* whether due to lack of information or of incentive is not known. Nevertheless, the nature of the market probably creates information breakdowns.

At first glance it seems improbable that the market reaction speed would be slowed by "the dominance of a relatively small number of firms" in the nurse market. Nationally, there are thousands of employers as well as employees in each field of nursing. However, an evaluation of the extent of competition in this market must be tempered by the evidence of the concentration of employment in hospitals and the low geographical mobility of registered nurses. The latter fact implies that the relevant market is local rather than national, and the former indicates that hospitals are likely to be the dominant nurse employers in most localities. Moreover, in most cases, hospitals are either monopsonists or oligopsonists. According to separate surveys of general hospitals in 1949 and in 1960-1962, more than 10 per cent of the hospitals were the only ones in their Hill-Burton Service Area, about 30 per cent were located in areas with one or two hospitals, 45 per cent were in areas with less than four hospitals, and over 60 per cent were in areas with less than six hospitals.[24]

Even in metropolitan areas the market for nurses is less competitive than might be expected. In a survey of the thirty-one largest metropolitan hospital associations, all but one association of the fifteen replying reported having established successful "wage-standardization" programs.[25] (The association that did not already have such a program asked for information on how to establish one.) The incentive to engage in such practices is quite strong, as unilateral wage changes are likely to evoke retaliation which will result in higher labor costs with little, if any, change in registered nurse employment. Because Arrow and Capron found no comparable situation for engineers, they did not explore its implications. They simply noted that the fear of precipitating a "wage war" tends to slow the market reaction speed. Since hospitals must be aware of their ability to influence local nurse salary scales, the typical nurse market undoubtedly has a slow reaction speed.

Although nearly all the evidence available favors the "dynamic shortage" hypothesis, not even its aggregate magnitude can be measured by the vacancy statistics in Table 4. In addition to the problems of measurement described above, a more fundamental difficulty exists at the theoretical level. Since monopsonistic and oligopsonistic employers will express the desire to hire

---

*One study found that 25 per cent of all married nurses made a geographical move when they changed jobs (probably because of a family move) but that only 5 per cent of the job changes of unmarried nurses involved a geographical move. Moreover, the same study disclosed that only 4 to 8 per cent of the nurses surveyed changed jobs because they were dissatisfied with their pay and only 10 to 15 per cent because they had found a better job.[23]

more workers at the equilibrium wage, vacancies will be reported even though there is no "dynamic shortage." If one does exist, its severity will be overstated by vacancy data. Thus, before one can test for a "dynamic shortage," the "equilibrium vacancy" level of the market must be determined. The first step is to specify theoretical models describing the equilibrium positions of such markets.

Model of an Imperfectly Competitive Labor Market

Under conditions of monopsony and oligopsony, firms face an upward-sloping factor supply curve. Consequently, since "the marginal cost of labour exceeds its average cost an employer who is maximizing his profits at the existing marginal cost will . . . offer no more, although he may report vacancies."[26]

Figure 5 shows a rising supply curve, S, and a corresponding marginal factor cost curve, MC, that is above S for all employment levels. An employer in this situation will hire workers until the value of their marginal product equals their marginal cost. Thus, in equilibrium, he will employ ON labor, pay wage OW, and report vacancies NM. He will not pay higher salaries, but he will be willing to hire more labor at the going wage. His reported vacancies do not represent "excess demand" and will not exert upward pressure on wages. An increase in demand will cause wages to rise and vacancies to increase. "Hence, given the two assumptions of [factor] market imperfection and profit maximization, *a large number of reported vacancies may be perfectly consistent with equilibrium in the labour market.*"[27]

This argument can be extended to oligopsony. The supply curve SS' in Figure 6 shows the response to wage changes by a single employer acting alone. If other employers are expected to retaliate, the supply curve will resemble GG'. If retaliation is expected to be "perfect," GG' will have the same slope as the aggregate supply of labor to the market. Further, if each

Fig. 5. Model of a monopsonistic market.   Fig. 6. Model of an oligopsonistic market.

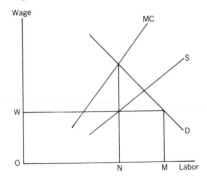

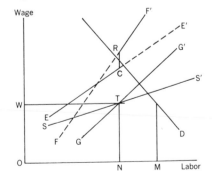

employer expects a wage increase (but not a wage cut) to result in retaliatory increases by the others, then the effective supply is the kinked curve STG'. The marginal cost curve FF' corresponds to the supply curve GG', and the marginal cost curve EE' corresponds to SS'. Thus the marginal cost curve for the kinked supply curve STG' is the discontinuous curve $ECRF'$. In order for equilibrium to exist, the demand curve D must pass through the vertical section CR of the marginal cost curve, yielding an equilibrium wage of OW and vacancies of NM.

Since vacancies NM do not represent "excess demand," they do not affect the equilibrium wage, and their size is determined by the demand curve slope and the point at which it passes through CR. Any increase in demand within CR will cause increased vacancies. No wage increase will occur until the demand curve cuts the marginal cost curve at a point above R. Below R employers know that they will not gain by raising wages, but they will continue to report vacancies in the hope that their efforts will cause a shift in the supply curve. Under these conditions, wage increases will probably come in "rounds," each being initiated by an employer who is temporarily strong enough (or hard-pressed enough) to act as the "leader." Other employers must follow suit. When the adjustment is over, relative stability will obtain until another employer is tempted to raise wages.

According to G. C. Archibald, "we will find oligopsony in the labour market whenever there are few employers of a given type of labour in an area and the cost of mobility is positive." This would explain "the apparent stickiness of the wages of many of the skilled and comparatively rare craftsmen.... The employer of skilled men who are limited in number will fear retaliation if he attempts to increase his share; the employer of casual labour will not." Thus excess demand may often " 'squeeze' the margin for skill." Moreover, if "solidarity" among employers exists and leads to collusion, it will "help to deter employers from making increased wage offers which . . . will, *in any case*, look doubtful and risky."[28]

Archibald, like Arrow and Capron, assumed that all employers are profit maximizers. Only a few employers of nurses are even profit seekers, much less maximizers. However, this strong assumption is not necessary. All that is required is that employers try to produce the output they desire as efficiently as possible, utilizing factors of production (including nurses) in the least-cost combination.[29] As a first approximation, it is not unreasonable to assume that hospitals — the major employers of nurses — behave in this fashion.[30]

Given the evidence that hospitals are monopsonistic or oligopsonistic nurse employers, the "shortage" might be explained by the increasing number of registered nurses concentrated in hospitals.* "Equilibrium" nurse vacancies

---

*It will be recalled that in 1946 salaries in all fields were more nearly uniform than at present. The dichotomous nurse salary pattern did not appear until hospitals became the dominant employers in local nurse markets.

may represent a misallocation of resources, but they are not likely to be "corrected" by normal market forces. This should not be interpreted as implying that there has been no "dynamic shortage" of nurses. The problem is that the vacancy statistics (Table 4), taken alone, measure neither "dynamic shortage" nor "equilibrium" vacancies. The author is currently engaged in research which, it is hoped, will lead to numerical estimates of both types of vacancies. To guide this effort, a model of the nurse market was developed which includes the dynamic factors brought out by Arrow and Canron as well as the effects of monopsony and oligopsony.

SUMMARY AND ECLECTIC MODEL OF THE NURSE MARKET

Since most nursing statistics are national in scope, it is tempting to think of the market in such terms. Actually, the data should be viewed as weighted averages of behavior in local markets that possess a high degree of autonomy because of low wage-induced geographical mobility and the site-specific nature of nurse services. Most local nurse markets are variants of two basic prototypes in the hospital sector. Conditions in the other fields of nursing exert little influence on salaries because hospitals are the dominant employers, and two-thirds of the nurses employed outside them have salaries directly tied to hospital scales, while the remainder work for employers who pay "above-scale." The more nurses in the latter category, or the greater the differential, the higher the average local wage will be. The same effect obtains with respect to the size of the hospital-related fields because, in the short run, they can increase only at the expense of the hospital supply, which would, of course, mean higher hospital salaries.

The ratio of hospital to all active nurses grew during the postwar period by almost the same amount (15 percentage points) as the drop in the proportion in private duty. This shift in the hospital supply curve undoubtedly contributed to the widening of the salary differentials between hospital-related and other nursing fields but in itself cannot explain the low level or slow rate of increase of the hospital nurse salaries. This trend is explained by the hospital's position in the structure of local markets. Since the Depression, hospitals have become either monopsonistic or oligopsonistic* and in recent years have tended toward collusion on employment policies. Nurses demonstrate little wage-induced geographical mobility, and, since positions in the highest paid non-hospital fields are scarce, they must often choose between hospitals and jobs outside of nursing. Few other occupations for which nurse

*During the 1920s and 1930s hospitals employed few graduate nurses, relying instead on students to provide most patient care. Offering free room, board, and small stipends, hospital nursing schools attracted girls in financial need. The steady stream of poorly trained graduates produced by this system was not absorbed into hospital employment. Those who could not find jobs in other fields went into private duty or became unemployed (often indistinguishable states).

training provides any advantage pay competitive salaries. In two studies, done in 1955 and in 1964, only 2 per cent of the nurses surveyed reported being employed in non-nursing positions.[31] It might be expected that the growth in the proportion of registered nurses holding baccalaureate degrees would increase this percentage.* Fragmentary evidence suggests that this has not been the case. The 1955 survey included both diploma-holding and degree-holding registered nurses, while the 1964 figure was for diploma graduates only. The fact that the two figures are the same would seem to indicate that nurses with baccalaureates do not have a significantly greater propensity toward non-nursing employment than others, perhaps because they hold a disproportionate number of positions in the highest-paid nursing fields.† Thus, interoccupational mobility is not likely to diminish monopsony or oligopsony in local markets.

As monopsonists and oligopsonists, hospitals normally report registered nurse vacancies at the going wage, indicating a "shortage" only in welfare theory terms (i.e., fewer nurses employed than at the competitive optimum). This situation could persist indefinitely because the market is in equilibrium, and no endogenous adjustment will "correct" the problem. However, this misallocation of resources is not what nursing authorities mean when they complain about the "shortage." They refer to a deficit of demand relative to "needs." The elimination of monopsony and oligopsony would undoubtedly result in higher registered nurse employment, but there is no reason to suppose that this increase would fully satisfy their criteria.

Monopsony or oligopsony increases the probability of a "dynamic shortage." When demand increases rapidly, salaries do not rise as much as they do in a competitive market. The smaller the increase in registered nurse salaries, the less the increase in the rate of return on training will be. Thus, to the extent that short-run supply shifts depend upon the number of new recruits, the lower salaries attributable to monopsony and oligopsony will work against increases in the supply of nurses. Monopsony and oligopsony also affect the other two factors responsible for dynamic shortages. The market reaction speed depends partly upon the availability of job information, the paucity of which accentuates the effects attributable to isolated local markets. Moreover, since monopsonists and oligopsonists "set" (rather than react to) the market wage, administrative delays will slow the market reaction speed even when job information is abundant. Monopsony and oligopsony

---

*Between 1956 and 1966 the percentage of active registered nurses holding baccalaureate degrees increased from 7.0 to 10.4.[32]

†In 1966, for example, 10.4 per cent of total nurses employed were baccalaureate graduates. By comparison, 33.8, 41.5, 30.4, and 18.7 per cent, respectively, of public health nurses, nurse educators, hospital nursing service directors, and hospital nursing supervisors held baccalaureates.[33]

further increase the probability of a "dynamic shortage," since it is inversely related to the elasticity of the marginal cost curve, and the latter is more inelastic than the average cost curve representing supply in a competitive market. Unfortunately, data on local nurse markets are insufficient to test this model. The national figures which are available must be interpreted as weighted averages of local statistics. This procedure presents no conceptual difficulties, but estimates of true "weights" would require considerably more knowledge of local markets than is now available.

From a policy standpoint, it is essential to distinguish between the two types of vacancies in the model. In equilibrium, all observed vacancies can be attributed to monopsony or oligopsony. Otherwise, some fraction will represent "excess demand." If the demand (or supply) function is continually shifting, it is extremely difficult to estimate the number of vacancies which would exist in equilibrium. However, such an estimate must be made before the size of the dynamic shortage can be measured.*

Although the relative numbers of each type of vacancy have not yet been estimated, their relationship to nurse demand and supply elasticities should be considered. Ceteris paribus, the lower the elasticity of demand, the higher the number of dynamic relative to equilibrium vacancies. Similarly, the lower the elasticity of supply, the greater the number of both types of vacancies. Thus if the initial distribution of the two types of vacancies were known, the effect of a change in either demand or supply elasticity could be predicted.

The fact that the separate sizes of the two types of shortage cannot currently be estimated would seem to preclude implementing remedial policies. This fact would not matter if only one type of shortage were "significant" or if the same remedies were invariably applicable to both. However, both types of shortage involve resource misallocation and, therefore, in the absence of quantitative information to the contrary, are equally worthy of policy consideration. The critical question is whether they respond to the same or to different policy measures.

SOME POLICY IMPLICATIONS

Table 5 summarizes the effect on vacancies of policy measures which would change the elasticity or the position of nurse demand and supply curves. The effects of alternative policies on both economic and "needs" shortages are given. Any measure which increases nurse employment (relative to "requirements") would reduce the size of the nurse "needs" shortage.

---

*As wages rise in response to disequilibrium, the number of dynamic vacancies will decline, but the number of equilibrium vacancies will rise. As a result of this process of transforming dynamic into monopsony vacancies, the difference between the ultimate level of equilibrium vacancies and the total number of current vacancies will underestimate the true magnitude of the dynamic shortage.

Table 5: Implications for Number of Vacancies of Alternative Policy Approaches to Alleviate Various Types of Nurse "Shortage"

Type of Vacancy	Effects of Policies Designed to Result in							
	Increase in Supply Elasticity[a]	Decrease in Supply Elasticity[a]	Increase in Demand Elasticity[a]	Decrease in Demand Elasticity[a]	Increase in Supply	Decrease in Supply	Increase in Demand	Decrease in Demand
"Equilibrium"	Decrease	Increase	Increase	Decrease	Increase	Decrease	Increase	Decrease
"Dynamic"	Decrease	Increase	Decrease	Increase	Decrease	Increase	Increase	Decrease
Total economic	Decrease[b]	Increase	Indeterminate	Indeterminate	Indeterminate	Indeterminate	Increase	Decrease
Relative to specified "needs"[c]	Decrease	Increase	Increase	Decrease	Decrease	Increase	Decrease	Increase

[a] The assumption is made that the elasticities are evaluated at the point of intersection between supply (average factor cost) and demand.
[b] If the elasticity of supply increase is due to collective bargaining, the introduction of long-term contracts may make the result indeterminate.
[c] The current employment level is assumed to be below the specified "needs."

The only policy which will reduce all vacancies simultaneously is one which will increase the elasticity of supply. Although decreasing the elasticity of demand reduces "equilibrium" and "needs" vacancies, it will increase "dynamic" vacancies. Any policy to decrease demand reduces all except "needs" vacancies. This is usually done by substituting less-skilled personnel for registered nurses, which, unfortunately, could have adverse effects on the quality of patient care. Nursing leaders have long advocated policies which would have the effect of increasing the short-run supply elasticity and to some extent shift the curve itself (e.g., flexible hours, more part-time personnel positions, child-care centers, refresher courses, non-discriminatory hiring, etc.). Except for the expansion of part-time employment (which I estimate was responsible for a 12 per cent increase in full-time-equivalent registered nurse employment between 1946 and 1964), hospitals have done little to implement any proposal which might involve higher costs. This behavior is, of course, not unexpected, as monopsonists will not incur higher costs to reduce "equilibrium" vacancies, but will institute "costless" measures to do so.

On the "seller's" side, collective bargaining is frequently espoused. Although the establishment of standard pay scales through such bargaining would reduce the *effects* of monopsony or oligopsony, it would not ensure their *elimination*, which would occur only if the negotiated wage were equal to the competitive wage.* Collective bargaining could even replace monopsony with monopoly resource misallocation, but experience indicates that this result is unlikely in the near future.† Its effect on dynamic vacancies is indeterminate because the introduction of a long-term contract decreases the market reaction speed at the same time that the reduction in monopsony power increases it. Moreover, collective bargaining may have a greater impact on hospital salaries than is indicated by the number of nurses directly involved. A negotiated settlement may cause other hospitals to offer higher salaries to forestall the spread of collective bargaining or as a response to the publicity which usually accompanies it.[35] This effect could be viewed as an increase in the market reaction speed, which, of course, decreases dynamic vacancies.

Professional registries offer an untried but potentially effective instrument for raising nurse salaries. Private duty fees are tied to general duty salaries and appear to be below market clearing rates. In an open market private duty

---

*The same could be said with respect to a special minimum wage for nurses, with the additional complication that a standard rate sufficient to eliminate all local market shortages would probably reduce registed nurse employment in some areas, thereby aggravating existing non-economic shortages.

†Between 1965 and 1967 the number of bargaining agreements in force as part of the ANA's Economic Security Program increased from 92 to 121. The number of nurses covered went from approximately 9,000 to 16,850. Some observers feel, however, that this rate of increase presages a bigger role for such bargaining in the future – especially if bona fide unions are formed and/or nurses are given the legally protected "right" to organize.[34]

earnings would rise, and, to the extent that hospital nurses were attracted by these higher earnings, hospital salaries would also rise and equilibrium vacancies would fall. (There would, however, be a temporary increase in dynamic vacancies.) The higher the proportion of private duty to hospital employment, the greater would be the increase in the hospital supply elasticity and the consequent decrease in both equilibrium and dynamic vacancies.*

At the national level, the establishment of a nationwide nurse registry would greatly improve the flow of information, which in turn would increase both the elasticities of supply and reaction speeds in local markets, simultaneously reducing equilibrium and dynamic vacancies.† "Moving cost" subsidies for the 35 per cent of all nurses who are primary wage earners would have the same type of effect.

Still another way to offset monopsony or oligopsony would be to pay subsidies to hospitals as an incentive for them to hire enough nurses to eliminate equilibrium vacancies. The size of the subsidy to a specific hospital would be the amount necessary to lower its marginal cost of nurses curve until it coincided with the pre-subsidy supply curve. Such a program would be difficult to implement and would have to be continued indefinitely, since, by itself, it would generate no forces which would continue to offset monopsony power if the subsidy were cut off. Moreover, the subsidy would have to be increased whenever the hospital experienced an increase in demand relative to supply.

It is most unlikely that Congress would pass legislation giving different subsidies to equivalent facilities facing different nurse market conditions. Experience suggests that legislators are more inclined to support demand for particular services. Medicare is a good example. By making it possible for hospitals to shift part of the burden of higher costs, the program had the same effect as would an increase in the elasticity of the supply of nurses. On the other hand, the resulting rise in demand for hospital services (approximately 5 per cent) meant some increase in relative demand for nurses as well.[37] The former would tend to decrease both equilibrium and dynamic vacancies, while the latter would have the opposite effect; thus nothing definite can be said at this time about the net result of Medicare.

---

*If registries became the standard source of placement in all nursing fields, it might be possible to eliminate equilibrium vacancies by breaking down the existing market segmentation. This would require, however, that three unlikely preconditions be met: each nurse would have to be willing to accept employment in any field at the market wage for her skill level; hospitals would no longer be able to identify their individual influences on supply; and registries would have to set salaries at market-clearing levels. By increasing the availability of job information, this plan might also increase the market reaction speed and thereby reduce dynamic vacancies as well.

†Although the ANA operates a "clearinghouse," its scale is too small to have much influence.[36]

The Nurse Training Act of 1964 (amended and continued in the Health Manpower Act of 1968) represents the major federal attempt to reduce the postwar nurse shortage. Not concerned with demand per se, the Act was an attempt to expand the supply of nurses, a policy which, if successful, would reduce both dynamic and "needs" shortages while increasing equilibrium vacancies. When the NTA was enacted, I criticized it on the grounds that any serious attempt to eliminate the nurse "shortage" would have to be addressed to its demand as well as its supply side. Moreover, within the bounds of its limited goals, I correctly predicted that student loans would not cause the increase in nursing school enrollments to be greater than was expected without them.[38] Therefore, the funds allocated for new building were excessive, although they did help to improve obsolete facilities and to build college-based programs to offset the decline in hospital schools.

In 1967 the NTA Program Review Committee recommended continuation of the same approach for another five years. As a dissenting member, I endorsed efforts "to improve the *quality* of both the existing and future supplies of nurses." However, in company with Frank Furstenberg, M.D., I took "exception to those aspects of the program designed to bring about a substantial increase in the *quantity* of professional nurses by 1975." We expressed our belief that "without a program to translate the nation's 'needs' into *effective* demand, the proposal to greatly increase the *supply* of nurses could cause large relative salary declines. Under such circumstances, nursing will become an even less attractive career than at present; and we will soon be faced with still another . . . 'shortage.' . . . If the determination of the supply of nurses is an appropriate Federal responsibility, so too is the assurance that effective demand will be sufficiently high to create employment opportunities at salaries attractive enough to eventually eliminate the discrepancy between the number of nurses 'needed' and those 'demanded.' " [39] Given the structure of the nurse market and the continuing increases in demand relative to supply, both equilibrium and dynamic vacancies are probably permanent phenomena, but it is doubtful that even economists would pay much attention to them if there were no longer a "shortage" of nurses, in the popular sense of the word.

NOTES

1. David M. Blank and George J. Stigler, *The Demand and Supply of Scientific Personnel* (New York: National Bureau of Economic Research, 1957), p. 24.

2. Donald E. Yett, "Lifetime Earnings for Nurses in Comparison with College-Trained Women," *Inquiry* 5 (December 1968):35–70.

3. In view of the well-known conceptual deficiencies of the internal rate of return as a criterion for investment decisions (Jack Hirshleifer, "On the Theory of Optimal Investment Decision," *Journal of Political Economy* 66 [August 1958]:350–52), estimates were also made of the present values and the rates of return over cost ("crossover

points") associated with each training option. The results were not substantially different from those obtained on the basis of internal rates of return.

4. Blank and Stigler, *Scientific Personnel*, p. 24.

5. Donald E. Yett, "The Supply of Nurses: An Economist's View," *Hospital Progress* 46 (February 1965):29.

6. Blank and Stigler, *Scientific Personnel*, p. 33.

7. *Ibid.*, p. 31.

8. W. Lee Hansen, " 'Shortages' and Investment in Health Manpower," *The Economics of Health and Medical Care*, ed. S. J. Axelrod (Ann Arbor: The University of Michigan, 1964), p. 80.

9. *Ibid.*

10. Kenneth J. Arrow and William M. Capron, "Dynamic Shortages and Price Rises: The Engineer-Scientist Case," *Quarterly Journal of Economics* 73 (May 1959):307.

11. *Ibid.*, pp. 293–94.

12. *Ibid.*, p. 299.

13. *Ibid.*, p. 300.

14. *Ibid.*, p. 293.

15. U.S., Department of Health, Education, and Welfare, Public Health Service, *Toward Quality in Nursing: Needs and Goals, Report of the Surgeon General's Consultant Group on Nursing*, Public Health Service Publication 992 (Washington, D.C.: U.S. Government Printing Office, 1963), pp. 15–17.

16. *Ibid.*, p. 9.

17. Arrow and Capron, "Dynamic Shortages and Price Rises," p. 302.

18. Hugh Folk and Donald E. Yett, "Methods of Estimating Occupational Attrition," *Western Economic Journal* 6 (September 1968):300.

19. Walter J. Johnson, "Public Health Nursing Turnover," *American Journal of Nursing* 57 (April 1957):465; Eugene Levine, "Turnover among Nursing Personnel in General Hospitals," *Hospitals* 31 (September 1957):52; and U.S., Bureau of Labor Statistics, *Employment and Earnings* 1 (May 1955):27; 2 (August 1955):31; 2 (November 1955):31; 2 (February 1956):31.

20. Yett, "The Supply of Nurses," p. 99.

21. Paul J. Feldstein and Ruth Severson, "The Demand for Medical Care," in American Medical Association, *Report of the Commission on the Cost of Medical Care* (Chicago: By the Association, 1964), 1:67–68; and Gerald D. Rosenthal, *The Demand for General Hospital Facilities*, American Hospital Association Monograph 14 (Chicago: By the Association, 1964), pp. 26, 35.

22. Arrow and Capron, "Dynamic Shortages and Price Rises," p. 303.

23. Phil M. Smith, *Influence of Wage Rates on Nurse Mobility* (Chicago: University of Chicago Graduate Program in Hospital Administration, 1962), pp. 8, 11.

24. See Dorothy P. Rice and Louis S. Reed, "The Nation's Needs for Hospitals and Health Centers, a Summary of Data from Plans Submitted by the States under the Hospital Survey and Construction Act," mimeographed (Washington, D.C.: U.S. Public Health Service Division of Hospital Facilities, 1949), pp. 88–156, for 1949 data. The figures for 1960–1962 were tabulated from unpublished information collected by the American Hospital Association from reports by individual states in these years.

25. Yett, "The Supply of Nurses," p. 100.

26. G. C. Archibald, "The Factor Gap and the Level of Wages," *Economic Record* 30 (November 1954):188–89.

27. *Ibid.*, p. 189.

28. *Ibid.*, pp. 193–95.

29. Donald E. Yett, "The Causes and Consequences of Salary Differentials in Nursing," *Inquiry* 7 (March 1970):91.

30. W. John Carr and Paul J. Feldstein, "The Relationship of Cost to Hospital Size," *Inquiry* 4 (June 1967):50–51; Judith K. Mann and Donald E. Yett, "The Analysis of Hospital Costs: A Review Article," *Journal of Business of the University of Chicago* 41 (April 1968):197.

31. See Irwin Deutscher et al., "A Survey of the Social and Occupational Characteristics of a Metropolitan Nursing Complement," mimeographed (Kansas City, Mo.: Community Studies, Inc., 1956), p. 56, for the 1955 figure. The 1964 figure was obtained from Margaret D. West and it represents one of the findings of her survey of the career patterns of all the graduates of the Hagerstown Hospital Nursing School during the period 1909–1963.

32. American Nurses' Association, *Facts About Nursing* (New York: By the Association, 1967), p. 11.

33. *Ibid.*, p. 10.

34. Archie Kleingartner, "Nurses, Collective Bargaining and Labor Legislation," *Labor Law Journal* 18 (April 1967):238; Karen S. Hawley, *Economics of Collective Bargaining by Nurses* (Ames: Iowa State University Industrial Relations Center, 1967), p. 149; and Daniel H. Kruger, "Bargaining and the Nursing Profession," *Monthly Labor Review* 84 (July 1961):704.

35. Memorandum from Evelyn B. Moses, Assistant Director of the Research and Statistics Department, American Nurses' Association, to Executive Directors of State Nurses' Associations, July 13, 1967; George L. Stelluto, "Earnings of Hospital Nurses, July 13, 1966," *Monthly Labor Review* 90 (July 1967):57–58.

36. American Nurses' Association, *Facts About Nursing*, p. 241.

37. Robert M. Ball, "Problems of Cost – as Experienced in Medicare," in U.S., Department of Health, Education, and Welfare, *Report of the National Conference on Medical Costs* (Washington, D.C.: U.S. Government Printing Office, 1967), p. 60.

38. Donald E. Yett, "The Nursing Shortage and the Nurse Training Act of 1964," *Industrial and Labor Relations Review* 19 (January 1966):200.

39. U.S., Department of Health, Education, and Welfare, Public Health Service, *Nurse Training Act of 1964*, Public Health Service Publication 1740 (Washington, D.C.: U.S. Government Printing Office, 1967), p. 3.

Sherwin Rosen
University of Rochester
and
National Bureau of Economic Research

COMMENT

Donald Yett's paper contains an extremely detailed examination of the presumed nursing "shortage" over the past twenty-five years. There have been widespread complaints about such a shortage from hospital administrators and others in the medical field during this period. What can be inferred about them from observed market data? Have we really experienced a nursing shortage, and if so, what can be done about it? The paper reflects considerable thought and a great deal of interesting and useful empirical work.

The major difficulty confronting Yett is in choosing a model with which to analyze this problem. There are two available candidates, and he chooses a modified version of one of them. My remarks will be confined to a critical discussion of these models and a sketch of an alternative that is not subject to the difficulties outlined.

The first model distinguishes short-run from long-run supply and presumes the former to be less elastic than the latter. Therefore, if an increase in demand results in a shortage (i.e., excess demand) at the old equilibrium price, the price must rise along the short-run supply curve to ration the relatively fixed number of nurses among eager demanders. The higher price calls forth new entry, which in turn reduces the price to its long-run equilibrium value. This analysis indicates that the new equilibrium price will most likely be higher than the old one, but the fact remains that long-run equilibrium values are not observed. As Yett recognizes, there will be a period when the price is falling, and this may dominate the observations; moreover, there can be no shortage except at the initial point.

Yett properly rejects such a model, primarily because of this defect. He adopts instead a modified version of the hypothesis that price changes are proportional to excess demand. There are some difficulties here, in that a dynamic structure is grafted onto what are otherwise equilibrium concepts. Supply and demand functions underlying the definition of excess demand do not apply when the market is out of equilibrium, for the conditions on which they are based do not hold. Yett's version is based on the fact that when the market adjustment is slow, demanders cannot hire as many nurses as they may desire at the going wage and conditions of work while the market is out of equilibrium; that is to say, they become monopsonists. It must be pointed out here that similar considerations hold on the other side of the market. In so far as this model is valid, the situation is more correctly described as "bilateral monopoly." Moreover, this situation can only be temporary, until the market gropes its way to the new equilibrium.

In order for the monopsony model to apply, there must be evidence of collusion on the demand side of the market. No persuasive evidence in this regard is presented. The importance of monopsony depends on the elasticity of supply, and there are several reasons for believing this elasticity to be high. Nurses currently employed in hospitals have the option of working in private duty and other nursing areas. In addition, the stock of potentially available nurses greatly exceeds the number employed because many trained nurses are engaged in non-market activities in their homes or are working in other occupations. The immense growth in market activities for women in general during this period undoubtedly produced a secular increase in the elasticity, and this has been manifested in the more general training of nurses. The evidence presented on the elasticity of supply is almost certainly biased and may very well reflect demand and other considerations, as can be inferred from the discussion below. Second, no evidence is presented for the existence of anti-pirating agreements. These must be present for collusive monopsony to characterize the nursing market. In this regard, it would be interesting to know the extent of turnover of nurses among hospitals within the same market area and the extent to which hospitals search other markets for nurses. However, even this knowledge would be inconclusive. We know that there is an enormous amount of labor market turnover for women, especially young women, and this situation must make policing collusive agreements difficult. Only small numbers on the margin are required to keep the system competitive. Third, it is difficult to understand the incentives for collusion. After all, hospitals, which are the major employers of nurses, are non-profit institutions. Even if a case could be established, for example, on the basis of effects on physicians' incomes, incentives to break such agreements are very large, as has been well documented in the literature.

In any case, the monopsonistic view of "shortages" has a superficial aspect. Excess demand cannot be defined for a monopsonist, since his demand function degenerates to a single point. It is certainly true that if the supply of nurses were somehow made elastic at the monopsonistic wage, more would be hired than are currently employed. In what sense is this a "shortage"? Would we be willing to make an analogous argument for monopolists and say that they exhibit "surpluses"? The argument attributes a certain degree of schizophrenia to hospital administrators. Given conditions of supply, they carefully find their optimum monopsonistic advantage, but then in reporting shortages they pretend that these supply conditions are different from what they truly are. If hospital decisionmakers wish that the supply conditions of some of the resources they buy were different, they are no different from most businessmen in that regard.

Another possible model produces an alternative interpretation of reported shortages. Inspection of the literature reveals that most complaints about labor market shortages in recent years concern classes of workers that embody a heavy component of human capital. In such markets adjustments on both demand and supply sides are likely to be costly and, in the face of uncertainty, will be distributed over time. It therefore becomes necessary to distinguish between long- and short-run responses on both sides of the market.

To simplify the presentation, I will use the simplest possible functional forms and discuss only a deterministic model. Monopsonistic elements could also be brought into it, but I do not do so here.

Let the long-run supply of nurses be

$$\overline{N}_t^s = a_{10} + a_{11} W_t - a_{12} P_t,$$

where W_t is an index of current wage conditions in nursing, and P represents a set of other variables affecting long-run supply, including alternative earnings in other occupations that nurses could enter and, since undertaking nursing training amounts to an investment, an index of expected future relative earnings. N^s is the number of nurses that would be forthcoming if W and P were constant for long periods of time. Short-run supply should be far less elastic. Suppose that after a period of stability W increases. A period of time will elapse before potentially active nurses discover how persistent the increase is: if it was not advantageous to enter nursing before, it will be disadvantageous to do so if the wage change is temporary. Thus temporary changes will call forth very few additional nurses. As the increased wage persists, more of it will be regarded as permanent, and this belief will eventually be sufficient to overcome the frictions and costs of changing jobs or re-entering the labor force for those already possessing nursing skills. It will also increase nursing trainees. A natural way of handling this delayed response is to postulate a lagged adjustment between actual and long-run supply:

$$N_t^s - N_{t-1}^s = \beta_1 (\overline{N}_t^s - N_{t-1}^s), 0 < \beta_1 < 1.0.$$

The change in the number of nurses actively engaged in the market is proportional to the difference between the number who would enter if conditions remained stable for long periods and the number who were previously in the market. This provides for gradual adjustment of supply to its long-run equilibrium with the speed of response governed by β_1. The higher it is, the faster the adjustment.

Now define a long-run demand curve for nurses:

$$\overline{N}_t^d = a_{20} - a_{21} W_t + a_{22} X_t,$$

where X is a conglomerate shift variable reflecting such things as the demand for medical care, technological changes in its production, prices of substitute inputs for nursing services, and future wage conditions. This is also interpretable as the total number of nurses demanded if existing conditions remained constant over time. Now suppose X rises after a long period of stability. There are substantial hiring, market searching, and training costs to employers to enter the market, and they will not undertake such costs if the change is regarded as temporary. Therefore, the immediate response is to utilize existing personnel more intensively and to turn to readily available, though inferior, substitutes. As they recognize the new conditions to be permanent, they will ultimately enter the market and increase employment. Therefore, specify a lagged response

$$N_t^d - N_{t-1}^d = \beta_2 (\overline{N}_t^d - N_{t-1}^d), \quad 0 < \beta_2 < 1.0.$$

The change in the number of nurses demanded is proportional to the difference between the number demanded in the long run and the number demanded in the last period. A term reflecting replacements of voluntary quits should also be added, but its omission does not alter the analysis in any important way.

Now that dynamic demand and supply functions have been specified, the model is closed by allowing current market price to serve its economic function of equating current market supply and current market demand. The market achieves short-run equilibrium in each period. If that is not identical to long-run equilibrium, market forces drive employment and wages to their ultimate stationary values.

A reduced form of this system is (ignoring constants) proportional to

$$N_t = -\beta_2 a_{21} P_t + \beta_1 a_{11} X_t + \rho N_{t-1}$$

$$W_t = \beta_1 a_{12} P_t - \beta_1 a_{12} (1 - \beta_2) P_{t-1} + \beta_2 a_{22} X_t - \beta_2 a_{22} (1 - \beta_1) X_{t-1} + \rho W_{t-1},$$

where ρ is a function of β_1, β_2 and the a_{ij}. Market stability is ensured by the requirement that $|\rho| < 1.0$. Let V_t denote the number of reported vacancies at the going wage. This is in fact the "shortage" and represents the difference between long-run demand and actual employment at existing conditions. It is the additional number of workers that employers are ultimately seeking to hire. The path of these dynamic shortages or unfilled vacancies is proportional to

$$V_t = a_{11}a_{22}\beta_2 (1 - \beta_1) (X_t - X_{t-1}) - \beta_2(1 - \beta_1)a_{12}a_{21}(P_t - P_{t-1}).$$

Suppose that it was agreed that a shortage existed, and the model indicated steadily increasing employment over time. It is still not necessarily true that wages will increase. That will depend on the relative values of the short-run elasticities of supply and demand and how rapidly these curves shift in relation to each other. The speed of response in the market depends on the magnitude of transaction costs on both sides of the market, while the actual course of prices, employment, and vacancies depends on initial conditions (roughly, the distance from long-run equilibrium), the course of X and P, and the *difference* between transaction costs on each side of the market, as well as their magnitude. With more complicated models of this sort it is even possible for reported vacancies to coexist with decreases in employment.

This is clearly not the place to discuss all the implications of this model. Suffice it to say that there may be some pitfalls in identifying the nature of shortages from isolated observations on market incomes and employment. This is recognized by Yett in his discussion of the first model. Indeed, this model will be recognized as an extension of the model which he rejects. However, it is not subject to the difficulties he lists, and, most important, it gives a clear and logical meaning to reported nurse vacancy or shortage statistics. It is a plausible and attractive alternative and can be estimated rather easily. Finally, its policy implications are sufficiently different from Yett's to more than warrant serious consideration.

REJOINDER

Sherwin Rosen states that in my "version" of an economic shortage model employers "become monopsonists" when, as a result of a slow market adjustment speed, they "cannot hire as many nurses as they may desire at the going wage and conditions of work while the market is out of equilibrium." This is not correct. The existence of monopsony or oligopsony does not depend upon the market adjustment speed. Any employer who *individually* faces an upward-sloping supply curve has some degree of monopsony or oligopsony power and will, therefore, report that he would like to hire more labor at the going wage. This is an equilibrium, not a disequilibrium, condition. In the paper I demonstrate that the "vacancies" resulting from monopsony and oligopsony are intrinsically different from those due to market disequilibrium.

If, indeed, it were true that market disequilibrium creates monopoly power, then Rosen's claim that "the situation is more correctly described as 'bilateral monopoly' " would be true. His definition is, of course, not the standard description of bilateral monopoly power. However, ample evidence is presented to show that *individual* nurses have little bargaining power, and that nurse collective bargaining is of minor importance at this time. Thus, applying the conventional definition of the term, it is apparent that the nurse market cannot be "correctly described as 'bilateral monopoly.' "

Rosen asserts that the monopsony model requires "evidence of collusion." This is incorrect. Monopsony is defined as the existence of one employer in a labor market. This may mean that only one employer exists, or that numerous employers collude so as to behave as a single employer. When I used the term monopsony it was always in the former sense. Evidence is presented in the paper that in some local markets a single hospital is effectively the only employer. In such cases monopsony applies so long as wage-induced mobility among markets is low.

An oligopsony model was developed to explain behavior in markets with several hospital employers, and evidence of collusive oligopsonistic (not monopsonistic) behavior is presented with respect to large urban areas. The element of collusion is not critical. So long as each employer can exert a noticeable influence over the market wage, a condition of oligopsony can be said to prevail. Evidence of overt collusion merely strengthens the argument by showing that each buyer explicitly realizes that he can affect the market price (wage), and that any attempt to outbid other buyers in the same market for the services of nurses will not go unnoticed but rather will initiate a "wage war" which will result in a higher total wage bill with little change in total employment. Under these circumstances, the typical hospital association seeks to minimize the probability of a wage war by acting as a wage policy coordinator. Its wage recommendations prevail because each member fears the consequences of a wage war, not because of overt "anti-pirating" agreements with effective "policing" on the part of the association.

Rosen rejects the evidence that the short-run elasticity of nurse supply is low, not on the basis of empirical estimates,* but rather on the grounds that

*Recent unpublished studies by Stuart Altman, Mario Bognanno, and Jesse Hixson all confirm my estimate that short-run nurse supply is inelastic within the range of observation.

nurses have other options (both within and outside of nursing) and that large numbers of nurses are professionally inactive. The tie between private duty, office, and hospital positions is clearly documented in the paper — as are the reasons why employment in other fields of nursing has little effect on hospital employment conditions. Evidence that only about 2 per cent of registered nurses work outside of nursing — and that this percentage has not yet been raised by "more general training of nurses" — is presented and discussed in the paper.

The fact that a large percentage of trained nurses do not work at all has little bearing on the situation unless they are all on the margin. In fact, the supply elasticity estimates generated using participation rate changes over the years confirm that few nurses are on the margin at, or near, the prevailing wage rate. Furthermore, high turnover rates are not inconsistent with the presence of monopsony or oligopsony (or even collusion) unless they are *wage-induced*. As is documented in the paper, all available evidence indicates that the high turnover rates observed in hospital nursing are not the result of wage differentials or other conditions deriving from competitive efforts on the part of hospitals as nurse employers. They are primarily the result of exogenous factors (e.g., marriage, child care, family relocation, etc.).

In many respects I agree with Rosen that "the monopsonistic view of 'shortages' has a superficial aspect." It is, of course, true that "excess demand cannot be defined for a monopsonist" or oligopsonist in equilibrium, but I did not make that assertion. "Excess demand" can exist only in a disequilibrium situation. However, monopsonistic vacancies are present in equilibrium situations and represent the difference between the amount of labor actually hired and the amount the monopsonist stands ready to hire at the prevailing wage. This is a "shortage" only in the sense that when explicitly asked how many additional workers he would *like* to hire at the prevailing wage, he would report a positive number. Whether such a shortage is deserving of policy consideration is another question altogether. If one asked a monopolist whether he would like to sell more output at the prevailing price, he would say "Yes," and would report a quantity which would represent the difference between the amount he is now selling and the amount corresponding to the intersection of his marginal cost curve and the prevailing price. The fact that demand is not sufficient to allow him to sell that quantity at that price is beside the point (and is never put into question). In the hospital nursing market the question *is* asked, and hospital administrators respond in a predictable manner. I have attempted to explain why they have responded in this manner for over thirty years, and why there is nothing "schizophrenic" about such behavior. It is not schizophrenic to say, if asked, that you would like to hire more labor at the existing wage even though you would not be willing to raise wages.

Rosen presents an "alternative interpretation of reported shortages" which bears a close similarity to one of the models I rejected. Specifically, his shortage "represents the difference between long-run demand and actual employment at existing conditions. It is the additional number of workers that employers are ultimately seeking to hire." The "actual employment at existing conditions" is described by the intersection of the short-run supply and demand curves — short-run equilibrium. Using this definition, all markets in a dynamic economy are always experiencing either "shortages" or "surpluses." Moreover, estimation of the size of the "shortage" is impossible without knowledge of the long-run equilibrium position. That these data are impossible to gather before the fact he would soon discover if he attempted to estimate the parameters contained in his model. Rosen is not entirely accurate in his contention that his model "is not subject to the difficulties" I identified in criticizing one interpretation of the Blank-Stigler model. No matter how "clear and logical" the meaning of reported vacancies in his model, it is readily apparent first, that they are not the type which are regularly reported by hospital administrators (which is the type I sought to explain) and second, that they do not measure a "shortage" in any of the several senses in which the term is currently employed by health manpower planners. In addition, his model suffers from the principal defect of the original Arrow-Capron model — namely, it requires an estimate of the amount of labor the employer would seek to hire after he had traced out all the implications of his decision.

In view of the above considerations, I question Rosen's contention that his model "is a plausible and attractive alternative" to mine, and I seriously doubt that he would continue to claim that it "can be estimated rather easily" if he actually tried to do so.

D. E. Y.

Charlotte F. Muller and Paul Worthington
City University of New York

FACTORS ENTERING INTO CAPITAL DECISIONS OF HOSPITALS

Interest in the provision of adequate community health facilities stems from a long tradition of egalitarian movements, a recognition of the social costs of ill health, and the desire to improve the stock of human capital. A part of this interest is focused on the problem of providing adequate capital for hospitals.

In the past the investment behavior of hospitals has received only a modest amount of attention. The investment behavior of commercial firms is explained in terms of familiar economic concepts: choosing among alternative amounts of capital, they base their decisions to add or not to add to capital stock on an evaluation of the expected productive contribution of the flow of services which can be attributed to each alternative and on the rate of interest, which is the cost of funds to the firm.[1] But little has been learned about factors which might systematically explain the investment decisions of voluntary hospitals.

The non-profit credentials of the voluntary hospital, surprisingly well preserved in the face of increased commercialization, have been largely responsible for this dearth of exploration. Capital has not been placed by hospital management under the same accounting rules as other inputs. Administrators have not sought to collect the full cost of capital services through pricing policy; i.e., depreciation expense and imputed interest on internal funds have been omitted. Before Medicare, inventories of capital assets were

This research was supported by Grant HM-00646-01, United States Public Health Service, and was carried out at the Center for Social Research, City University of New York. We should like to acknowledge the cooperation of the United Hospital Fund of New York and of Hortense Dillon. Acknowledgments are due also to Anne Picker, Data Management, Clara Federschmid, Secretary, and Dr. Leonard S. Kogan, Statistical Consultant.

rare. There have been no systematic and accepted means of funding capital accumulation within institutions and within a group of institutions in a region. There has been little expectation that charges would cover capital costs — indeed, even meeting non-capital operating costs was not assured. The organizations made a virtue of their lack of business orientation with respect to capital, and to a considerable extent this is still the case.

Since 1945 the separate treatment of capital has become more and more difficult to maintain. Conventionally calculated allowances for depreciation, as distinct from a fixed percentage of operating cost, have come to be included as elements of reimbursable costs in Blue Cross hospital contracts. Similar allowances are provided in Medicare regulations.[2]

Concern with the adequacy of resources for meeting expanding commitments for care has directed attention to the way in which hospital and health capital is and could be formed. The belief has been current that capital accumulation depends on availability of capital funds, and that this availability, in turn, depends on government decisions (exogenous) and philanthropy (essentially fortuitous).[3] These assertions leave unexplained the basic reasons why voluntary hospitals seek additional funds.

In a study conducted in New York City it was hypothesized that an evaluation by the hospital of the productive contribution of alternative stocks of capital is a determinant of desired investment, and thus of the level of investment activity. On this basis, it should be possible to predict a substantial portion of investment behavior from the movement of variables which reflect hospital services currently produced and demanded.

The relationship between such variables and actual investment data was tested on data for twenty-one years of operation of forty voluntary hospitals in New York City. These data were made available by the United Hospital Fund. Annual reports were examined, and time series were developed for investment in plant and equipment, extensive and intensive aspects of services provided, and extent of teaching commitment and activity.* (Teaching services form part of the productive activity of hospitals and impose diverse demands on facilities.) A full twenty-one-year time series for member hospitals in 1965 was constructed. Necessary adjustments were made in the data to estimate missing observations, to separate buildings and equipment from land in asset accounts, to reconcile differences in accounting practices, and to combine the experiences of parties to a merger.

The principal findings were as follows: when annual aggregates for the forty hospitals were treated as variables, 68 per cent of the variance in annual real investment† was explained by three factors: yearly changes in an output index, yearly changes in the ratio of semiprivate days to admissions, and an

---

*UHF data were supplemented by AMA directories of internships and residencies.
†The deflator used was the Dow Construction Cost Index.

allowance for a distributed lag in carrying out desired investment projects. In a cross-section of means for each variable, the lag disappeared, and somewhat different variables stood out as predictors. Of the variance in mean annual real investment per hospital, 56 per cent was explained by mean annual differences in admissions and in the extent of teaching commitment. This is a brief summary of the results of our work, which involved several trials with modifications of the hypothesized relationship.

CAPITAL IN THE HOSPITAL ECONOMY

In the course of their operations, hospitals are obliged to choose among alternative uses of resources, and they do in fact select some option from the array presented. The selection itself implies a preference and can reasonably be interpreted as implying comparison and evaluation of outcomes of the various alternatives.

This statement is applicable to any resource, and in this sense hospital capital is homogeneous with hospital labor. We are familiar with discussions of shortages of both capital and labor in hospitals. The fact that a hospital can calculate a shortage of any resource presupposes that, given its demand conditions and the state of technical knowledge, the hospital knows the number and types of personnel that it wants and the size and design of the plant and equipment that it wants. The reference to what "the hospital wants" is deliberate: it is not assumed that the conditions considered by the hospital in determining its demand for factors of production are necessarily an expression of society's needs. The services of resources are demanded because they contribute to some outcome that is a final objective of the institution making the decision. Certain authors have suggested that hospitals operate so as to "maximize" output, however defined. In a somewhat different argument,* Baumol and Bowen describe the typical non-profit organization as being in pursuit of quality services as an end in itself. Citing research, the performing arts, and adequate hospital facilities as examples, they say: "These [quality] goals constitute bottomless receptacles into which limitless funds can be poured."[4] The notion of "bottomless receptacles" implies that a non-profit hospital will always have a list of projects which it would like to finance in the event that funds were available.[5] The idea captures a facet of the non-profit style but does not provide insight into the mechanism by which the hospital chooses among "eligible" projects.

One must assume that changes in the conditions which provide the basis for evaluating the outcome of various alternatives do influence the target goals of hospitals in seeking out funds, and thus the amounts eventually received and spent; that is, hospital initiative and demand take on an auton-

---

*Theirs is a different but not a contrasting view, since production of health services at a higher level of quality is in some ways an increase in output.

omous role in the capital allocation process. Factors which are believed to be influential in evaluating alternative allocations include the hospital-doctor relationship.[6] Admitting privileges of doctors stem from private arrangements with hospitals. Doctors are therefore disposed to go where they will have the greatest possible array of services and facilities to support their private practices. The hospital thus acquires a motive for taking into account the capital it will require both for the patient load it anticipates and for satisfaction of the requirements of the physicians admitting the patients. The basis is laid for an investment policy – a planned response to new technology and to the expansion of services and the treatment of more patients. The hospital must respond because the doctor can withdraw his affiliation if he becomes dissatisfied with the hospital's services. Implicit in this reasoning is the fact that doctors at levels of skill and range of specialization that the hospital would like to retain or attract are relatively scarce.

What are the economic considerations which lie behind the doctor-hospital arrangement? A productive factor that can claim the value of its marginal product as its rate of return, which is possible in fee-for-service pricing, can increase its return with no increase in price by raising its productivity. This can be achieved by increasing the input of other factor services relative to its own. Consequently, doctors in hospital-oriented medical practice can increase their incomes without cost to themselves and without raising fees by arranging for the hospital to increase the personnel, beds, and facilities at their disposal.[7] Thus, the amount of capital which the hospital desires to invest in plant and equipment will be determined by the ability of that capital to contribute to the production of services in two ways: (1) delivery of the anticipated type and amount of care, and (2) ability to attract and hold medical staff. These two functions may be served by the same unit of capital.

The tendency of hospitals to duplicate facilities[8] flows from their competition for doctors. The result is that unmet needs coexist with excess capacity, and the community loses services. The present relationship, in which doctors, although neither owners nor employees, have a voice in management decisions, may pass into history as a transitional form of hospital organization as more doctors assume full-time posts at hospitals. However, given the relative scarcity of doctors, the incentive for hospitals to try to provide doctors with technically optimal facilities will remain.

The teaching hospital offers a special case of the general proposition. Its patient composition differs from that of community hospitals; care is consequently different, and more demands are made on its facilities. Management desires to attract doctors with specialized qualifications, and these doctors have extra requirements; indeed, management itself has special requirements in a strong teaching hospital. Certain laboratories and other facilities are needed for the specific purpose of carrying out the teaching function. In addition, both present and future teaching status would be expected to have a bearing on the hospital's demand for facilities.

TEACHING STATUS

Planning of hospital capital spending is probably influenced both by past experience and by future expectations. It is aimed either at maintaining an established position within the broad ranking by teaching status of the city's institutions or at increasing the hospital's activity in teaching and related clinical services as part of the general upgrading of health and welfare services in the surrounding community. Data available in our study made it possible not only to classify hospitals on the basis of teaching status in 1965 but also to observe changes in this status over the preceding twenty years. During the years 1946–1965 the forty voluntary hospitals in our survey invested more than $340 million, at current prices, in plant structures and equipment. It was part of our original hypothesis that teaching commitment of hospitals would be associated with strength of demand for plant and equipment. It was both convenient and plausible to use end-of-period (1965) teaching status in assigning a rank to individual hospitals.

For our purposes four classes were defined, the highest having a major medical school affiliation, and the second having five or more approved residencies. Hospitals in the third class were approved for internship, but had fewer than five approved residencies, and the fourth and lowest class includes hospitals with no internship approval. The two upper groups were combined into one to create a dummy variable; the two lower groups were similarly treated.

Hospitals in different teaching ranks maintain distinctly different medical styles, which are reflected in resource requirements as well as in variations in patient mix. An illustrative example from the 1965 data is given below.

Activity in Hospitals by Teaching Status

Functional Ratios	Teaching Status			
	1 (High)	2	3	4 (Low)
No. of hospitals	8	13	12	7
Operations/admission	0.46	0.66	0.53	0.32
X-ray films/admission	9.33	10.79	8.80	2.95
Laboratory tests/admission	27.01	33.47	31.32	12.79
Semiprivate days/admission	4.22	7.54	6.48	4.19
Interns and residents/bed	0.15	0.19	0.14	0.03
Special/general professional staff	0.29	0.39	0.36	0.22

The second class of hospitals in several ways showed more intensive activity than the rest.

Of the forty hospitals studied, twenty-one held the same teaching status in 1945 and in 1965, with no change in status in the intervening years. Seven hospitals changed status during the interval but ended in their original class. These seven were mostly upward-strivers if not upward-movers. Another ten hospitals moved up in status. Two hospitals, each with fewer than five approved residencies, merged to produce a hospital with a major medical school affiliation. Two hospitals moved down in status by losing their approval for internship. In 1945 fifteen of the forty hospitals were in the upper two classes and twenty-five were in the others. By 1965 there were twenty-one in the upper classes and nineteen in the lower classes.

Movement in Teaching Status, 1945-1965

Categories	*Teaching Status*			
	1 (High)	2	3	4 (Low)
Same status, 1945–1965	6	4	7	4
Beginning and ending status the same, with temporary change	–	2	4	1
Ending status of upward-movers	2	7	1	–
Ending status of downward-movers	–	–	–	2
All hospitals, 1945	7	8	19	6
All hospitals, 1965	8	13	12	7
Average investment per hospital (millions)	$20	$9	$4	$2

These data, collected from AMA directories,[9] reveal an unmistakable upward movement in teaching commitment. The record probably understates this movement for two reasons. First, the categories are broad. For example, an increase in the number of residency programs would not lift a hospital out of class 2. Second, with advances in medical knowledge and social expectations, the input content attached to teaching programs probably has gone up. In summary, 1965 teaching status was a good predictor during the period 1945–1965 of "expected future status," and in over half the cases was identical with "current status."

Of the total investment ($340 million) of the forty hospitals in the period, major medical school affiliates spent 46 per cent and hospitals with five or more residency programs another 35 per cent. Average investment per hospital was $20 million at the highest teaching level and $2 million at the lowest.

METHOD OF REGRESSION ANALYSIS

Investment data on an annual basis are presented in Table 1, along with measures of the extensive and intensive changes in services provided. The rate

Table 1: Total Gross Investment, Admissions, and Selected Functional Ratios for Forty Hospitals, 1945–1965

Year	Gross Investment	Admissions	Functional Ratios					
			Operations/ Admissions	X-Ray Films/ Admissions	Laboratory Examinations/ Admissions	Semi-private Patient Days/ Admissions	Interns and Residents/ Beds	Professional Care: Special Staff/ General Staff
1945	$1,261,379	278,379	.533	2.525	8.516	3.706	.062	.220
1946	2,367,903	303,252	.568	2.981	9.292	3.449	.082	.226
1947	2,367,903	323,492	.550	3.253	9.827	3.388	.084	.229
1948	4,425,011	324,434	.549	3.545	10.743	3.587	.087	.232
1949	7,762,421	325,927	.550	3.821	11.652	3.578	.092	.242
1950	10,282,013	334,154	.547	4.103	11.660	3.740	.091	.246
1951	15,375,865	341,394	.543	4.008	11.647	3.774	.093	.247
1952	10,410,972	344,960	.525	4.247	12.010	3.927	.095	.246
1953	14,279,434	354,161	.526	4.434	12.506	4.175	.095	.254
1954	11,929,146	364,058	.508	4.674	12.703	4.656	.102	.254
1955	21,926,987	371,280	.509	4.996	13.726	4.553	.106	.253
1956	8,788,423	383,909	.512	5.274	14.553	4.763	.113	.259
1957	14,519,396	391,845	.503	5.258	15.769	4.805	.124	.248
1958	20,641,059	398,515	.499	5.540	17.436	4.806	.125	.255
1959	17,675,633	408,745	.503	5.808	18.751	4.927	.128	.262
1960	15,404,627	410,872	.499	6.152	19.043	5.087	.127	.266
1961	26,480,726	415,042	.496	6.422	19.755	5.252	.129	.276
1962	28,889,981	421,653	.515	6.763	22.148	5.264	.127	.278
1963	36,625,322	428,318	.522	7.199	23.805	5.314	.139	.284
1964	38,333,310	438,990	.521	7.737	24.904	5.386	.143	.281
1965	32,954,581	448,497	.518	8.457	27.393	5.491	.144	.309

of investment per year in current prices is defined as the annual change in adjusted book value of plant and equipment, as reported by the hospital to the United Hospital Fund.

Because it was believed that the estimates of annual investment often understate gross investment, it was decided to take them as approximations of net investment in current prices. These figures are deflated by the Dow Construction Cost Index provided by McGraw-Hill Services. This index does not include equipment and, by definition, does not take into account changes in productivity. The downward bias imposed by these factors is in opposition to the possible upward bias inherent in assuming that the investment is net. The deflated figures serve as approximations for the rate of real net investment. The hypothesis about factors influencing this rate is as follows: observed investment by hospitals can be predicted to a considerable extent from observations of annual changes in variables reflecting hospital services currently produced and demanded. The original design called for trial of this relationship in three forms. *Model 1*, yearly aggregate data for all hospitals combined for the years 1945-1965; this approach yielded 19 observations.* *Model 2*, a pool of 760 (40 × 19) observations of annual investment by individual hospitals, matched with values of the predictor variables. *Model 3*, average annual rates of investment per hospital and average annual change in predictor variables over twenty years, that is, 40 observations, one for each hospital.

Seven variables were selected to account for investment in the period These were the increment between periods (*t*-2) and (*t*-1) in the following areas: (1) *admissions* (this was taken as a measure of extensive demand for hospital services); (2) *operations per admission*; (3) *X-rays per admission*; (4) *laboratory tests per admission*. These ratios were taken as measures of intensive demand for hospital service. Also studied were (5) *semiprivate days per admission*, a measure of the hospital's shift away from ward care to care of solvent insured patients; (6) *interns and residents per bed*, a measure of teaching activity, a major service product of metropolitan hospitals; (7) *ratio of special to general professional staff*, a general measure of the relative intensity of services. Special professional staff includes those in such departments as X-ray, laboratory, and operating room. General professional staff includes interns, residents and nurses on inpatient service, pharmacists, social workers, etc. A final predictor variable, investment in period (*t*-1), was included to take care of the lag arising from the fact that an investment plan, a desired adjustment, takes several years to complete.

---

*Since differences in capital stock from year to year constituted the measure of investment, there were 20 observations of investment. However, to match 1947 investment, 1945-1946 changes in predictor variables were used, and a similar procedure was followed for each subsequent year; therefore, there were 19 observations to use in the equation.

TRENDS IN THE VARIABLES

The twenty-one-year trends in the values of the variables show a note-worthy increase in the various aspects of hospital service. Admissions rose from 278,000 to 448,000. X-rays per admission went up from 2.5 to 8.5, and laboratory tests per admission more than tripled, going from 8.5 to 27.4. The number of interns and residents per bed rose from 0.06 to 0.14 and the ratio of special to general professional staff rose from 0.22 to 0.31. Semiprivate days per admission went up 50 per cent (from 3.7 to 5.5) in the period.

The one exception to the rise in the "functional ratios" was the ratio of operations to admissions, which remained at 0.5. (AMA figures show an actual decline between 1946 and 1961, from 0.49 to 0.43 nationally, and a slightly smaller decline for the northeast region.[10]) It would appear that the transformation of admissions into highly active work sessions was partially brought about by non-surgical modalities. In addition, since the "mix" of surgery became more complex, the number of operations in different years fails to measure the number of inputs required.*

Table 2: Real Investment, Changes in Semiprivate Patient Days
per Admission (Lagged One Period), and Changes in
Average Output Equivalent: Annual Aggregate, Forty
Voluntary General Hospitals

Year	Real Investment (00 omitted)	Change in Semiprivate Patient Days/ Admission	Change in Average Output Equivalent
1946	$1,261.3	–	–
1947	2,097.3	-.257	32,947
1948	3,624.0	-.061	19,029
1949	6,290.4	.199	19,601
1950	8,597.0	-.009	19,007
1951	11,560.8	.162	5,159
1952	7,804.3	.034	13,222
1953	10,593.0	.153	23,585
1954	8,720.1	.248	20,680
1955	15,441.5	.481	32,674
1956	5,878.5	-.103	38,014
1957	9,452.7	.210	23,028
1958	13,273.9	.042	39,764
1959	11,144.7	.001	43,121
1960	9,456.4	.121	20,153
1961	15,952.2	.160	26,172
1962	17,044.2	.165	58,755
1963	21,232.0	.012	52,779
1964	21,854.7	.050	57,699
1965	18,400.1	.072	83,139

*Because operations per admission *was* a static ratio, the output variable was recalcu-lated with this component omitted, without prejudice to the correlation presented on p. 410 (annual aggregates for forty hospitals).

The trend of investment in the time period studied was upward. At current prices, investment by the forty study hospitals rose from $1,261,000 in 1946 to $32,955,000 in 1965 (deflated value, $18,400,000; see Table 2). Six hospitals which closed their doors during the study period had a mean annual rate of investment of $36,370 over eighty-six hospital-years of observations and had a total investment of a little over $3 million, or less than 1 per cent of the investment by the forty hospitals which survived the two decades in original or merged form. The average annual rate of investment was far below the $425,418 rate for the forty hospitals included in the regression analysis.

ADJUSTMENT OF CAPITAL STOCK

Behind the relationship between investment and the predictor variables described lies a supposition about the dynamic process of adjusting capital stock from some historical level toward some desired level. Both levels are continually changing. The size of desired capital stock is related to the anticipated future levels of its determinants, to which the present and the recent past serve as guides.[11]

Letting X_i represent the ith determinant and $\hat{K}$ the desired stock of capital, and letting the subscript t denote the year for all flows and the end of the year for all stocks, the basic hypothesis, assuming linearity and using seven determinants, can be stated as follows:

$$(1) \qquad \hat{K}_t = \sum_{i=1}^{7} \delta_i X_{i_{t-1}}.$$

Changes in the determinants, as described previously, set in motion the dynamic adjustment process. Desired real investment $(\hat{I}_t)$ is the difference between desired and existing capital stock.

$$(2) \qquad \hat{I}_t = \hat{K}_t - K_{t-1},$$

and by substitution

$$(3) \qquad \hat{I}_t = \sum_{i=1}^{7} \delta_i X_{i_{t-1}} - K_{t-1}.$$

On the assumption that only a (constant) fraction of a desired adjustment is completed in each period,* the *observed* rate of investment is

$$(4) \qquad I_t = \beta \left(\sum_{i=1}^{7} \delta_i X_{i_{t-1}} - K_{t-1} \right).$$

---

*This is an expression of the stock adjustment principle used widely in empirical economic analysis.[12]

By writing this equation for t-1 and making appropriate substitutions, one puts the investment equation in a form useful for empirical testing, as follows:

$$(5) \qquad I_t = \text{constant} + \beta \sum_{i=1}^{7} \delta_i(X_{i_{t-1}} - X_{i_{t-2}}) + (1-\beta)I_{t-1}.$$

FINDINGS OF VARIOUS TRIALS

Model 1: Yearly Aggregate Data

The eight predictor variables were used in an early trial of the first version of the relationship with yearly aggregate data. Over half the variance was explained.* However, intercorrelations between three pairs of variables were found and the large number of variables imposed a high threshold for statistical significance. Accordingly, a revised version of this equation was created. An average output equivalent was developed, combining the influence of admissions and the ratios of operations, X-ray films, and laboratory tests to admissions. An output equivalent was calculated for each ratio variable in each year, using the value of the ratio in 1945 as a base. For example, in 1945 there were 2.5 X-ray films per admission. For each succeeding year an output equivalent was calculated for this variable by dividing actual total X-ray films by 2.5. For each year admissions and the output equivalent calculated for the three service ratios were summed and divided by 4. The year-to-year changes in the resulting variable were substituted in the regression equation for variables 1–4. The effect of using this variable is to give more weight to an absolute increase in services when the base year intensity (ratio to admissions) is low. The output equivalent is an admittedly rough attempt to amalgamate the impact of growth of various services, and so to reduce the number of predictor variables.

---

*R^2 is .56. The equation, as estimated, is as follows (investment in hundreds of dollars), with t statistics in parentheses below each regression coefficient:

$$I_t = 23,380.2 - 1.14 \, \Delta X_1 + 311.30 \, \Delta X_2 + 50.26 \, \Delta X_3$$
$$\quad (0.6515) \quad (-0.5775) \quad (0.2815) \quad (0.6761)$$

$$+ 17.33 \, \Delta X_4 + 157.04 \, \Delta X_5 + 698.28 \, \Delta X_6$$
$$\quad (0.8958) \quad (2.1432) \quad (0.3216)$$

$$- 1,198.81 \, \Delta X_7 + 0.56 \, I_{t-1} \quad (n = 19).$$
$$\quad (-0.5640) \quad (2.9015)$$

The coefficient for the change in semiprivate patient days per admission (ΔX_5) is significant at the .10 level, and the coefficient for the lagged value of investment (I_{t-1}) at the .02 level. Their last order partials are .56 and .67, and they are not associated.

Variables X_6 (interns and residents per bed) and X_7 (professional staff intensity ratio) were deleted because they showed no association with investment. Furthermore, since a preliminary trial indicated that the response of investment to output changes was more rapid than originally assumed, output change from $(t\text{-}1)$ to (t) was matched with investment in t. It was assumed that changes in output and changes in emphasis on semiprivate days were independent, so that the time subscript of the latter was not affected. The resulting equation is

(6) I_t = constant + $\beta \delta_5 \Delta X_5 + \beta \delta_8 \Delta X_8 + (1 - \beta)I_{t-1}$.

The results of the multiple regression analysis based on this equation are as follows:

(6a) I_t = 20,022.41 + 136.80 ΔX_5 + .94 ΔX_8 + .49 I_{t-1} (n = 19).
  (1.19)   (2.74)   (1.52)   (2.41)

The multiple R^2 is .68. The coefficients of changes in semiprivate days per admission (X_5) and of previous year investment I_{t-1} are significant at the .05 level, but the coefficient of the average output equivalent is significant only at the .15 level. These results show that over two-thirds of the variance in investment is predictable by the combined effect of changes in output, changeover to semiprivate (insured) care, and a distributed time lag. Multicollinearity is indicated by the simple correlation between ΔX_8 and I_{t-1} * (see Table 3).

The implied values for the basic parameters of the equation — δ_5, δ_8, and β — can be derived from equation 6. $\beta = 1 - .49$, or .51.† β is the fraction of a given desired addition to capital stock that is accomplished in a given period. Thus, the value .51 implies that about five years of investment activity would be required to complete a desired addition to capital stock.

For community planning purposes, the value of β establishes an *average* expected time between initiation of facility projects and their readiness to deliver service. For very rough comparison, New York City's municipal hospital sector shows a mean completion time for projects of 70.5 months in much the same historical period, with the first month in which design progress was reported counted as month 1.[13] (This is about one-sixth longer than the voluntary sector time.) This information helped to define the lead time required for planning inputs to materialize in service capacity at a desired date.

---

*However, the determinant of the matrix of independent variables is increased from .086 in the trial with eight variables to .401 in the present version, implying a reduction in multicollinearity.

†This by division gives a value of 267.39 for δ_5 and 1.84 for δ_8.

Table 3: Matrix of Zero-Order Correlation Coefficients for Selected Variables: Annual Aggregates, Forty Voluntary General Hospitals, 1947–1965

Variables	Real Investment (t)	Change in Semiprivate Patient Days per Admission $(t-1)$	Change in Average Output Equivalent (t)	Real Investment $(t-1)$
Real investment (t)	1.0000	0.3547	0.6531	0.7634
Change in semiprivate patient days per admission $(t-1)$	—	1.0000	0.1352	0.0371
Change in average output equivalent (t)	—	—	1.0000	0.7563
Real investment $(t-1)$	—	—	—	1.0000

Model 2: Pooled Data

The correlations just reported did not carry over to a trial of the second version of the hypothesis based on pooled data for forty hospitals. A dummy variable, teaching status, was added as a predictor in order to use a measure of teaching commitment as a determinant of desired investment which would be more revealing of facility requirements than the ratio of house staff to beds. This trial of the general model produced a trivial R^2 of .08 and was inundated with small but significant correlations between the various independent variables.

These results at the disaggregated level are consistent with similar trials in commercial sectors of the economy. Robert Eisner offers an explanation: capital expenditures are influenced by expected changes in demand, and the firm, in estimating future demand, considers only those variations in past demand which it interprets as permanent. Alternative groupings of the data produce alternative observed proxies for the estimates of changes in future demand, with different "permanent" components.[14] On the basis of this reasoning, a hospital turns less to short-run movements in its own service variables than to the experience of its reference group (hospitals with a similar level, mission, and regional location) as an indicator of its own future prospects. Transitory fluctuations in individual hospital experience tend to cancel each other out when the mean experience of a hospital over time is calculated, so that a cross-sectional comparison of hospital means would reflect the permanent component in average annual differences among hospitals.

Model 3: Annual Averages per Hospital

The foregoing serves to introduce the trial of the relationship expressed in terms of average annual investment per hospital and annual averages for the predictor variables (version 3). The lagged value of investment did not enter into this formulation, but the dummy variable for teaching commitment was retained. A preliminary trial showed a substantial R^2 (adjusted) of .55 but also revealed significant* intercorrelations between six pairs of variables. These were:

	Admissions	X-Rays/ Admission	Interns and Residents/Bed
Teaching status	.4532	.3627	.5140
Interns and residents/bed	–	.5212	–
Semiprivate days/ admission	–	–	–.4014
Laboratory tests/ admission	–	.4598	–

*When $r = .3128$, $t > 2.02$ (significant at $p = .05$).

To overcome the effects of multicollinearity, another test was made using only two predictors, average annual change in admissions $(\overline{\Delta X}_1)$ and teaching commitment (D). The equation and the results are as follows:

$$(7)\, I = -257,325.8 + 10,053.1\, \overline{\Delta X}_1 + 1,620.2D \quad (R^2 \text{ [adjusted]} = .56).$$
$$ (-.5042) \quad\quad (4.8851) \quad\quad\quad (2.4847)$$

The coefficients of both average admission changes and teaching commitment are significant at the .02 level. The constant term is not significantly different from zero, and the equation explains more than half the variance in the average annual rate of investment.*

CONCLUSION

A hypothesis that the rate of investment in voluntary hospitals is influenced by anticipated changes in future demand was tested in three versions, with affirmative results in two. The tests showed that more than one-half the variance in real investment can be explained by selected variables describing changes in services, which stand as proxies for anticipated changes in demand.

In the time series analysis these proxies were the current change in an average output equivalent, and the change in semiprivate days per admission. To take account of the adjustment process, which explains some of the actual investment in a given year, a lagged value of investment was used as one of the predictors of current investment. The least-squares estimate of the coefficient for lagged investment was .49, which implies that on the average a complete adjustment of capital stock to a desired level takes about five years. The coefficient for the change in semiprivate patient days per admission passed a high test of significance. Increase in the value of this variable reflected the increased dependence of hospitals on insured (solvent) patients. It is suggested that the reaction of hospitals to this situation reflected conditions of supply of medical staff and even of management, i.e., facility requirements that are regarded as a minimum. In the cross-sectional analysis of hospital averages, more than half the variance in average annual investment among hospitals was explained by average annual changes in admissions and teaching status.

The focus of this analysis was on demand factors; future research is planned to consider the effect of variations in the supply of capital funds. Discussions of policy concerning health capital increasingly assume that autonomous decisions of voluntary hospitals cannot be relied on to assure a socially optimal allocation.[15] Actually, the concern is far from new. The

---

*Some evidence that multicollinearity has been reduced is provided by the fact that the determinant of the matrix of independent variables rose from .151 to .798.

Hospital Survey for New York in the 1930s referred to excessive autonomy, resulting in poor location, duplication, and uneven standards of care.[16] Rorem in 1930 called for better control by the public over capital investment in hospitals.[17]

Proposals have been made for pooling depreciation allowances in a community fund under control of a planning agency.[18] To a growing extent this source of funds represents direct or indirect support* by government, as, of course, is true of grants. The Secretary's Advisory Committee on Hospital Effectiveness recommended that federal grant funds be disbursed only to those hospitals which adopt annual financial budgets and service plans.[19] A position paper prepared for the committee recommends a community planning agency whose jurisdiction would include capital spending for expansion of existing services and introduction of new services[20] but would exclude improvement of quality. This type of suggestion represents a distinct departure from the assumption that philanthropic willingness, as stimulated by some form of "community endorsement,"[21] is sufficient validation of the community need for a given hospital.

The observed importance of demand factors in the process of allocation of capital stock to hospitals implies that if from the social point of view there is a misallocation of capital mere provision of more capital funds is not a solution. Even if the effective cost of funds to each hospital were reduced to zero, there could still be duplication, underutilized facilities, and shortages.

NOTES

1. See Kenneth E. Boulding, *Economic Analysis* (New York: Harper and Bros., 1948), pp. 816–23. There is more agreement on the variables on which the investment decision is based than on the specific criteria for choosing an alternative. See also Billy E. Goetz, *Quantitative Methods: A Survey and Guide for Managers* (New York: McGraw-Hill Book Co., 1965), pp. 299–301, a guide to computation of alternatives within the framework of a "master planning budget," following the principle of maximizing present value.

2. U.S., Department of Health, Education, and Welfare, Social Security Administration, *Principles of Reimbursement for Provider Costs and for Services by Hospital-Based Physicians* (Washington, D.C., 1967).

3. Millard F. Long, "Efficient Use of Hospitals," in *The Economics of Health and Medical Care*, ed. S. J. Axelrod (Ann Arbor: The University of Michigan, 1964), p. 213.

4. W. J. Baumol and W. G. Bowen, "On the Performing Arts: The Anatomy of Their Economic Problems," *American Economic Review Papers and Proceedings* 55, no. 2 (May 1965):497.

5. See Douglas J. Colman, "The Key Issues," *Hospitals* 39 (January 1963):30.

6. See Melvin W. Reder, "Some Problems in the Economics of Hospitals," *American Economic Review Papers and Proceedings* 55, no. 2 (May 1965):472–80.

---

*Direct as far as Medicare and Medicaid reimbursement are concerned and indirect as far as Blue Cross and commercial third parties are concerned because industrial group insurance benefits are subsidized by favorable provisions of the income tax law affecting business enterprises.

7. See Roy Penchansky and Gerald Rosenthal, "Productivity, Price and Income Behavior in the Physicians' Services Market – A Tentative Hypothesis," *Medical Care* 3, no. 4 (October–December 1965):244.

8. The President's Commission on Heart Disease, Cancer and Stroke, *A National Program to Conquer Heart Disease, Cancer and Stroke* (Washington, D.C.: U.S. Government Printing Office, 1965), 2:52–53, 55–56.

9. American Medical Association Council on Medical Education and Hospitals, *Directory of Internships and Residencies*, annually, 1962–66. (For 1946–1961 the directory was published with the Education Number of the *Journal of the American Medical Association*.)

10. American Medical Association, *Report of the Commission on the Cost of Medical Care*, vol. 4: *Changing Patterns of Hospital Care* (Chicago: By the Association, 1964), p. 27.

11. See Robert Eisner, "A Permanent Income Theory for Investment: Some Empirical Explorations," *American Economic Review* 57, no. 3 (June 1967):364–65.

12. See Michael J. Hamburger, "Interest Rates and the Demand for Consumer Durable Goods," in *ibid.*, no. 5 (December 1967):1131–53; William R. Bryan, "Bank Adjustments to Monetary Policy: Alternative Estimates of the Lag," in *ibid.*, no. 4 (September 1967):855–64.

13. Charlotte Muller and Paul Worthington, "The Time Structure of Capital Formation: Design and Construction of Municipal Hospital Projects," *Inquiry* 6, no. 2 (June 1969):42–52.

14. "A Permanent Income Theory for Investment," p. 387.

15. See Manuel Gottlieb, Discussion of Melvin W. Reder, "Some Problems in the Economics of Hospitals," *American Economic Review Papers and Proceedings* 55, no. 2 (May 1965):503.

16. United Hospital Fund, *The Hospital Survey for New York*, Report of the UHF Study Committee (New York: By the Fund, 1938), p. 41.

17. C. Rufus Rorem, *The Public's Investment in Hospitals* (Chicago: University of Chicago Press, 1930), p. 216.

18. Robert M. Sigmond, "Hospital Capital Funds: Changing Needs and Sources," *Hospitals* 39, no. 16 (August 1965):52.

19. U.S., Department of Health, Education and Welfare, *Report of the Secretary's Advisory Committee on Hospital Effectiveness* (Washington, D.C.: U.S. Government Printing Office, 1968), p. 21.

20. R. M. Grimes, R. D. Gregg, and J. M. Armstrong, "Sources of Capital in Hospitals" (Paper prepared for the *Report of the Secretary's Advisory Committee on Hospital Effectiveness*, 1968), p. 25.

21. American Hospital Association, *Guides to Capital Financing of Hospitals*, Proceedings of an Institute Conducted by the Association, Chicago, April 5–7, 1961 (Chicago: By the Association, 1962), p. 18.

Judith R. Lave
Carnegie-Mellon University

Robert M. Sigmond
University of Pittsburgh

COMMENT

In their paper Muller and Worthington attack the problems of determining which factors affect the hospital investment decision. Little work has been done on this important area. Although the availability of capital from philanthropy and government usually has been considered the only determinant of investment, this bit of conventional wisdom is incorrect because hospitals increasingly are using the capital markets. Muller and Worthington supply the other side of the Marshallian scissors, arguing that demand conditions significantly affect the investment decision. They discuss a number of factors which are likely to affect the demand for capital, formulate some hypotheses, and use United Hospital Fund (UHF) data to test them.

First and foremost, the authors deserve to be highly commended for attacking such a difficult problem, and even more so for their willingness to get their hands dirty in their attempt to construct an investment series. (We are not aware of other comparable capital series for hospitals.) As they indicate, the data on capital for hospitals are usually inadequate. In gathering their data, they were faced with problems of missing observations, overly aggregate data, and inconsistent and different accounting procedures across time and hospitals. The data had to be extensively adjusted before they were suitable for testing anything. However, their results must be viewed with some skepticism.

The data represent an investment series for some hospitals belonging to the UHF which are, in turn, only some of the hospitals in New York City. They are not representative of the hospitals in that city or in the nation. There are certain possible biases that could be further detailed. For example, one would

416

think that the investment series for large teaching hospitals are more likely to be complete than those for small hospitals. If this bias is important, the estimated coefficients (particularly in Model 3) would be biased. We would like to focus our criticisms on three aspects of the paper: the somewhat misleading nature of the introduction, the authors' use of data, and the nature of the conclusions.

The introductory sections of the paper, although interesting and informative, are somewhat deceptive. One is led to believe that the problem of central concern is the allocation decision of a particular hospital. How does a hospital determine which of many possible investment projects to undertake? This interesting problem is not the focus of the empirical investigation. Rather, the paper is concerned with hospitals' total investment behavior: what factors affect the total investment of a hospital or group of hospitals. Naturally, as the authors indicate, these two problems are interrelated.

In passing we would like to draw attention to an interesting matrix which is presented on page 403. Here certain measures of hospital activity are classified by the hospital's teaching status. The authors note that hospitals representing the second highest level of teaching have the highest level of intensive activity. However, examination of the data indicates that, in four out of the six measures, hospitals of type 3 have more intensive activity than the most advanced type 1 teaching hospitals. This is certainly not what one would have expected a priori.

Muller and Worthington spent a considerable amount of time and effort in constructing an investment series for the UHF hospitals. One might well ask whether they made the best possible use of their data. In two out of the three reported models the data were either aggregated or averaged. Why was this procedure used? Were there errors of observation or short-run disequilibria so large that this approach was necessary? Much is lost in these aggregation and averaging procedures. One looks for some tests to determine that this procedure was necessary or that it did not lead to information loss. It is somewhat irritating that the authors did not follow established convention in reporting their work or, indeed, in deciding which statistics to report. We would also like to note that the independent variables were listed but not defined. In most cases they are self-explanatory, but what is meant by the ratio of special professional to general professional staff (not defined in the original paper)?

In estimating two of the three regressions, the authors discovered a significant amount of multicollinearity among the independent variables. They tried to circumvent this problem in Model 1 by constructing an output equivalent index, and in Model 3 by dropping some of the variables. Neither of these approaches eliminates the problem caused by multicollinearity. By dropping variables, for example, one can bias the estimated coefficients of the remaining variables.

Many investigators have tried to find an appropriate measure for hospital output. The proposal put forward here is worth brief consideration. The authors determined an output measure for hospitals by determining first an output equivalent for admissions, X-rays, operations, and laboratory tests by dividing the relevant yearly figure by the ratio of its 1945 value to 1945 admissions. These are then summed and divided by 4. Neither a medical nor an economic justification for this procedure is given. We find it difficult to provide either. Note that what they are doing, from a statistical viewpoint, is constraining the coefficients of each of the adjusted variables to be identical.

We would like now to focus on the conclusions of the paper. Although we believe that they are probably correct, we do not believe that they follow from the empirical analysis. We will consider the two most important conclusions. First, in two of the three models, the rate of investment appears to be influenced by variables one would consider important a priori. One can hope that the failure to demonstrate this type of relationship in Model 2, the cross-sectional time series model, can be attributed more to the crudeness of the data and the specification of the variables than to the crudeness of those who demand and supply capital. However, we would question whether or not the empirical analysis does affirm, as the authors assert, that the rate of investment is influenced by changes in demand. The question can well be raised whether the variables measure supply or demand influences. For example, in Model 1 the most significant variable is lagged investment. One could argue, however, that the distributed lag form of the investment function is susceptible to interpretation as a supply theory of investment. If hospitals are successful in raising capital in one period, they are likely to be successful in raising capital in the next period. In Model 3 the two significant variables are admissions and a dummy variable for teaching status. The teaching variable also could be interpreted as a surrogate for a supply variable: teaching hospitals have more "luck" in getting capital from government and philanthropic sources. The admissions variable also could be construed as part of a supply model; hospitals which are increasing their admissions are more likely to be able to attract capital from philanthropists and government. As the authors indicate, the single-equation method of analysis is inadequate.

Second, the authors argue that their finding that demand conditions are an important determinant of investment implies that the provision of additional capital cannot be relied upon to bring about a socially desirable allocation of capital. This implication does not follow from their empirical tests; it follows from the generally accepted argument presented in the introduction with respect to the duplication of hospital facilities. It has been hypothesized that hospitals tend to invest in capital projects which will attract physicians with particularly desired skills and who, they hope, will bring patients with them. Whether a capital project is socially desirable is irrelevant to the hospital making the decision.

In concluding these notes, we would like to be somewhat more positive and to offer a number of general and specific suggestions for modifications of the authors' work. They assert that hospitals in a city such as New York City perform specialized roles in treating patients. This observation has often been made but never tested. In developing this investment model, supply and demand factors cannot be separated unless both cost and demand functions are specified. Some specific suggestions follow. First, individual time series analyses on each hospital could be performed, and the coefficients of the independent variables could then be compared to see if the hospitals should be aggregated. Second, dummy variables for time could be included. Third, one might test the hypothesis suggested by the authors on p. 412 that hospitals are more influenced by the experience of some reference group than by their own direct experience. This could be tested by inserting into the time series regressions for the individual hospitals variables which represent the experience of the relevant reference group. For example, if one were looking at the demand for capital by a teaching hospital, one could include as an independent variable not its own admissions but the admissions to New York City teaching hospitals as a group.

LIST OF PARTICIPANTS

Second Conference on the Economics of Health
December 5–7, 1968, Baltimore, Maryland

STUART H. ALTMAN
Department of Economics
Brown University
Providence, Rhode Island

RONALD ANDERSEN
Center for Health Administration Studies
University of Chicago
Chicago, Illinois

ODIN W. ANDERSON
Center for Health Administration Studies
University of Chicago
Chicago, Illinois

RICHARD M. BAILEY
Graduate School of Business
University of California
Berkeley, California

LEE BENHAM
Center for Health Administration Studies
University of Chicago
Chicago, Illinois

SYLVESTER E. BERKI
Department of Medical Care Organization
School of Public Health
The University of Michigan
Ann Arbor, Michigan

RALPH E. BERRY, JR.
Department of Economics
Harvard University
Cambridge, Massachusetts

AGNES W. BREWSTER
Leonard Davis Institute of Health
  Economics
University of Pennsylvania
Philadelphia, Pennsylvania

IRENE H. BUTTER
Bureau of Hospital Administration
School of Public Health
The University of Michigan
Ann Arbor, Michigan

CARL CHRIST
Department of Political Economy
The Johns Hopkins University
Baltimore, Maryland

HAROLD A. COHEN
Department of Economics and Statistics
The University of Georgia
Athens, Georgia

PETER E. DE JANOSI
The Ford Foundation
New York, New York

DAVID F. DRAKE
American Hospital Association
Chicago, Illinois

DAN ELDOR
National Bureau of Economic Research
New York, New York

RASHI FEIN
Center for Community Health and
  Medical Care
Harvard University School of Public
  Health and Medical School
Boston, Massachusetts

MARTIN S. FELDSTEIN
Department of Economics
Harvard University
Cambridge, Massachusetts

PAUL J. FELDSTEIN
Bureau of Hospital Administration
School of Public Health
The University of Michigan
Ann Arbor, Michigan

CHARLES FLAGLE
The Johns Hopkins University
Baltimore, Maryland

EDGAR W. FRANCISCO
Department of Epidemiology and
  Public Health
Yale University School of Medicine
New Haven, Connecticut

VICTOR R. FUCHS
National Bureau of Economic Research

The City University of New York
New York, New York

VICTOR GARLIN
School of Public Health
University of California
Berkeley, California

JEREMIAH J. GERMAN
Department of Economics
Loyola College
Baltimore, Maryland

ELI GINZBERG
Conservation of Human Resources
  Project
Columbia University
New York, New York

RICHARD GOODE
Fiscal Affairs Department
International Monetary Fund
Washington, D.C.

HARRY GREENFIELD
Health and Hospital Planning Council
  of Greater New York
New York, New York

MICHAEL GROSSMAN
National Bureau of Economic Research
New York, New York

CHARLES P. HALL, JR.
Department of Insurance
School of Business Administration
Temple University
Philadelphia, Pennsylvania

W. LEE HANSEN
Department of Economics
The University of Wisconsin
Madison, Wisconsin

D. BRIAN HELLER
Division of Research
Blue Cross Association
Chicago, Illinois

NORMAN HOLLY
Health Services and Mental Health
  Administration
Department of Health, Education, and
  Welfare
Arlington, Virginia

A. G. HOLTMANN
Institute for Social Research
The Florida State University Graduate
  School
Tallahassee, Florida

MARY LEE INGBAR
Department of Health, Hospitals and
  Welfare
Cambridge, Massachusetts

HELEN H. JASZI
School of Hygiene and Public Health
The Johns Hopkins University
Baltimore, Maryland

JAMES R. JEFFERS
Department of Economics
University of Iowa
Iowa City, Iowa

SANDER KELMAN
Bureau of Hospital Administration
School of Public Health
The University of Michigan
Ann Arbor, Michigan

WILLIAM KISSICK
United States Public Health Service
National Institutes of Health
Bethesda, Maryland

HERBERT E. KLARMAN
School of Hygiene and Public Health
The Johns Hopkins University
Baltimore, Maryland

JUDITH R. LAVE
Graduate School of Industrial Administration
Carnegie-Mellon University
Pittsburgh, Pennsylvania

IRVING LEVESON
The RAND Corporation
New York, New York

MELVIN LURIE
Department of Economics
The University of Wisconsin at Milwaukee
Milwaukee, Wisconsin

WILFRED MALENBAUM
Wharton School of Finance and Commerce
University of Pennsylvania
Philadelphia, Pennsylvania

ALEX R. MAURIZI
Department of Economics
The University of Iowa
Iowa City, Iowa

JOEL MAY
Center for Health Administration Studies
University of Chicago
Chicago, Illinois

KENNETH MCCAFFREE
Department of Economics
University of Washington
Seattle, Washington

FREDERIC C. MENZ
School of Business Administration
Temple University
Philadelphia, Pennsylvania

EDWIN S. MILLS
Department of Political Economy
The Johns Hopkins University
Baltimore, Maryland

GEORGE N. MONSMA, JR.
Department of Economics
Amherst College
Amherst, Massachusetts

CHARLOTTE F. MULLER
Center for Social Research
City University of New York
New York, New York

JOSEPH P. NEWHOUSE
The RAND Corporation
Santa Monica, California

MARK V. PAULY
Department of Economics
Northwestern University
Evanston, Illinois

ROY PENCHANSKY
Department of Medical Care
   Administration
School of Public Health
The University of Michigan
Ann Arbor, Michigan

MARK PERLMAN
Department of Economics
University of Pittsburgh
Pittsburgh, Pennsylvania

R. D. PETERSON
Department of Economics
Colorado State University
Fort Collins, Colorado

NORA PIORE
Association for the Aid of Crippled
   Children
New York, New York

ARNOLD H. RAPHAELSON
School of Business Administration
Temple University
Philadelphia, Pennsylvania

ELTÓN RAYACK
Department of Economics
University of Rhode Island
Kingston, Rhode Island

LOUIS REED
Social Security Administration
Department of Health, Education, and
   Welfare
Washington, D.C.

DOROTHY P. RICE
Social Security Administration
Department of Health, Education, and
   Welfare
Washington, D.C.

K. K. RO
National Bureau of Economic Research
New York, New York

ROBERT L. ROBERTSON
Department of Economics
Mount Holyoke College
South Hadley, Massachusetts

SHERWIN ROSEN
Department of Economics
University of Rochester
Rochester, New York

National Bureau of Economic Research
New York, New York

GERALD ROSENTHAL
Department of Economics
Brandeis University
Waltham, Massachusetts

JEROME ROTHENBERG
Department of Economics
Massachusetts Institute of Technology
Cambridge, Massachusetts

SIMON ROTTENBERG
American Bar Foundation
Chicago, Illinois

DONALD RUCKER
Social Security Administration
Department of Health, Education, and
    Welfare
Washington, D.C.

A. PETER RUDERMAN
School of Hygiene
University of Toronto
Toronto, Canada

LEONARD G. SCHIFRIN
Department of Economics
College of William and Mary
Williamsburg, Virginia

ROBERT E. SCHLENKER
Department of Social Services
Lansing, Michigan

ANNE A. SCITOVSKY
Palo Alto Medical Research Foundation
Palo Alto, California

GEORGE A. SILVER
The Urban Coalition
Washington, D.C.

MORRIS SILVER
National Bureau of Economic Research

City College of New York
New York, New York

JENS SORENSEN
Statistical Department
National Health Service of Denmark
Copenhagen, Denmark

ALAN SORKIN
The Brookings Institution
Washington, D.C.

HENRY B. STEELE
Department of Economics
University of Houston
Houston, Texas

H. LOUIS STETTLER III
Department of Political Economy
The Johns Hopkins University
Baltimore, Maryland

CARL M. STEVENS
Department of Economics
Reed College
Portland, Oregon

VINCENT TAYLOR
The RAND Corporation
Santa Monica, California

CHRIST THEODORE
Department of Survey Research
American Medical Association
Chicago, Illinois

MURRAY A. TUCKER
Washington, D.C.

HUGH D. WALKER
Management and Operations Research
    Unit
Ontario Hospital Services Commission
Toronto, Canada

GERALD WEBER
The Brookings Institution
Washington, D.C.

PAUL WEINSTEIN
Department of Economics
University of Maryland
College Park, Maryland

JEFFREY H. WEISS
Office of the Assistant Secretary for
  Program Coordination
Department of Health, Education, and
  Welfare
Washington, D.C.

GROVER C. WIRICK
Bureau of Hospital Administration
School of Public Health
The University of Michigan
Ann Arbor, Michigan

PAUL WORTHINGTON
Center for Social Research
City University of New York
New York, New York

DONALD E. YETT
Human Resources Research Center
University of Southern California
Los Angeles, California

INDEX

427